BEHAVIORAL APPROACHES
TO COMMUNITY PSYCHOLOGY

(PGPS-63)

PERGAMON GENERAL PSYCHOLOGY SERIES

Editors: Arnold P. Goldstein, *Syracuse University*
Leonard Krasner, *SUNY, Stony Brook*

TITLES IN THE PERGAMON GENERAL PSYCHOLOGY SERIES
(Added Titles in Back of Volume)

Vol. 1.   J. WOLPE–*The Practice of Behavior Therapy, Second Edition*
Vol. 2.   T. MAGOON *et al.–Mental Health Counselors at Work*
Vol. 3.   J. McDANIEL–*Physical Disability and Human Behavior, Second Edition*
Vol. 4.   M.L. KAPLAN *et al.–The Structural Approach in Psychological Testing*
Vol. 5.   H.M. LaFAUCI & P.E. RICHTER–*Team Teaching at the College Level*
Vol. 6.   H.B. PEPINSKY *et al.–People and Information*
Vol. 7.   A.W. SIEGMAN & B. POPE–*Studies in Dyadic Communication*
Vol. 8.   R.E. JOHNSON–*Existential Man: The Challenge of Psychotherapy*
Vol. 9.   C.W. TAYLOR–*Climate for Creativity*
Vol. 10. H.C. RICKARD–*Behavioral Intervention in Human Problems*
Vol. 11. P. EKMAN, W.V. FRIESEN & P. ELLSWORTH–*Emotion in the Human Face: Guidelines for Research and an Integration of Findings*
Vol. 12. B. MAUSNER & E.S. PLATT–*Smoking: A Behavioral Analysis*
Vol. 14. A GOLDSTEIN–*Psychotherapeutic Attraction*
Vol. 15. F. HALPERN–*Survival: Black/White*
Vol. 16. K. SALZINGER & R.S. FELDMAN–*Studies in Verbal Behavior: An Empirical Approach*
Vol. 17. H.E. ADAMS & W.K. BOARDMAN–*Advances in Experimental Clinical Psychology*
Vol. 18. R.C. ZILLER–*The Social Self*
Vol. 19. R.P. LIBERMAN–*A Guide to Behavioral Analysis & Therapy*
Vol. 22. H.B. PEPINSKY & M.J. PATTON–*The Psychological Experiment: A Practical Accomplishment*
Vol. 23. T.R. YOUNG–*New Sources of Self*
Vol. 24. L.S. WATSON, JR.–*Child Behavior Modification: A Manual for Teachers, Nurses, and Parents*
Vol. 25. H.L. NEWBOLD–*The Psychiatric Programming of People: Neo-Behavioral Orthomolecular Psychiatry*
Vol. 26. E.L. ROSSI–*Dreams and the Growth of Personality: Expanding Awareness in Psychotherapy*
Vol. 27. K.D. O'LEARY & S.G. O'LEARY–*Classroom Management: The Successful Use of Behavior Modification, Second Edition*
Vol. 28. K.A. FELDMAN–*College and Student: Selected Readings in the Social Psychology of Higher Education*
Vol. 29. B.A. ASHEM & E.G. POSER–*Adaptive Learning: Behavior Modification with Children*
Vol. 30. H.D. BURCK *et al.–Counseling and Accountability: Methods and Critique*
Vol. 31. N. FREDERIKSEN *et al.–Prediction of Organizational Behavior*
Vol. 32. R.B. CATTELL–*A New Morality from Science: Beyondism*
Vol. 33. M.L. WEINER–*Personality: The Human Potential*
Vol. 34. R.M. LIEBERT, J.M. NEALE & E.S. DAVIDSON–*The Early Window: Effects of Television on Children and Youth*
Vol. 35. R. COHEN *et al.–Psych City: A Simulated Community*
Vol. 36. A.M. GRAZIANO–*Child Without Tomorrow*
Vol. 37. R.J. MORRIS–*Perspectives in Abnormal Behavior*

The terms of our inspection copy service apply to all the above books. A complete catalogue of all books in the Pergamon International Library is available on request.

The Publisher will be pleased to receive suggestions for revised editions and new titles.

BEHAVIORAL APPROACHES

TO COMMUNITY PSYCHOLOGY

Michael T. Nietzel

Richard A. Winett

Marian L. MacDonald

William S. Davidson

Foreword by L. P. Ullmann

Pergamon Press

New York/Toronto/Oxford/Sydney/Frankfurt/Paris

Pergamon Press Offices:

U.S.A.   Pergamon Press, Inc., Maxwell House, Fairview Park,
                  Elmsford, New York 10523, U.S.A.

U.K.   Pergamon Press, Ltd., Headington Hill Hall,
                  Oxford OX3, OBW, England

CANADA   Pergamon of Canada Ltd., 207 Queen's Quay West,
                  Toronto 1, Canada

AUSTRALIA   Pergamon Press (Aust) Pty. Ltd., 19a Boundary Street,
                  Rushcutters Bay, N.S.W. 2011, Australia

FRANCE   Pergamon Press SARL, 24 rue des Ecoles,
                  75240 Paris, Cedex 05, France

WEST GERMANY   Pergamon Press GmbH, 6242 Kronberg/Taunus,
                  Frankfurt-am-Main, West Germany

Library of Congress Cataloging in Publication Data

Main entry under title:

Behavioral approaches to community psychology.

Bibliography: p.
1.   Community psychology. 2. Community mental health
services. 3. Behavior modification. I. Nietzel,
Michael T.
RA790.5.b36   1977   362.2'2   77-30566
ISBN 0-08-020376-0

Printed in the United States of America

Table of Contents

Preface   vii

Foreword   ix

1 Behavioral Community Psychology   1

2 Problems in the Schools   13

3 The Juvenile Justice System   57

4 Adult Corrections   97

5 Drug Abuse   145

6 Alcoholism   183

7 Community Mental Health   228

8 Social Skills Training for Psychiatric Residents   263

9 Aging   284

10 Unemployment   299

11 Environmental Problems   310

12 The Behavioral Paradigm and Community Change   345

References   361

Index   427

THE AUTHORS

Michael T. Nietzel (Ph.D. University of Illinois, 1973) in 1973 joined the faculty at the University of Kentucky where he currently is an Assistant Professor of Psychology. His major research interests are the evaluation of community mental health interventions, the effects of the criminal justice system, and the role of nonspecific factors in psychotherapy.

Richard A. Winett (Ph.D. the State University of New York at Stony Brook, 1971) is currently with the Institute for Behavioral Research in Washington, D.C. and The American University. His primary research interests involve the application of behavior analytic procedures to community needs such as educational innovation, child care, and environmental protection.

Marian L. MacDonald (Ph.D. University of Illinois, 1974) is currently an Assistant Professor of Psychology at the State University of New York at Stony Brook. Among her major research interests are behavioral assessment and behavior modification with the aging.

William S. Davidson (Ph.D. University of Illinois, 1975) joined the faculty of Michigan State University where he is an Assistant Professor of Psychology. His major research commitment is the development and evaluation of approaches for the juvenile system.

PREFACE

One characteristic which appears to have unified many community psychologists is their attitude of disfavor toward "traditionalism" in clinical psychology or mental health disciplines in general. There is no doubt that this objection has been associated with numerous innovations in assessment and interventions. Along with such service innovations, there have been more decisive changes at the theoretical level with "mainstream" concepts of maladjustment and behavior change being discarded for models more consonant with the environmentalist, nonmedical, activist attitudes that are denotative of the modal community psychologist.

While the importance of community psychology's nontraditional spirit should not be underestimated, it is our belief that this attitude has been transformed infrequently into actual operations, interventions, or programs capable of mitigating the social problems which plague most American communities and prevent the growth of what Sarason has termed the "psychological sense of community." The field of community psychology is at a historical point where the continued recitation of objections to traditional clinical theory and practice will yield diminishing returns and detract from the more crucial business-at-hand: the development of effective, social problem interventions and the empirical evaluation of the impact of such interventions. It is to this objective that we wish to direct the current volume.

The following chapters attempt to review and evaluate the extension of social learning procedures to several demanding community problems. It is our feeling that an integration of community psychology with behavior modification and/or behavior therapy techniques provides a potential operationalization of community psychology which has been lacking in previous conceptualizations of the field. Such an integration is accomplished by consideration of the applied behavior analysis paradigm from several perspectives: a preventive emphasis, the ecological setting of the application, prospects for institutional rather than individual change, and enrichment of behavioral approaches by attention to sociological, political, and systems variables. Applications of the behavioral paradigm are presented for the following social problems: problems of the schools, environmental protection, juvenile delinquency, adult offenders, drug addiction, alcoholism, community mental health, aging, unemployment, and psychiatric residence.

While the book is intended primarily for a graduate student or upper level undergraduate seminar in community psychology, it should be a useful supplementary resource for courses in abnormal psychology, social work, mental health, and community psychiatry. We also have intended it to serve as a comprehensive resource book for applied researchers and practitioners in community mental health settings.

This book is partly the product of many individuals whose contributions to it have been indirect but very influential. We would like to express our appreciation to the teachers, colleagues, clients, students, and friends whose influences are reflected here. We hope that they are able to recognize their influence on us with approval. A number of individuals have made direct and solicited contributions which strengthened both the contents of the book as well as our enthusiasm for writing it. We would like to express special gratitute to Len Ullmann, Len Krasner, Ray Martorano, E. Scott Geller, Charles Kondo, Deedra Benthall-Nietzel, and Sheila G. Winett for the comments, insights, agreements, and disagreements. Finally, we would like to thank Bridget McFarland, Mary Griffith, Peggy Hood, Rebecca Mulholland, Elsa Reyna, and Denise Slaughter for their skillful and patient preparation of the manuscript, and Mrs. Sylvia Halpern, Chief Manuscript Editor at Pergamon Press, for her skillful supervision of the manuscript's production.

FOREWORD

by Leonard P. Ullmann

Behavioral Community Psychology
Implications, Opportunities and Responsibilities

There is a story that Willie Sutton, after being caught robbing a bank, was asked why he chose such difficult targets. He answered that that was where the money was. Applying the concept to psychologists, the idea is to go where the variance is. If we wish to have impact, we must seek the greatest benefits for the least cost, and this implies working with the largest and most easily influenced sources of variance in people's behavior. It is in this context that the present volume is so very welcome: it indicates a new and exiting way for psychologists to influence, have impact, and benefit their community, their clients, their students, their profession, and their own lives. It combines the "where" of behavioral science with the "how" of an "educational," "behavioral," "socio-psychological," or "social learning" model. The name is not important, but the orientation away from an internal psychodynamic orientation to an active, responsible, data-based and data-generating effort is vital. In short, by working on the interface of behavioral therapy and the community arena, the present authors have helped define a new field, its methods, its research, its promise, and its benefits to all.

From a Medical to a Behavioral Model

Given the obvious need served by the present volume, one may wonder what took so long. I think the answer stems from the change of models that underlies the present volume, and growing from the model it presents, the demands that are made on those who choose to work within it. This section will deal with the historical and intellectual context which is challenged by the present book and a later section will deal with changes in the psychologist's role.

Every society and every individual within a society must have some method for coping with breakdowns and deficiencies in the social contract that is implicit in the day-to-day construction of reality. This contract may be called expectancies or contingencies or custom and morality. With the breakdown of religious influence from the Renaissance to the Rationalists, a medical orientation was used to explain people who acted differently than expected and who, in their difference, created a changeworthy burden for themselves or others. Actions which had been sins against God became sins against health. The physician was used not to discover new contractual items, but rather to provide a justification for existing ones. In all models, religious, medical, or behavioral, there is an enterprising act of adding new items to the list of changeworthy behaviors due to interpretations of and deductions from the dominant model. In our own day we have seen various idiosyncracies and role conflicts added to the domain (for example, existential problems), while other acts have become assimilated after considerable political maneuvering (for example, victimless sexual preferences and arrangements).

The dominant paradigm provides a seeming explanation for contractual limitations and disruptions. It permits intervention, especially intervention for a target person's own good. This is indeed having one's cake while eating it—one may feel virtuous while acting tyranically. A good example is the parent who feels it his duty to physically abuse his child for the child's own good.

The medical model, both in its physiological aspects such as chemical intervention and its interpersonal aspects such as the psychoanalytic approach, placed the difficulty as a deviation from *natural occurrence within the individual*. There was something wrong within the person, and the area for investigation—where the variance was—was within the person. The person was isolated from the environment within which behavior took place. At most, the environment was a source of stress which led to a deviation from natural processes. But the natural processes were unchangeable and given, even though across times and across cultures there was considerable evidence that such natural behavior was far from universal.

At a community level, this led to a concept of "miasma," a condition that was generally sick and sickening. The measures of the sickness—like fever for a physical problem—were indices such as divorce, crime, abortion, unemployment, and the like. It is interesting how many of the indices of a "sick" society may, within even a decade, become indicants of a forward-looking, liberal one; for example, no-fault divorce, variation of lifestyle arrangements, legal abortion, and realistic evaluation of marijuana. The indices of a good person or a good life change rapidly in a communicating, media-swamped society—from an inner-directed to an outer orientation, from hoarding worldly goods to gaining worldly experiences, from gaining power over others to doing one's own thing.

The medical model broke down for many reasons during the early 1960s. Some of the pressures were economic—the pressure of "paramedical" groups to assert an independent role and fill a need for service (it is ironic that the group benefiting most from efforts to free psychology from medical dominance is today, for economic reasons, rushing to a medical model of professional remuneration—private practice with a register of "health" care providers to share in "health" insurance payments). Another influence was data that "sick" people did not act the way they should but rather were responsive to environmental situations, data that treatment efforts were more effective in the era of moral treatment prior to adoption of the medical model, and data that direct intervention was rapid, teachable, measurable, inexpensive, and, most important, effective and without symptom substitution. For some inexplicable reason, my favorite references for efforts bringing such data together and building a new model are by Ullmann and Krasner (1965, 1969).

A new model leads to collection of new data and, in turn, a new profession. There was a shift from the difficulty being within the individual to a focus on the interaction between person and psychological environment—contracts, constructions, contingencies, etc. An associated result was a movement away from categorization and traditional diagnosis along trait and/or illness patterns to a functional analysis of behavior, its antecedents and consequents. This work was and is done within an educational model which seeks to designate target behavior and conditions that will lead to changes in frequency.

Running throughout was an increasing recognition that with the very limited exception of brain syndromes, changeworthy behavior was socially and societally defined.

Here the medical and educational models came to a major difference in application. If there were contracts that in themselves were "sick" or "miasmal," then it was legitimate for a physician to intervene and even dictate social relations. Healthy relations were ones that were "natural" in the manner defined by the physician, usually a psychoanalyst. The results were probably most devastating to women, but men who were told what was natural and healthy, for their children as well as themselves, were not left out. At one extreme, screening of public servants by psychiatrists (despite the failures of the OSS assessments) was seriously suggested for the world's ills. At another, a group suggested that violence was equivalent to catharsis—hence healthy and therefore valuable. If the group that was to become violent, for its own good mental health, did not act in the manner prescribed, the professional raised the subjects' consciousness and programmed crises in order to politicize.

It is possible to identify numerous other examples of the medical model applied to social behavior in psychologists' practice. There is the "red-tagging" or diagnosis of children as being "high-risk." High-risk of what? The definition is given in terms of the goals of the dominant group represented by the people doing the labeling; it is interesting how high-risk and minority status overlap and the psychologist who red-tags adds to the burden and self-fulfilling prophecy that works against these children. Such derivatives of the medical model use tests and standards that are not appropriate to the target groups and offer no validated service to the people whom they mark. Fundamentally, there is an error when epidemiology, which has served medicine well, is applied to social behavior: people are far more reactive than spoiled water or specific bodily organs; the designation in medicine is made reliably and is not biased by the judge's values or the subject's personal characteristics; diagnosis does not carry a stigma that is applied generally and permits service providers to rationalize their failures; and, an effective amelioration may be present in medicine that is discrete to the target and does not disrupt the person's social patterns. In short, a method that is appropriate for medicine may be destructive in the realm of social behavior.

Another example of the medical model is that type of family therapy which views the family as an organism or physical system rather than an organization of individuals. In the medical view of family therapy there is a site of abnormality or illness; if one person changes for the better, some other person must deteriorate. In short, there is an idea of symptom substitution within the group as well as within the individual. Considering how thoroughly the symptom substitution hypothesis has been discredited, its application in this context is particularly offensive. The dogmatic assertion that all members of the family must be involved and that there must be communication that is feeling rather than task-oriented does not tailor treatment to client need; while absolving the professional of the need to do an evaluation, it puts the family members one-down as sick and unaware of the things that the professional "knows."

Another example of the medical model in psychological practice is labeling disagreement with the professional as "sick." This may be either a failure to be properly radical (the person is rigid and suppressed and one wonders what keeps the person from doing what is natural) or a failure to be properly submissive and accepting of established authority whether male or medical (the person has a poor attitude and is covertly aggressive).

A final example of medical thinking in the behavioral area is a concept of "stress inoculation" similar to inoculation against a disease. The idea is that presentation of some stress will aid the person in overcoming unwanted effects when faced with difficulties in the future. Where a disease is a specific entity, stress is not well defined. Further, the stress inoculation is without context and implies a general trait model rather than a repertoire of responses to specific situations. Stress inoculation does not teach the person what to do in future difficult situations.

To summarize the medical way of thinking as applied to behavioral and social problems, the person is passive and protected by the superior knowledge of the professional and "stress" is removed; the context is ignored; there is categorization rather than analysis of the situation; the person is dehumanized and treatment is based on a label or category rather than individually tailored; the person is not taught skills that are relevant to tasks, and there is an ideal of normal functioning, natural acts, or optimal mental health from which the person deviates; the individual is the locus of difficulty and treatment is within the individual; the professional institutes a process and the client is blamed for failure; and the system is closed and the professional does not program in evaluation of the impact of the intervention. Finally, therapist personal qualities (age, race, sex) rather than activities become the focus for there is no differentiation of treatment based on individuals. In the medical model the target is the "diseased" personality, and overt behavior is merely "symptomatic."

From the very beginning, the medical model and its psychoanalytic analogue met with criticism. To the extent that psychoanalysis tried to formulate all human behavior with a single set of concepts, was optimistic in its emphasis on the possibility of change, focused on life experiences rather than genetic endowment, and was unique in its exciting, motivational analysis, it was a major step forward. While discrepancies were noted as well as failures of treatment, there was no strong opposition to the model because there was no alternative available. Psychoanalytic thinking provided a method for psychologists to move from psychometric exercises to dynamic personality evaluation (projective techniques) and later to treatment. Social workers found in psychoanalysis a rationale for the case approach and enrichment of their jobs in the same way as had psychologists; they moved from people who described to ones who treated. Finally, psychoanalysis was a system closed to data that might contradict it: on the one hand, the critics were evaluated in terms of underlying suppressed problems that kept them from the natural and healthy condition of accepting psychoanalytic theory, while on the other hand, the system itself provided only one clearly testable hypothesis—that of symptom substitution. All other inconsistent data could be rationalized by reaction-formation, repression, displacement, or some other intrapsychic mechanism.

The key concept is that not only data but also an alternative for professional and personal activity were required before there could be a move away from the medical model and its analogues. This alternative is detailed throughout this volume.

An Alternative Model

There are many ways to start a presentation of the alternative model embodied in the combination of behavioral and community concepts. The major question is how we think of people and ourselves. What are the variables that will best permit us to describe, understand, predict, and influence behavior? Having this information, we must ask if we can influence behavior, in what direction should we endeavor to do so, and with what restrictions on our own efforts as influencers. We need to have ethics of influence and rights of clients—the two are faces of the same coin.

If we were to understand, describe, or predict a person's activity, probably the most useful, rapid, and easily obtained information would deal with age, education, race, socioeconomic status, religion (especially whether observant or not), place of residence (rural-urban, nationality, ghetto or middle class), political-economic orientation (liberal-conservative), record of interaction with social institutions (hospitals, prison, military, research grants, elective offices), and to close associates on and off the job (Krasner & Ullmann, 1973). This type of information is quite different from either the traditional concepts of personality traits as measured by personality inventories and projective tests on the one hand, and goes beyond the functional analysis of explicit behavior-in-situations on the other. The upshot of the clinical-actuarial controversy of the late 1950s and early 1960s was that such face-sheet information more frequently than not did significantly better than traditional test measures, and, more importantly, traditional psychological testing accounted for little additional variance. It should also be noted that traditional tests were unreliable, lacked clear validities, and, very importantly, were costly in terms of time spent for training professionals and later for time spent in interpretation. The clear work of the late 1960s and early 1970s was that behavior was situation specific rather than organized in terms of dimensions or traits across situations.

The value of face-sheet information was recognized by traditional test procedures—this information was required as a context for the interpretation of projective tests. This was an advantage over analysis of behavior which was limited to specific responses. The grave error in this approach was that the professional forgot that *the target is behavior-in-reaction-to-situations, and not responses per se. The genuine target is to have the person deal effectively with situations, and frequently traits such as "anxiety" were the result of ineffectiveness which made the situation realistically aversive, rather than the cause of ineffectiveness.*

Demographic, "face-sheet," or biographical information gives information about what the person's behavioral environment is likely to be. That is, who are likely to be the actors, what options are available, what changes are likely to be consistent and feasible. It is a very rough but rapid and inexpensive way of designating the likely contract; the specific situation should then be investigated. But lists of target behaviors without a context of who the subject is leads to many errors: the first is that the list of target responses are seemingly conservative and defined by the powerful adult or dominant social group; a second is that instead of people, we are likely to think of abstract categories designated by responses (the overweight, the blind, the school-child, the retarded, the sexually different); a third reason is that the approach may indeed partake of the stereotype of the behaviorist as unthinking and mechanistic; and a final, fourth problem is that the person remains the passive recipient of treatment and at best adjusted to a situation.

We need to know what options are open to people, and how they are perceived by these people as well as others. Sometimes we will be able to offer new options which had not been investigated. At other times we will find that the situation requires change. But we must always start where the person is and this means not only capabilities and current acts, but also the situations and contingencies available to each person.

Altering contingencies alters the situation. Contracts both in personal and in social terms are the conditions under which acts are emitted, and we must specify these conditions.

At times we will alter not only the contingencies, but the very contract. It is in this context that the psychologist will strive for change of the situation-contract (at its broadest, laws and economic policy). Examples are definitions of acceptable behaviors (abortion laws), types of treatment (equality of opportunity based on merit), and retirement based on capability rather than age. To make liberal laws which are not used because there are few people who can make effective use of them is a chimera—a striving for image that placates rather than substance that achieves. The concept of black capitalism is a recent example.

A look at the contingencies on people based on age, sex, socioeconomic status, and the like provides us with an insight into areas for social change. We must next look, as do a number of the chapters in this volume (for example, those on work and on the older person), at the match between actual capabilities and current contingencies. Social policy here may work towards suppression of prosocial responses, as with the aged and the female, and not only encourage and maintain activity but deny opportunity for its expression. To prepare a person for an activity that is not available is as fearful a violation of trust as to provide an opportunity that the person cannot utilize.

We need to know both what currently exists and what the people whom we serve see as the reality. Only when we have solid knowledge of what exists in terms of options for behavior and service can we move forward. Much of the present volume is devoted to providing this information. Only when we have a basis of information rather than sentiment, can we as professionals act effectively.

After evaluating competencies and contingencies, a functional analysis of behavior, both for individuals and groups, is required. The strategy will be one of progression based on what is feasible and what individuals may use. To move to an ideal immediately presumes that we can identify such an ultimate ideal, and also runs the risk of a frozen rather than flexible society.

We must recognize that people are reacting to social systems. The person in the power structure or "establishment" is as much trapped in that web of interpersonal organization, options, and contingencies as the person who is outside that organization or "served" by it. One method of service is to find out what the options and contingencies are and to change the behavioral environment for the professional worker. We must never forget that there are no entities such as organizations, establishments, or systems other than those embodied in people and how they have contracted and been shaped to live together. To depersonalize the "organization" is as severe an error as to depersonalize the aged, the young, the addict, or the female. Rather, we have people: civil servants, teachers, women, children, and people who at specific times and under certain specified conditions ingest more of a substance than is expected by society with results that are overt and aversive to some group within that society.

There are a number of crucial points related to this concept. The first is that economic and social policy becomes a major concern and arena for psychologists. These concepts define the psychological situation, the options for both client and therapist. The most crucial problem, then, is to select the direction of change and, thereafter, the methods by which change is to be achieved.

In an earlier era (Ullmann, 1969a), I addressed this problem as an outgrowth of the overthrow of the medical model. If there were no natural behavior that was based on biological givens as in Freud, then the therapist-psychologist was faced with problems of defining the very population to be served, the methods that were legitimate, and the goals to be attained. The psychologist could no longer claim to be a part of a healing process, a midwife as it were, but rather had to recognize a responsibility and a position as a bargaining agent contracting with both clients and the larger society which the psychologist implicitly represented. At that time, the guidelines were that of (a) increasing the range of reasonable options for the client, which (b) were consistent with the client's values and perceptions, and (c) might deviate, as in the case of victimless crime, from absolute legal standards, but did not violate the fundamental methods of the society for changing itself and did not increase the likelihood of harm to other individuals. In short, at that point, the idea was that the therapist was analogous to a leader of a social movement. Not only were the steps in therapy similar to those of religious and political conversion, but the limits of legitimate activity were similar to those imposed on political, religious, and social leaders. Today, after a decade which has seen the development of an arrogant, social activism and a withdrawal from responsibility to others of a sensational and sensual "existentialism," I would add a clear need to adhere to professionalism. By professionalism, I refer to the idea that a person has specialized knowledge which requires long and arduous preparation, such that a layperson cannot be privy to it or accurately evaluate it, so that the client takes the professional's judgment on faith. This requires that the professional, to be acting in good faith, must be impersonal, which in turn means that decisions are based on the specialized knowledge and not the professional's personal sentiments or interests. The professional is permitted behaviors or privileges that are not usual—confidentiality is a prime example—but, in turn, is expected to live up to a special code of ethics that is enforced by fellow professionals. If as behavioral scientists we wish to be listened to with more respect than lay people, our obligation is to be professional in the sense of not using our status for our own personal, sentimental, financial, or political ends. Our goals and our methods must be open and available for inspection by our fellow professionals and by consumers. It is in this area that there can and must be informed consent. Just as data presumes honesty by the investigator, so informed consent demands honesty. There can be no hidden agendas, no surprises, even if the professional believes that it is for the client's own good. The ethical standards adopted by the American Psychological Association for research with human participants are a valuable example.

Along with methods, we have goals, and the two cannot be separated. A concept that because violence (frequently defined idiosyncratically) has occurred, a professional may engage in any counterviolence from slandering his colleagues to misleading his clients so that they engage in acts ranging from sexual intercourse to physical acts of aggression and terrorism must be rejected on the basis that the engagement of violence legitimizes violence.

Our goals must incorporate a respect for ourselves as professionals, our clients as individuals, and our social fabric as a human product and contract that may and should be changed but must not be destroyed. In searching for fundamental values, a starting place is that of honesty of data and as accurate a conception of people as possible. Next, given open and honest statement of methods and goals, I would urge the value of an increase in the range of actions possible to individuals. By this I mean valid and possible acts, not ones that give the image of freedom without the possibility of its attainment. I think much of what I am groping to say may be covered by the phrase "increasing ability to deal with situations." It is a goal of an active person. At an abstract level, it is an attempt to overcome helplessness that is depressing and debilitating. At the level of models of activity, it is a counteraction to the passivity engendered by medical approaches of community intervention.

We have noted that there are broad, undefined concepts of "stress" similar to that of a sickening miasma. If we change conditions to reduce stress—that is, place the individual in a sterile protective environment—we keep the person passive, receptive, and eventually helpless.

There are two aspects to this. The first is that change cannot be of an attitudinal, trait, or psychodynamic nature. That is, we cannot change the person in general, but rather need to train the person to deal with situations. For substance abusers, this means preparation for dealing with situations and conditions under which the abuse previously took place, rather than a limitation to the substance itself. If strengthening the person needs operational definition, it should occur in the realm of dealing with stimuli, both from the social environment and what people provide by speaking to themselves or reacting to physiological changes. After one has effectively dealt with situations that previously led to aversive consequences, including self-labeling as helpless and ineffective, one may obtain changes in self-esteem, and these concepts are based on realistic evaluation of one's own activities. To raise self-esteem without training in those acts which are role expressive is likely to lead to disappointment in both oneself and the helping agent.

The second implication of the present view is that to alter a situation in order to avoid stress on individuals is a poor policy in terms of effectiveness and one that denigrates the very person who presumably is to be helped. The proper route is to prepare the person to deal with situations effectively and to create situations in which active coping and interaction will be supported. An example of the sterile, stress-avoiding approach may be found in excusing students from mastery of material that a special group considers "irrelevant" but that is a prerequisite for social skills. Mathematics is an example; if it is not considered relevant to a "woman's role," women as a group will not be proportionately represented in professions calling for mathematical skill. The "kindness" of alleviation from stress because task-mastery is not relevant is in reality an ultimate of stereotyping. To say that a skill is irrelevant for a particular group, but not for others, means that the group so "privileged" is eventually barred from an area of activity if criteria of merit are employed, or will become second-class citizens providing second-class service if they enter the activity unprepared.

The erosion of competence in the short-term view of stress-avoidance not only deprives groups of opportunity but has a bad consequence for the total society. At a first level, there is the loss of the talent of groups of people and a systematic deterioration of the pool of potential talent. At a second level, we may see a deterioration of the concept of merit, a matter to which I shall return. Demographic quotas, seniority, and other guidelines that focus on who the person is rather than what the person can do, when applied for long periods of time, will deprive society of reward for competence and hence for levels of effective performance. The minimal performance, the sufficing or adequate one, rather than the enterprising, innovative, effective one, will become the standard. Our progress towards increasing options for all depends on excellence to provide new resources and options, not on stagnant mediocrity. Psychologists altering social systems and environments must view long-term consequences for social groups just as formerly they viewed ultimate consequences for individuals.

The goal is competence, dealing effectively with situations, and not adjustment, the avoidance of "symptoms." We need to increase skill rather than lower requirements.

We may then start the search for conditions that foster competence, that encourage creativity and problem solving, that lead to feelings of worth rather than helplessness and dependency. We will look for the teaching of reactions to situations, for increasing the range of valid situations, and teaching strategies for entering and mastering new situations. We will seek ways for both the person and the group to foster change. The following chapters address this task and provide a wealth of ideas, methods, and strategies.

Some Additional Comments

Throughout the following material the authors frequently point out implications of their work for therapeutic procedures, theoretical formulations, required research, and social and ethical patterns. At the risk of being redundant, I would like to highlight some issues.

When a person is trained in one environment and moves to another, there is a change of both discriminative and reinforcing stimuli. In this circumstance, it is reasonable to expect that the newly developed behavior may not be maintained.

A major task facing behavioral community psychology is how to prepare a person so that there will be stability of emission of *appropriate* behavior in a changing environment. It should be explicit that emission of a single type of behavior when conditions change may well become stereotyped and self-defeating. The challenge is to teach clients to become their own therapists (Ullmann, 1969b) and this leads to the current work teaching strategies for self-programming. We are moving to training for independence and this skill will become a reinforced class of behavior.

The alternative to such procedures may be seen in programs that do not train *individuals* in skills. At the point of discharge, the entire group or system must be moved to a new locale rather than permitting individuals to be fully reintegrated as individuals in the larger community.

Another solution stems from the need to provide opportunities and consequences for behavior learned during treatment in the environment from which the person originally came to treatment. It is tempting in this situation to design communities so that they support the pro-social behavior that was the target of the therapist. While this option is an important one, it must be clear that clients are but a small portion of the total population and care is needed that we do not design a total society to serve but one segment. Such a situation would lead to the disequilibria which may have provided a background for the original treatment group.

In this context, we must do functional analyses of behavior for larger units of behavior than has so far been the case. We must determine what are the antecedents and consequences of the behaviors we consider pro-social and those we consider counterproductive. We must ask what are we reinforcing and what are the probable consequences of our interventions. If we are striving for a concept of community, should we reinforce disruptive behavior and give oil to the squeaking wheel? What do we teach when we give in to violence, especially in view of our belief that modeling and social learning are effective procedures? What do we show others when we reward people for who they are rather than what they do? The point here is that if we are behavioral psychologists, *we will apply functional analyses of behavior to our own activities and not only to those of our clients or the people whom we hope to influence.*

As in direct service, when working in larger social contexts, we must look for unintended consequences of our programs. Some of these effects may be predicted, especially if we engage in programs that assert the predicate. For example, if we find that delinquents come from broken homes with few children, will we endeavor to reduce delinquency by making divorce or birth control more difficult? While this example is obviously ridiculous, the reader may wish to think of programs that strive to eradicate general conditions associated with a category of target behavior without first specifying how the general condition altered the target behavior of individuals. We must remember that frequently behaviors that are our focus are ones emitted by a minority of the group from which the client is drawn. One point is that we may have much waste and many false alarms if we deal with groups rather than tracking problems and finding out the effects on individuals.

Another aspect of this idea is that we may do well to study people of the same population as our clients but ones who do not need our services. For example, what are the antecedents and present contingencies for the aged, the blind, and the members of "disadvantaged groups" who are socially successful. It is a remnant of the medical model that there is a focus on pathology. If we aspire to "primary" prevention, we will do better to look at successes in the system as a source of ideas, rather than the rehabilitation of failures of that system.

Failure to specify how a general condition affects individuals' actions and omission of data about the conditions that lead to success may be the root of the disappointing results of many ambitious social programs. We must identify and stringently test our formulations prior to major social investments lest the funds for such efforts become unavailable due to our very own actions. Legislators, even as other mammals, may extinguish pressing a level which provides little benefit after considerable cost. Poorly formulated interventions, although fast and easy, in the long run reduce the chance for interventions of genuine worth.

From our analysis of current "successes" we may also determine what stylistic and behavioral strategies seem most generally useful. Self-modification, assertion, problem-solving orientations, and creativity in approach to interpersonal situations may be such general behaviors, and we may be able to ascertain the conditions that already exist that lead to and maintain such acts for the majority of the population. As behaviorists, it would be congruent for us to shape acts for which there is already a baserate rather than for us to instigate totally new ones.

This idea that we should apply the same functional analysis of behavior that we use with clients to ourselves as professionals leads to concepts of training for both professionals and paraprofessionals that are similar to those advocated for parents and hospitalized patients. It also means that we must look to our own activities rather than being able to absolve ourselves by blaming either the victim or some abstract and "sick" system. Finally, it means that the ends are acceptable only if the means are acceptable. Just as we would consider a successful criminal an unacceptable goal for a correctional system, so falsification of data is an unacceptable procedure no matter how beneficial it may be in obtaining a short-range goal.

The present volume cannot cover all the areas of impact. It offers, however, a large sample of field-tested methods and provides the reader with many answers to what and how questions for application to target populations, acts, and situations. If there is a group that I would have wished to have seen included, it probably would have involved women or sexual minorities. If there is an area that I think is missing that will be increasingly important in behavioral community psychology, it is recognition that much of a person's environment lies within the confines of that person's body. The area making the most use of this concept at present is in the abuse of alcohol. Biofeedback, it seems to me, will have its greatest use not in conditioning levels of somatic activity per se but rather in helping individuals to be alert to their own bodily environments and to use these cues as discriminative stimuli. For example, the feeling of "anxiety" may be used adjustively when it is taken as an indicant that there are social stimuli requiring a functional analysis and a new, skillful response, rather than a maladaptive cue to escape or avoid the situation itself. In line with this, self-modification programs of all sorts seem to be particularly important.

It is a strength of the present book that pro-social activities and skills are brought into the realm of psychologists' professional concern. When dealing with concepts such as staff and organizational use, we will probably be most effective when we think of changing social environments rather than physical ones. A table of organization is even more an outline of behavioral interaction than the floorplan of a new college or office building.

There are many implied effects on graduate education for professional psychology. The present orientation reduces the importance of the laboratory analogue and deduction from a medical, psychoanalytic, or psychopathological model. The laboratory is likely to be located in the community with independent variables of interventions with people whose changed social acts will become the dependent variables. The distance between data gathered scientifically and the area to which it will be generalized will be reduced. The behavioral community psychologist will be a person specializing in applied behavioral science—economics, political science, anthropology, and history—as well as psychology and sociology. The mainstays of traditional clinical psychology will change from "testing" to functional analysis of overt behavior, and evaluation will change from measures such as self-report and attitudes to behavior emitted in social situations. While the form of treatment will be based on learning concepts and social psychology, the behavioral community psychologist will remain a person who is skilled in both the theory and practice of intervention. A person who is all theory and no skill cannot model for students or shape colleagues and consumers.

Steadily, we will see an emphasis away from the personal characteristics of the psychologist to emphases on skills emitted in situations with social implications. As interventions increase in effectiveness, the amount of the variance accounted for by characteristics of either the therapist or client will decrease. The questions will steadily move towards what will be done for particular people with particular problems and away from therapist or client characteristics that are irrelevant.

Finally, while behavioral community psychology fosters many new features of service deliverers, of target populations, of target behaviors, and of intervention procedures, its basis is a way of formulating people's behavior. All surface aspects of behavioral community psychology may be duplicated by other approaches. Even if some people use behavioral language or technology, they are not behavioral community psychologists until they apply behavioral concepts routinely and systematically to all their work and especially to their own behavior. There is no separate creation, not even for psychologists.

What Is the Core of Behavioral Community Psychology?

Behavioral community psychology is not a matter of more of the same, but of a different, new, nonmedical way of formulating how people interact. It is not a restriction to what makes people "sick" or a new definition of "stress." It matters little where—community, hospital, or clinic—service is delivered. It matters much what people do and how they formulate their actions and their relations. It matters less what populations are served than what is done for these people. We must look to professional and psychological models and then to what deductions and acts are made within these models. The alternative of doing whatever we wish and then rationalizing our acts later, whether through a psychoanalytic, behavioral, or physiological model, is destructive of the very basis of professionalism.

What will be the most fruitful direction for further activity? In the opening remarks, it was noted that the variance is in the environment and not within the individual. Suggestions have been made as to various paths and effects of this viewpoint. For the future, I wish to note that there needs to be much more emphasis on the delivery system and the people delivering the service, but not in terms of who delivers so much as *what* is delivered, and *how* it is delivered, and for what measurable *results*.

Influencers Are Influenced

The people in a delivery system are as much under control of the conditions under which they labor as the people who are served. This point has been presented in terms of a system of psychiatric hospitals (Ullmann, 1967). What people were paid off for and how they maneuvered within formal channels, and when frustrated developed informal, reciprocal obligations, were used to explain results of a study of 30 psychiatric hospitals. A key feature of such work, which should be taken to heart by future community psychologists, was the possibility of displacement of goals in which the ostensible aim of an organization is changed by the employees to their own—that is, to gain security of employment, to manipulate professional staff and supervisors, to maintain the status quo and avoid trouble, and to obtain promotion by the guidelines established for their jobs. In larger measure, the organizations responded to the conditions of funding (increased or decreased positions), which in turn led to changes in workloads and number of supervisees.

In short, one of the major topics of behavioral community psychology in the future will be an analysis of the influencer and his (her) interaction with the people served. Such work will draw on sociology and industrial psychology. We will look for the conditions that increase service to people, and we will measure this by results such as people released from hospitals or people returned to employment or developing new skills, rather than the feelings of either the workers or the clients.

Organizational patterns and systems analysis will become important tools for the community behavioral psychologist. The behavioral community psychologist will ask what conditions lead to what useful acts by the staff. It will be in this context of service and outcome that we will be able to determine whether similarity among worker and client of race or sex is a crucial variable, or whether the important variance lies with how the person performs: what is done, when, how often, etc. My own experience in the multi-ethnic setting of Hawaii indicates that acceptance has a paradoxical effect on many mainland minority members. The behavior for which they had been reinforced is that of being a minority member, and suddenly they are faced with people who say to their minority status, "so what?" The focus becomes what does the person know how to do and a repertoire of identification and rationalization of acts based on minority status is extinguished. The person is no longer a minority member but a person who is expected to have professional knowledge.

If we focus on who rather than what, we deprive the people we train of skill and the people who they will serve of assistance. The effect on the staff person is to keep that individual forever a member of a minority and out of the status of professional. A person whose stock in trade is being a woman rather than a psychologist is forever a woman if that is all she has to offer clients. Again, the Hawaiian experience indicates how ridiculous is the emphasis on "who" rather than "what" skills: serving Caucasians, Chinese, Japanese, Samoans, Filipinos, Koreans, and native Hawaiians, across different social classes and generations in the islands, makes a match of therapist and client on demographic bases impossible.

People who serve need to learn the values of their clients; they are also alert to the problem of culture conflicts where different values are observed for the same person in different situations, such as going to a modern high school during the day and returning to a traditional Shanghai culture in the evening, with "success" demanded in both settings. A person who believes that there is one ideal set of human interactions is likely to damage the client in all settings.

In a different manner, much of our effort as a democratic group will be to make age, sex, race, and ethnicity irrelevant so that we can honestly focus on what people do and respond to them on the basis of their individual accomplishments rather than their demographic stereotypes.

I believe that there will be an increase in evaluation of clients. This will not be in terms of traditional diagnostic categories of illness that have been used to justify intervention, or underlying trait descriptions that are measured by test situations that lack stimulus differentiation (e.g., are "you anxious" rather than "when are you anxious") or overgeneralize from response to irrelevant stimuli (e.g., TAT which makes an isomorphic fallacy and sees the world of fantasy as indicative of the world of reality). Rather, there will be scrutiny of what skills need to be developed in order to deal with specific situations. The focus will be patterns of reinforcement-in-reaction-to-acts and not providing reinforcement per se. We will not strive for warm parents, but rather ask in response to what behaviors is the parent warm? In the same manner as noted for service deliverers, we may note that children should be reacted to on the basis of what they do and not because they are children per se. By being equally warm to all acts, we do not help people differentiate their behaviors; by universal unconditional positive regard we do the greatest disservice of all; we do not treat the person's acts as meaningful and we abrogate our responsibility—at times even our own legitimate humanity—by teaching nothing.

Ethical and Professional Behavior

There needs to be an open recognition that a problem of values exists for all behavioral psychologists (Ullmann, 1969a). We cannot claim that any act is sick or in itself a deviation from an ideal of normal. Further, many people in the field of community mental health use good words in an emotional and poetic rhetoric aimed at swaying rather than documenting. This effort is political rather than professional; it may be appropriate for the private citizen but not one who claims legitimacy and respect as a psychologist—i.e., a profession based on specialized knowledge impersonally applied. We find, in many people who use emotional rather than data appeals, a day-to-day exploitation of clients, students, and colleagues whom they denigrate from the pedestal of their self-designated sanctity. These people are willing to sacrifice others for their own "cause."

The way to avoid such a trap is to define operationally what we mean and to make our values explicit and measurable. It is a method of accountability, and this is a fundamental obligation and crucial characteristic of a behavioral community psychologist and not a slogan to be applied to others, Again, industrial psychology and systems analysis proceed only when there is a measure—cost per item, absenteeism, accidents, etc. With task-relevant criteria, we can determine whether assumptions are correct: that likability is associated with productivity, that demographic status rather than knowledge is associated with effectiveness in service delivery. Only when we have criteria can we ascertain the conditions that are associated with effectiveness.

If we wish to use words such as "freedom" or "dignity" or "community" or "equality" or "morale," we must define them explicitly and then and only then can we determine the conditions under which they are more likely to occur for the people we hope to serve. Dogmatic statements without data partake of religious belief at best; at worst, they are the refuge of the unthinking, self-serving scoundrel who strives for power over others.

Methodology is *not* a luxury. Data must always be the test of actions. A person who would manipulate others without a knowledge base for the act, engages in a paternalistic, nonprofessional act, which in no manner can be legitimized as a profession based on science.

How Do We Make a Start?

In simple words that may yield to operational definitions, first, we may strive to prepare people and multiply situations in which they may realistically increase their range of choices. This means that people have the skills to make use of opportunities as well as that such opportunities exist. Ability and opportunity cannot be separated, for they reciprocally make each other meaningful. To provide a situation without ability to deal effectively with it is a tease; a development of ability without opportunity for use is a source of frustration.

Second, we will seek to increase activities and stimuli that have positive outcomes for people. This means not only making available situations and rewards more broadly, as in the immediately preceding goal, but utilizing media and behavioral technology to increase the range of stimuli and activities that people find valuable and pleasant. Such stimuli may involve active human interaction and participation in work that gives a feeling of accomplishment, worth, and value rather than passive consumption of physical objects and resources. Another way of putting this is that we need to facilitate the redefinition and expansion of outcomes for which people will strive, and such outcomes do not have to be material goods. In fact, other than basic survival needs, many of the status symbols and "needs" of our culture are unnecessary and partake of substitutes for interpersonal relations and ways of demonstrating worth to others and hence to self.

Third, associated with increased choice, there should be a reduction of actions maintained by avoidance of aversive stimuli or escape from such unpleasant stimuli. Reality poses aversive stimuli, but competence, in the manner outlined above, is the major method of offering alternatives. It is in the increase of options of activities and outcomes that are realistic that we may strive to reduce activity under control of aversive stimuli.

Fourth, and associated with avoidance of irrelevant stimuli limiting opportunity for skill development and usage (opportunity and ability), we should note that people of equal ability and effort should have equal opportunity for skills training and usage. That is, equals are to be treated equally, and if this is not done, either unequal people are treated equally (share similar outcomes for dissimilar performance) or equals are treated unequally (receive different outcomes for similar performance). Equal performances should receive equally valuable (but not necessarily identical) outcomes in terms of values such as pay, promotion, and recognition. This means defining and measuring ability and performance, and monitoring activity. Equality is not legislated; it is a result of active work by both the professional and the person served. A correlate is that inequality based on irrelevancies such as age, sex, ethnicity, likability, or family connections destroys the community's fabric of fairness.

To recapitulate, knowing people by their acts is a fundamental tenet which makes a person a behaviorist. As deductions from this position, one must measure in order to evaluate where people are, what learning experiences will be of benefit, how well programs serve clients, how programs should be organized and articulate with each other, what conditions prevail and how they may be altered to increase success, and what outcomes are effective in increasing people's activities.

A crucial guideline that was mentioned before is that the person's acts have impact on altering conditions and consequences. It is of equal import that such impact be just and equitable. If one's acts have no meaningful consequences (that is, if outcomes are determined by irrelevancies such as age, sex, or the like), then one is helpless. Even if the consequences are pleasant, as long as the person's acts have no impact, the person's life is not under that person's control but rather dependent on an external and eventually uncontrolled source. Capricious reinforcement is a denigration of the individual as a worthwhile, significant actor in his or her own life, and we may see evidences of such in people who may be recipients of considerable quantities of the good things of life and who yet manifest "existential" problems. Inequality of reinforcement eventually leads to helplessness.

How May We Define Community?

We need to strive for competence rather than clamor; we want reciprocal support for performance and people who care for each other rather than ones who hurt each other as they compete for limited values. We wish to avoid having people gain pleasure through destroying others who are seen as barriers. To develop a community, we must have people see themselves as having an equitable opportunity and viewing other people as partners rather than competitors. This means increasing personal competence. Community is not, "I'll get mine from you," but rather "we'll get ours by working together," and we can feel secure in our positions because they are earned. Operationally, we wish to shift from aggression to assertion, from isolation to cooperation, from hoarding to sharing. These six topics have all been subjects of psychological research (Krasner & Ullmann, 1973; Ullmann & Krasner, 1975).

In contrast to such an approach, we may note the current popularity of "power" and "intimidation" books which represent self-serving behavior developed in situations in which it is assumed that competence and performance are irrelevant to personal advancement and attainment of values. Such power and intimidation tactics are used to gain ascendancy over others and exploit them. The popularity of these books is an indication of where we now are, and the situation which needs to be changed. These books also indicate a tearing of the web of interpersonal reciprocity in a community which is not perceived as based on equitable consequences for performance.

In broad economic terms, if we wish to increase the slice of the pie for all, we must increase the whole pie. The task is not defining who gets what of a limited store of value, but increasing the supply of values itself. Confrontation and conflict in the long run are counterproductive for all.

In Summary

We are behaviorists because we focus on activity and the conditions which increase or decrease it. *Behaviorists* are interested in behavior; this sounds tautological but from this view stem deductions which differ markedly from the medical-psychoanalytic and the radical-existential models. We define *community* as a web of human interactions, ones of reciprocal reinforcement, of cooperation, sharing, support, and value, which lead to feelings of competence, security, and personal worth. *Psychologists* are professionals engaged in the scientific study and application of concepts. They collect relevant data to measure the effects of their interventions. Scientific method is a safeguard against error, and particularly against interventions which harm people both as individuals and as groups. Science is not a luxury; it is a necessity against a developing mental health industry which at best is only wasteful but at worst a source of promises that will not be fulfilled and hence a source for the dissolution of community.

Behavioral community psychology is an interface of complex ideas. The present volume, as with work with individuals, starts from where we are. From this effort, there follows a wealth of ideas as to how and where we may go. This book is an effort at community through behavioral psychology; it provides the reader with a realistic and realizable opportunity. It is up to each reader to judge and to act.

REFERENCES

Krasner, L., & Ullmann, L. P. *Behavior influence and personality*. New York: Holt, Rinehart, & Winston, 1973.

Ullmann, L. P. *Institution and outcome*. New York: Pergamon Press, 1967.

Ullmann, L. P. Behavior therapy as social movement. In C. M. Franks (Ed.), *Behavior therapy: Appraisal and status*. New York: McGraw-Hill, 1969(a).

Ullmann, L. P. Making use of modeling in the therapeutic interview. In R. D. Rubin & C. M. Franks (Eds.), *Advances in behavior therapy, 1968*. New York: Academic Press, 1969(b).

Ullmann, L. P., & Krasner, L. (Eds.), *Case studies in behavior modification*. New York: Holt, Rinehart, & Winston, 1965.

Ullmann, L. P., & Krasner, L. *A psychological approach to abnormal behavior*. Englewood Cliffs, N. J.: Prentice-Hall, 1969.

Ullmann, L. P., & Krasner, L. *A psychological approach to abnormal behavior, 2nd edition*. Englewood Cliffs, N.J.: Prentice-Hall, 1975.

Chapter 1
BEHAVIORAL COMMUNITY PSYCHOLOGY

A common identifying belief of most community psychologists is that the development and patterning of human behavior is the result of a transactional process between the person and the environment (Kelly, 1966), and as a consequence efforts to alleviate social problems necessarily entail modification of *both* environmental events and human behavioral repertoires (Cowen, 1973). While the field continues to exhibit major differences in preferences for social change tactics—for example, social action versus working "within the system" or person-oriented versus system-oriented intervention (Bloom, 1973; Cowen, 1973)—there appears to be both a historical and consensual endorsement of the need for interventions with the focus and ability to change both individual skills and the environmental-social systems within which such skills are to be enacted. This position is exemplified in numerous descriptions of the conceptual foundations for community psychology:

> Community psychology . . . is devoted to the study of general psychology processes that link social systems with individual behavior in complex interaction. Conceptual and experimental clarification of such linkages were seen as providing the basis for action programs directed toward improving individual, group, and social system functioning. (Bennett, Anderson, Cooper, Hassol, Klein, & Rosenblum, 1966, p. 7)

> The vanguard of the community approach to mental health seeks ways in which aspects of people's social environments can be changed in order to improve mental health significantly through impact on large groups. (Smith & Hobbs, 1966, p. 501)

> Community psychology is regarded as an approach to human behavior problems that emphasizes contributions made to their development by environmental forces as well as the potential contributions to be made toward their alleviation by the use of such forces. (Zax & Specter, 1974, p. 3)

The application of the physical and biological sciences alone will not solve our problems because the solutions lie in another field. Better contraceptives will control population only if people use them. New weapons may offset new defenses and vice versa, but a nuclear holocaust can be prevented only if the conditions under which nations make war can be changed. New methods of agriculture and medicine will not help if they are not practiced, and housing is a matter not only of buildings and cities but of how people live. Overcrowding can be corrected only by inducing people not to crowd, and the environment will continue to deteriorate until polluting practices are abandoned.

. . . we need to make vast changes in human behavior, and we cannot make them with the help of nothing more than physics or biology . . .

What we need is a technology of behavior. (Skinner, 1971, pp 4-5)[1]

Unfortunately, as suggested by the quotation from B. F. Skinner, the conceptual conformity of community psychologists has not been accompanied by a compatible technology capable of delineating principles or procedures for the modification of environmental, social, and physical structures in ways which could reliably influence important human behaviors. A continuing deficiency of the community psychology movement has been this inability to operationalize its rhetoric into specific, programmatic methods for bringing about measurable social change. For the most part, community psychologists are distinguished by the attitudes about how social problems should be conceptualized and not by their development of an effective intervention technology for preventing or treating such problems.

One possible source of such an intervention technology is the applied behavioral paradigm which, within the last 15 years, has achieved a wide circulation and prominent status among mental health professionals (Davison & Neale, 1974; Franks, 1969; Rimm & Masters, 1974; Ullmann & Krasner, 1969, 1975). The appeal of behavioral methods has been attributed to several of their distinctive characteristics. First, there is behavior modification's (the generic term for behavior therapy and applied behavior analysis) empirical and conceptual groundings in operant and classical conditioning theory (Skinner, 1953; Wolpe, 1958), general learning theory (Bandura, 1969), and experimental and social psychology (Goldstein, Heller, & Sechrest, 1966). Second, while behavioral extensions to applied work have involved some conceptual and practical adaptations (London, 1972), many procedures—particularly the adherence to objective data and the "scientific method"—can be traced to their historical origins in experimental research. However, the conceptual foundations of behavior modification are currently being extended by the decreasing reliance on simplistic conditioning explanations and concomitant emphases on

---

[1]Skinner, B. F. *Beyond freedom and dignity*, 1971. New York: Alfred A. Knopf, Inc.

self-control (Thoresen & Mahoney, 1974), cognitive processing (Bandura, 1974), and physiological psychology (Schwartz, 1973). Another trend involves the examination of linkages between macro-level (economics, physical settings, "culture," etc.) influences and behavior (Krasner & Ullmann, 1973). Thus, in its broadest historical and contemporary perspectives, behavior modification resides within Western "mainstream" psychology. In addition, its environmentalist position in many ways parallels the conceptual basis for community psychology.

Behavior modification is also an action-oriented, problem-solving approach. Behavior is "understood" when it can be demonstrated that particular processes or procedures (generally, environmental events) are responsible ("functionally related") for specified behavior changes (Mischel, 1968, 1976). A simple, descriptive account of behavior and its context is considered an inadequate level of understanding. Thus, a behavioral approach is not a highly developed hypothetico-deductive theory, but rather a framework and a set of principles and methods for changing human behavior (Zifferblatt & Hendricks, 1974).

This experimental tradition also has been transferred to applied work and represents probably the most unique aspect of behavior modification (Kazdin, 1975b). Experimental methodology is used to provide data validating the effects of different procedures on specified target behaviors (Kazdin, 1975a). These data also serve as feedback to the change agent and client. Ideally, there is *not* a clear demarcation between service/intervention and research. Data collection is an integral and inherent part of the change process itself. Optimally, service and research are thoroughly integrated (Winett, 1976b).

Besides the conceptual and procedural linkages to experimental and general psychology and the reliance of applied work on validated data sources, behavior modification methods provide another utilitarian advantage when compared to other "traditional" behavior change approaches. The relative simplicity of the terminology and procedures has enabled other professionals (O'Leary & O'Leary, 1972) and non- or paraprofessionals to use behavior modification techniques with documented success (Tharp & Wetzel, 1969). In addition, the behavioral approach seems to be effective with a broad range of clients and problems on a "short-term basis (Rimm & Masters, 1974), suggesting that clinical services need no longer be limited to those persons who fit the "YAVIS syndrome" (Zax and Cowen, 1972). This ability to train large cadres of paraprofessionals effectively or to consult with other professionals so as to reach diverse groups of persons with "problems in living" was one of the original goals of the community mental health act (Zax & Cowen, 1972).

While the initiation and development of the behavioral paradigm and the community psychology movement have shared both the same temporal context and some common objections to alternative models of deviance and treatment (Ullmann & Krasner, 1975), they have only recently evidenced any attempts to comprehensively integrate their unique and extremely complementary strengths into a decisive science of social change (Winett, 1974). Intuitively, such an integration has much appeal. The contributions from a collegial alliance of community psychology and the behavioral paradigm are likely to exceed those derived from either model in isolation from the other.

While clinical applications of the behavioral paradigm have grown rapidly in stature and the scope of problem behaviors addressed has expended ambitiously (Stolz, Wienckowski, & Brown, 1975), this movement is at a critical stage which parallels the development and problems of community psychology. Behavior modification has primarily been used in ways that mirror most other forms of mental health interventions. Behavior therapists essentially have adopted the modes and mores of other clinicians by working within a structure that emphasizes one-to-one treatment with mildly distressed individuals who possess the personal and financial resources required by traditional psychotherapy (Rappaport & Chinsky, 1974). On the other hand, programmatic efforts with large groups of people (e.g., token economies) have generally focused on individuals with chronic, recalcitrant problems in closed institutional settings. Regardless of the effectiveness of both of these types of rehabilitative processes, it has been emphasized for over 15 years that this mode of service delivery can neither generate enough person-power to deal with all individuals who will require help nor ameliorate social conditions that may be responsible for many problems which people develop or encounter (Albee, 1959, 1967; Zax & Cowen, 1972). These same social conditions seriously constrain the effectiveness of many clinical interventions (Kelly, 1966).

Behavior modification techniques remain wedded to the existing mental health structure, which has had long-standing and severe limitations in addressing both the causes of and eventual solutions to human problems. Further, the environmentalist position of behaviorists has not usually been translated into active efforts at changing social-environmental determinants of human problems. Rather, a person's "deficits" and "excesses" are modified to fit the prevailing social system. This has been particularly true for institutionally based programs (Atthowe, 1973a).

On the one hand, behavior modifiers need to demonstrate that their principles and methods can be effectively used on a broader scale with a diversity of problems that are treated in less circumscribed settings and modalities than has been the usual case—for example, in clinics, well-controlled hospital wards, classrooms, etc. (Reppucci & Saunders, 1974; Winett, 1974). While behavioral methods have been shown to produce change in highly controlled, well-funded demonstration projects, their application for the most part has not been organized around system-level interventions that attempt to be preventive in nature and focus on large groups of people who often have only marginal social standing.

From a different perspective, community psychologists need to develop, adapt, or embrace a technology that provides empirically based methods for promoting these system-oriented changes. Currently, the rhetoric of the community psychology camp has not been matched by validated, concrete demonstrations of effective changes. While the political climate and fiscal cutbacks for social programs during the 1970s may have contributed to the relative impotence of this movement (Hersch, 1972), one solution to the disparity between words and deeds rests with the merging of perceptive social analyses with a technology of human behavior change.

This book attempts to survey the synthesis of the behavioral paradigm with community psychology—behavioral community psychology (Briscoe, Hoffmann, & Bailey, 1975)—by reviewing the recent extension of behaviorally based procedures to a number of community problems. This integration will be accomplished by an evaluation of these extensions on such criteria as preventive emphasis, ecological setting of the application, prospects for institutional rather than individual change, attention to generalization of changes across settings and time, and enrichment of behavioral approaches by investigation of sociological, political, economic, and systems variables. Applications will be presented for the following problem areas or settings: schools, juvenile offenders and adult offenders in institutions and community settings, drug abuse, alcoholism, community mental health programs and community organization, social skills training, programs for the aged, unemployment, and environmental protection.

Besides providing a content review, a methodological evaluation, and an ethical critique of the work in a given area, each chapter reflects several significant trends in the behavioral community psychology field. Hopefully, discussions of behavior modification and/or behavior therapy techniques will provide specifications of social interventions and services that often have been lacking in other summaries of community psychology. In addition, the systematic and relatively exhaustive coverage of behavioral applications to "nontraditional" mental health problems should illustrate the potential suitability of these procedures for problems which often have been considered too complex or pervasive to allow significant modification.

The specific content and emphasis of each chapter is summarized below:

Chapter 2—Schools

Behavioral research in school and child-care settings is the most developed area in terms of quantity of studies, methodological sophistication, and procedures and variables investigated. Because of the great number of projects involving school and child-care environments, this chapter is restricted primarily to a review of research completed within recent years. The review is divided into sections that include: the use of children in various therapeutic roles, self-control techniques, group change procedures, the problem of maintenance of treatment effects, ecological considerations involved in response generalization, curriculum development, basic skills and creativity, investigation of common classroom practices (homework, question asking, etc.), controversial areas (such as drug control of hyperactivity, racial integration, and self-government), influence of ecological variables, and consultation to teachers and other school personnel. While these studies provide a rich empirical foundation for school and child-care programs, the reviewed work consists primarily of demonstrations of functional relationships and not evaluations of programs. For this reason, the effects of behavioral interventions on long-standing school problems remain unclear as do the effects of dissemination and utilization efforts. However, the trends established by this work suggest that these questions as well as concerns about altering social and economic structures to assure high quality educational environments will soon be addressed. In addition, the scope of this chapter's research indicates that in the future the effective school interventionist will have an interdisciplinary preparation.

Chapter 3—The Juvenile Justice System

Chapter 3 discusses the historical development of the juvenile justice system and the conceptual basis for the enthusiastic incorporation of behavioral techniques into juvenile corrections. Behavior modification programs are reviewed according to the setting in which the intervention was delivered. Each of these categories is segmented further into the type of research design employed: case studies, single-group studies, A-B-A studies, and control-group studies. It is concluded that these investigations indicate an overall pattern of positive results, although interpretive confidence is restricted by several recurring methodological weaknesses (e.g., unstable baselines, lack of essential controls, failure to obtain multiple measures of outcome). Furthermore, programs conducted in nonresidential community settings tend to be associated with the most comprehensive levels of behavior change. A central concern of this chapter is a consideration of the larger impact which behavior modification may have on social policy decisions and the various social systems that affect youth who become "official" delinquents.

Chapter 4—Adult Corrections

Chapter 4 reviews the application of behavioral principles to adult offenders. Programs have been organized according to the correctional setting in which they have been implemented. While behavior modification techniques most frequently have been conducted in penal institutions (e.g., Alabama's Draper Correctional Center, Virginia's Contingency Management Program, and the Federal START Program), other intervention settings such as community-based residences, nonresidential treatment, and probation are reviewed. In the remainder of the chapter, correctional behavior modification is evaluated in terms of methodological, legal, ecological, conceptual, and ethical criteria. It is concluded that the ecological restriction of these techniques to institutional settings has prevented the behavioral paradigm from attaining either conceptual maturity or methodological rigor. In addition, suggestions are offered in response to the numerous legal and ethical challenges to correctional behavior modification which have been formulated recently. For the most part, these emerging legal-ethical requirements are compatible with the needed conceptual-methodological innovations. Hopefully, simultaneous responsiveness to both sets of demands will yield new procedures with a greater capacity for influencing criminal conduct than heretofore has been the case.

Chapter 5—Drug Abuse

Chapter 5 provides an overview of the diverse strategies of drug abuse control which have been attempted. These efforts have included legal controls, moral injunctions, and numerous attempts at therapeutic modification involving detoxification, civil commitment, therapeutic communities, methadone maintenance, opiate antagonists, heroin maintenance, psychotherapy, and drug education. Emphasis is placed on behavior therapy techniques which have been applied increasingly to a wide range of drug abuse problems. Specific treatments have followed one of the five therapeutic paradigms: aversion, systematic desensitization, contingency contracting, token economies, and multimodal treatment combinations. Despite the rapid proliferation of social-learning treatments for drug abuse, it is concluded that an unconfounded assessment of intervention efficacy would be premature at this point. In addition to the methodological inadequacy of the existing literature, most behavioral approaches to drug abuse have involved methods whose suitability is limited to a narrow range of clients, treatment settings, and therapeutic personnel. Recommendations for more ambitious empirical and intervention objectives are formulated.

Chapter 6—Alcoholism

Following a discussion of general assessment and theoretical approaches to alcoholic behavior, a review of social-learning therapies for alcoholics is presented. It is concluded that a continuation of the historical reliance on aversion treatments of alcoholics will yield outcomes that are neither comprehensive nor durable enough to exert a substantial impact on a community's drinking problems. For this reason, the chapter emphasizes the development of three treatment dimensions which are less concerned with suppressing drinking or nullifying the positive valence of alcohol and are more concerned with increasing the probability of alternatives to uncontrolled drinking in high-risk situations. One trend has been to select goals that are likely to be supported maximally by post-intervention social networks. The choice of controlled drinking as a treatment objective reflects the decision that some alcoholics can learn a pattern of moderate drinking that will be more easily maintained by natural contingencies than abstinence. A second development has been the bolstering of social contingencies which would maintain sobriety in the community. Regulation of familial, legal, social, and vocational consequences of drinking has proven that maintenance of either controlled drinking or abstinence can be accomplished through the contingent mobilization of these resources. A final trend is the use of "broad-spectrum" behavior therapies which seek to reduce alcohol abuse by the combined establishment of interpersonal behaviors, vocational skills, and general problem-solving abilities and/or the modification of frequently suspected elicitors of alcoholic drinking such as anxiety.

Chapter 7—Community Mental Health

The rationale for presenting a selective group of topics and studies in this chapter rests on a number of considerations. First, there is a need to provide empirically based, accountable mental health services, criteria often ignored in many mental health systems. Second, the continuing problems of maintaining marginal people in communities and the public prejudice against community treatment indicate the significance of demonstrating that carefully planned programs can provide mechanisms for community maintenance. Third, innovative community mental health often has relied on the development of (1) training programs for paraprofessionals and (2) technologies for organizational change. Finally, there is a general awareness that community mental health must move beyond the provision of outpatient services to areas that include community development and organization, primary and secondary prevention, and large-scale systems' change. Behavioral and nonbehavioral studies are reviewed in each of the above areas. While it is concluded that the chapter presents an idealized version of community mental health, it is noted that the research was selected to show the rich potential for developing an accountable community mental health based on organizational, community, and social change.

Chapter 8—Social Skills Training for Psychiatric Residents

Behavioral researchers and clinicians increasingly have been concerned with developing programmatic treatments that effectively promote pro-social interpersonal skills. While the primary research populations for this work have been college students, Chapter 8 describes the extension of this research to hospitalized psychiatric residents who typically are characterized by inadequate interpersonal adjustment and severe social skill deficiencies. A number of treatment approaches applied to both collegiate and psychiatric populations are reviewed and organized according to the following levels of research strategy: investigation of isolated behavioral treatment elements, examination of the effects of complex treatment packages involving more than one presumably active treatment ingredient, and evaluation of the comparative effectiveness of alternative behavioral programs applied to matched or randomly assigned participants. While numerous and apparently effective techniques and treatment packages are identified, this chapter emphasizes the necessity of modifying both hospital structures and post-residential environments so that they contribute to the maintenance of previously existing or treatment-instigated social skills. Recommendations for the design of supportive environments are presented.

Chapter 9—Aging

Numerous problems faced by the aged are discussed in Chapter 9. From a sociopsychological perspective, the origin of these problems can be attributed to several sources including cultural myths about aging, environmental impediments to full functioning, limited financial resources, self-fulfilling social expectations, and the passivity-inducing nature of traditional "treatments" for being old. A series of programs intended to reverse such influences are presented with special emphasis devoted to interventions that encourage maximal retention of recipients' independence and dignity, provide increased access to psychological and health services, involve a multiservice orientation, and promote improved patient functioning in old age facilities. Recommendations for future directions in geriatric services are presented with the suggestion that aging be conceptualized not in personal, individual-centered terms but as an environmental-social problem which requires structural and social redesign.

Chapter 10—Unemployment

Psychology, as a profession, has had little impact on the condition of unemployment or the numerous personal and social consequences with which it is associated. Following an analysis of factors contributing to chronic or cyclical unemployment, Chapter 10 reviews the programs that have been intended to increase employment rates. A prominent example of such programs is found in the series of legislative actions that have mandated funded manpower development and job training programs. In addition, a description of the few behaviorally based employment interventions that have appeared recently is provided. While the methodological infancy of this work does not permit cause-effect conclusions, it is encouraging to observe that psychologists' legacy of neglect is beginning to be replaced by social learning programs that attempt to develop basic behaviors functional in obtaining and maintaining employment—for example, soliciting prospects, interviewing skills, and solving on-the-job problems. In addition, this chapter examines and details some needed modifications in the economic system to reduce the problem of unemployment.

Chapter 11–Environmental Problems

Interest in environmental problems and in the more general area of the impact of the physical environment is burgeoning. However, most work in this area has been descriptive, correlational, and theoretical. Recent behavioral research presents a contrast to many of the studies in environmental psychology in that the behavioral paradigm dictates active attempts to prevent or ameliorate environmentally destructive behaviors. Research in litter control, recycling, energy conservation, transportation, architectural design, and population change is reviewed. This work is methodologically sound and advances research techniques appropriate to community-wide programs by employing "open field" methods. There is also a concern in these studies for developing practical, cost-effective procedures. In addition, some of the projects involved multiple measurement techniques and collaboration with researchers from other disciplines. All these developments indicate that behavioral-environmental research can have a significant impact on environmental problems and can broaden the conceptual and methodological base of behavioral community psychology.

* * *

There are several important trends that emerge in these chapters. It is apparent that interdisciplinary training or multidisciplinary teams are needed for these endeavors even when such work entails only minimal change in educational, legal, media, economic, or political systems. It is especially clear that the behavioral community psychologist's "content" will not be restricted to typical mental health concerns, nor will it suffice to be simply conversant with behavioral methodology or principles (Winett, 1976a).

It is probable that future roles of the behavioral community psychologist (particularly at the advanced degree level) will not involve "direct service" but rather will include job descriptions such as "educator" or "trainer" of other professionals and paraprofessionals, "organizational and management consultant," "program developer and evaluator," and "environmental designer." It also seems that these broader frameworks and roles will prompt, if not directly require, the development of strategies and active efforts to disseminate procedures or programs that have been favorably evaluated in (a) selected site(s). All of these discernible trends suggest that the label "behavioral community psychology" is a tentative, impermanent term which will quickly be replaced by others that become more appropriate (Winett, 1976b).

While the synthesis of behavior modification and community psychology seems timely and promising, the subsequent chapters also identify several limitations and sources of caution. The diversity of material that is presented indicates that behavioral methods can be applied in many new areas (e.g., environmentally destructive behaviors, unemployment, evaluation of physical settings, and population control), but there undoubtedly will be settings and problems that are inappropriate for behavioral analyses and applications. In addition, many proposals and projects that seem to be logical extensions of the behavioral model may be shown to be shortsighted, impractical, misused, or simply ineffective. There are many such examples in the studies and projects reviewed in this book.

It is hoped that the feedback provided from successful and unsuccessful projects will modify and expand the behavioral paradigm by leading to the incorporation of other data sources, principles, and concepts, and when necessary will result in the abandonment of earlier cherished but dysfunctional notions. These constructive developments will be made possible if the major tool of the behavioral approach—experimentation—is rigorously retained and strengthened by the inclusion of multiple assessment sources. We are firmly advocating an "open systems" model so that behavioral community psychology does not become a new but cloistered social problem school (Kazdin, 1975b). Behavioral community psychology can stimulate excitement and provide solutions to some aspects of social problems but by itself cannot provide the panacea to either current or future social problems.

Aspiring to acquire knowledge from diverse disciplines, working cooperatively with other professionals and paraprofessionals, and developing and disseminating effective programs for institutional change are ambitious goals for behavioral community psychologists. While the fulfillment of these ambitions will be welcomed, the means by which they are pursued require our constant and deliberate scrutiny. The following chapters should reflect the growing necessity for public and professional monitoring of social interventions. The means for such monitoring may take the form of codes of ethics appropriate for these social programs (Braun, 1975), guidelines for social experimentation that include informed consent from both individuals and communities (Ullmann & Krasner, 1975), procedures that assure input and control from citizens (Winett, 1974), and increased clarity concerning the political and social values that are inherent components of our work (Winett & Winkler, 1972; Zax & Specter, 1974).

Chapter 2
PROBLEMS IN THE SCHOOLS

This chapter examines recent research being conducted in public school settings,[1] an area that has received the most concentrated attention by behaviorists during the last decade. This literature has been organized around a number of procedural innovations or problem areas, including: children as agents of change in the classroom, self-control procedures, group-change and other methods to increase the practicality of behavioral programs, the maintenance and generalization of treatment effects, positive and negative "side effects" (response generalization) of behavioral programs, curriculum development, social issues (e.g., the use of drugs for behavior control, IQ testing, racial integration, peer management), ecological variables, and consultation to teachers and other school personnel.

This brief overview of topics to be covered should apprise the reader of the great breadth of work currently being done in school settings. The magnitude and diversity of public school projects are amplified further by noting that the large body of research reviewed in this chapter has been limited to publications of the last several years. Though this research is not without its limitations, it does exemplify how a field can develop quickly and progress conceptually given a sound methodological base. Following this review is a summary of the principles and problems suggested by the literature. This review should provide a rich empirical foundation for persons working in a variety of school settings.

The status of behavioral approaches to educational problems warrants an initial caveat. The studies reviewed in this chapter are essentially demonstrations of functional relationships. They are not programs. While the program designer now has a vast research literature to use as a basis for structuring programs, it remains unclear how either the outside change agent or the researcher gains entry to schools to implement programs or how internal change agents function (Reppucci & Saunders, 1974). This is not a criticism restricted to behavioral work per se because little experimental data is available to clarify this issue as it relates to any orientation or system. A recent study by Fairweather, Sanders,

---

[1] For analogous work at the collegiate level, the interested reader should consult the *Journal of Applied Behavior Analysis*, 1968 to present.

and Tornatzky (1974; described in detail in Chapter 7, this volume) indicated that many theories about entry into systems were not substantiated by actual attempts at implementing a program in 255 mental hospitals where the level and mode of approaching these hospitals and persuasive efforts to have the hospitals adopt the program were varied systematically. Rather, the data suggested that a shaping strategy for entry and organizational change would probably be the most successful approach.

It is also uncertain how behavioral literature and methodology are incorporated by most teachers and other school personnel into programs. Specific questions would be concerned with how the procedures are adapted and adopted; by what kinds of teachers, schools, and systems; under what conditions and for what purposes; with how much time lag from publication of a finding to its implementation; and how such procedures might be misused (Stein, 1975).[2]

It also remains unclear whether the use of specific procedures or packages or the behavior analytic process itself makes any real difference compared to other traditional or nontraditional approaches in ameliorating such recalcitrant problems as the failure of schools to educate many lower class or minority children (Bereiter & Englemann, 1966). Answers to this type of question call for a shift to a comparative experimental methodology (Winett & Edwards, 1974) that examines the relative worth of different educational models on diverse measures of different types of children and school settings. These are, of course, questions of dissemination and utilization (Fairweather et al., 1974). The time is ripe for examining such issues, but, as this chapter will indicate, the development of maximally effective education programs will require continuing, basic, micro-level evaluation of behavior change strategies. Indeed, it is because of the behavioral paradigm's strong tradition of experimentation, replication, and gradual accumulation of knowledge and technology that concerns about dissemination are now relevant.

Children as Agents of Change in the Classroom

Effects on Peers

While the use of children in the classroom as helpers and tutors is not innovative, the attempt to delineate and evaluate potentially therapeutic behaviors is a relatively new area of investigation. If children can learn some behavioral techniques and/or be shown to be effective in a number of

---

[2]The innumerable behavior modification books and courses for teachers and other school personnel do not necessarily indicate that behavior change procedures are applied correctly. Further, the data on teacher consultation suggest that information about behavior modification does not usually lead to behavioral changes.

educational capacities, such research can have great impact in solving the "mini-max" problem of service delivery (Reppucci & Saunders, 1974)—that is, how to provide the maximum service at the minimum cost.

A few studies and case reports have shown that retarded children can serve as reliable observers in behavioral studies (Craighead, Mercatoris, & Bellack, 1974), that children can dispense tokens for appropriate behaviors to other children in a token economy (Winett, Richards, Krasner, & Krasner, 1971), and that normal and retarded children are able to use other simple reinforcement procedures effectively with their peers (Drabman & Spitalnik, 1973; Suratt, Ulrich, & Hawkins, 1969).

Recent research has become increasingly diverse and sophisticated. Drabman (1973), working with 22 extremely disruptive children (ages 11-15) in a state psychiatric hospital, compared the effectiveness of two types of token economies—one in which the teacher decided how many tokens each child earned for in-class social behaviors and dispensed the tokens, and a parallel system in which these duties were performed by an elected peer captain. Drabman's results indicated that the peer captain system was as effective as the teacher-monitored system in sharply reducing disruptive behavior.

Solomon and Wahler (1973) demonstrated that peers can both maintain and change inappropriate behavior. Five disruptive sixth-grade boys were the participants. Their peer therapists were selected because of their high reinforcement value (based on sociometric ratings) and their willingness to cooperate with the teacher and experimenter in change programs. The peer therapists were given brief training in identifying appropriate and inappropriate behavior, and in the use of social contingencies and differential attention. This intervention produced a gradual reduction in the disruptive behavior of all five participants.

During the initial baseline, all peer attention directed to the five boys followed disruptive behavior. The peer therapists were partly responsible for maintaining the deviant behavior originally and were totally responsible (the teacher's behavior did not change) for modifying the inappropriate behavior. However, the peer therapists accomplished the successful changes primarily by ignoring problem behaviors rather than by providing approval for pro-social behaviors. These data suggest that any pro-social behavior by the deviant boys was ignored during baseline and intervention periods. This study thus illustrates that children often unwittingly maintain problem behavior in their peers but are capable of supporting more acceptable behaviors when instructed in simple procedures of contingency management.

Greenwood, Sloan, and Baskin (1974) investigated methods of training peer mediators to perform behaviors that would differentially affect the work of other children in a special classroom. Children were divided into four small groups. A peer manager was elected from each group with eligibility based on high rates of school attendance and correct responding on programmed mathematics material. The study sought to compare the performance of the peer

manager with *minimal* and *more thorough* training and two types of contingencies—a *manager performance* maintenance contingency (manager received
points contingent on his performance) and a *group performance* maintenance
contingency (manager received points contingent on the group's behavior).

The results indicated that with minimal training, the four managers'
performance (giving points and praise) was inferior compared to the teacher's.
More thorough training led to large increases in appropriate dispensing of praise
for three of the four managers, but had variable effects on appropriate point
dispensing. In general, the training procedure modified the managers' behaviors
so that their performance approximated the teacher's. Also, the manager
performance contingency tended to produce more appropriate behavior of the
other students than the group performance contingency.

This study is important in again demonstrating that children who were judged
to be "unmanageable, uncontrollable" (Greenwood et al., 1974, p. 113) could
be trained effectively as change agents for their equally disruptive peers.
However, more data are needed on the behavioral changes of the managers' peers
and the longevity of changes associated with these kinds of interventions.

A much more formal procedure involving peer tutoring was investigated by
Harris and Sherman (1973a). Such procedures are important for programs that
cannot afford to decrease the student-teacher ratio (Winett, Calkins, Douglas, &
Prus, 1975). Fourth and fifth graders were asked to arrange themselves in groups
of two and three for a 15-minute period and to help each other with math work.
Following the tutoring session, the children worked independently on math
problems. The study was designed to evaluate the effects of tutoring on
problems correct, problems worked on, and correct problems per minute. In
addition, the effects of an academic contingency, extra study time, and prior
exposure to the materials on which the children would be working were
examined. The most effective procedures involved tutoring with the same
problems to be used in the regular period or same-problem tutoring combined
with the contingency. Moreover, improvement associated with tutoring using
only similar materials suggested that the children were not just receiving answers
but were learning general skills. The informality and ease of this type of peer
tutoring makes it an important adjunct to various forms of classroom teaching.

Johnson and Bailey (1974) have performed a systematic study of cross-age
tutoring. Tutors were fifth graders who were selected on the basis of their
superior academic performance, good behavior, and interest in being a tutor. Ten
kindergarten children who could not count objects or name numerals were the
tutees. These students were matched on arithmetic ability and placed in an
experimental or control group. Arithmetic was chosen as the subject area
because arithmetic tasks can be defined in behavioral terms and are well suited
to drill and review exercises, precisely the type of instruction that tutors can
perform with minimal training.

Tutor instruction consisted of only three 30-minute sessions in which proper principles of modeling, social reinforcement, and data recording were described, role played, and practiced. Tutoring sessions were 20 minutes long for 26 sessions; each session was followed by a 10-minute reinforcement-activity period contingent only on reasonable social behavior. The tutoring program was based on the mastery concept of instruction. During each session, specific tasks were the focus of instruction. At the end of a session, a test was given on the tasks; a perfect score on three consecutive tests allowed the student to progress to the next task. Participants also were rated on categories that included social reinforcement, academic responding, and instructional behaviors.

The experimental and control group initially scored about the same on a test designed to assess number skills. However, on three successive tests, the experimental subjects consistently outscored controls. Individual data revealed that children gained only in those areas in which they were tutored and that children who received the least praise from the tutors gained the least. A wide range of differences was found in the rate of learning from this small group of children, further suggesting the need for individualized instructional programs supported by tutors.

In addition to the benefits accrued to the tutee, there also is evidence that the tutor gains as much if not more than the tutee (Cloward, 1967; Dineen, Clark, & Risley, 1976 in press). Therefore, tutoring procedures have at least four advantages when adopted by educational systems: (1) tutors allow a greater individualization of instruction; (2) teachers' time can be spent in such activities as program planning rather than drill work, for example; (3) tutees can gain academically; and (4) tutors can gain academically. There is also the need to document nonacademic gains that can be attributed to tutoring programs. Finally, in the Dineen et al. (1976 in press) study tutoring was performed by same-age children; further work needs to examine optimal matches and gains associated with different ages and ability levels of tutors and tutees.

Effect on Teachers

Another area involving children as change agents is found in recent work showing that children can modify the behavior of their teachers. For example, Graubard, Rosenburg, and Miller (1971) taught retarded children to use contingent eye contact, requests for extra help, and complimentary comments to increase a teacher's positive contacts and decrease negative contacts. In general, the effects that student behaviors have on elementary teachers have received little empirical attention. Sherman and Cormier (1974) instructed two very disruptive fifth graders on appropriate and inappropriate classroom behavior. Following this, the children planned behavior change strategies and received feedback on their efforts. In another part of the study, they received tangible reinforcement for the reduction of inappropriate behavior. Measures included a wide range of observed teacher and student behaviors.

The data indicated that the children's behavior became more appropriate only during the tangible reward condition. During this manipulation, they also received more teacher attention to their appropriate behavior, fewer negative and more positive verbal responses by the teacher, and more positive behavioral ratings. Thus, changes in the students' behavior produced consistent changes in the teacher's behavior.

Although this study primarily examined the changes which student behavior produced in the teacher as opposed to the more usual program involving teacher influence on students, the focus was still unidirectional. This kind of orientation tends to ignore the inherent two-way quality of social interactions and may be one of the reasons behavioral programs often have failed to show maintenance of behavior change (Kazdin, 1973b). For example, a triadic model of consultation with teachers (Tharp & Wetzel, 1969) suggests that reciprocal reinforcement systems must be developed wherein changed teacher behavior is reinforced by changed student behavior, changed student behavior is reinforced by changes in the teacher, specific consultant behaviors reinforce the teacher (Cossairt, Hall, & Hopkins, 1973) while the consultant is reinforced by changes in both students and teachers. Abrupt withdrawal of the consultant or lack of reciprocal changes at any point may cause the system to break down. This broader, "ecological" perspective will be discussed further in subsequent sections of this chapter. However, the research reviewed in this section indicates that children can be effective agents of change in their classrooms and schools. It is likely that the range of potential therapeutic roles for children will be expanded greatly in the future.

Self-Control and Self-Evaluation

Self-control procedures are important for numerous reasons. They represent an important synthesis between humanistic and behavioral approaches (Thoresen & Mahoney, 1974; Winett, 1973), may be one method to increase generalization, and may reduce professional and other staff time needed to produce change.

Typical self-control procedures involve several components (Glynn & Thomas, 1974), including self-assessment, self-recording, self-determination of reinforcement, and self-administration of reinforcers. However, in the studies to be reported, all of these aspects of self-control are performed within a framework provided by an external agent (teacher, experimenter). The student generally does not decide what sorts of behavior(s) he deems appropriate or inappropriate.

In an early study, Lovitt and Curtiss (1969) found that a 12-year-old pupil in a class for children with behavior disorders performed at higher academic rates when he arranged the contingency requirements rather than the teacher specifying them. A subsequent study with the same pupil indicated that his higher rate of performance was not related to the magnitude of reinforcement but to the person serving as contingency manager.

Glynn (1970) used four heterogenously grouped classes of ninth-grade girls to examine the effects of experimenter-determined, self-determined, and chance-determined token reinforcement systems compared to a no-token control. The task in this experiment consisted of a daily reading of different passages followed by a multiple choice test. Tokens were assigned in the experimenter-determined condition by a predetermined criterion of tokens per correct response; in the self-determined condition, students were given no explicit guidelines to follow in rewarding themselves for correct answers. The chance-determined treatment involved a yoked design wherein each child was randomly matched to a student in the self-determined condition and received the same number of tokens that day.

Both the experimenter and self-determined systems were effective in improving daily test performance, while the chance and no-token conditions did not show improvement. Students in the self-determined condition placed more stringent requirements on themselves than those developed by the experimenter.

The Lovitt and Curtiss (1969) and Glynn (1970) studies are procedurally similar in that limited self-assessment and self-recording were involved. The students could control only how much reinforcement they should receive for certain tasks which were preselected by teachers without any input from students.

In the context of a study involving a comparison of reward and response-cost token reinforcement procedures with pupils in a psychiatric hospital, Kaufman and O'Leary (1972) examined the feasibility of a self-evaluation technique as a method to increase generalization once an external reinforcement system was terminated. Following O'Leary's previous work (O'Leary, Becker, Evans, & Saudargas, 1969), students in the reward condition received ratings from the teacher based on their behavior during special reading classes. Ratings were based on how well students followed the classroom rules, and ratings were convertible to tokens. In the cost condition, students began with the number of tokens equivalent to the greatest number that could be earned by a student in the reward condition. Based on their ratings, they lost tokens for less than full adherence to classroom rules. The results revealed that the two procedures were equally effective in decreasing the frequency of disruptive behavior. Withdrawal of either system resulted in a marked increase in disruptive behavior.

After 3 months in which the main part of the study was conducted, self-evaluation procedures were introduced into the reward class for 6 days and into the cost class for 7 days. In both classes students gave themselves high ratings and their behavior did not deteriorate as it had during the withdrawal stage of the study. Surprisingly, the data indicated no correspondence between the students' evaluations and the ratings made by the teacher.

Santogrossi, O'Leary, Romanczyk, and Kaufman (1973) examined the effectiveness of self-evaluation procedures over a longer time period and also attempted to ascertain the importance of several elements of the self-evaluation procedure. Participants were nine adolescent residents in a psychiatric hospital who were involved in a remedial reading program. The study was conducted over a 3-month period and included the following sequence of experimental conditions: baseline, self-evaluation alone, teacher-determined points with back-up reinforcers, self-determined points with back-ups, matching of self and teacher's ratings with the reward of three bonus points over the teacher's rating if the residents were within one point of the teacher (or a loss of three points if they were not), teacher-determined points with back-ups, and self-determined points with back-ups. Data consisted of observations of the residents' disruptive behavior.

Initially, the residents were very disruptive. Self-evaluation (alone) proved unsuccessful, with the children giving themselves very high ratings for very disruptive behavior. The teacher-determined system decreased disruption, while the self-determined system was not successful. During the matching phase, the residents openly revolted against the system and became extremely unruly and refused to cooperate. A return to the teacher-determined system was not as successful as it had been before, and a final attempt at self-determined reinforcement was not successful. This study should indicate caution for practitioners interested in the promotion of student self-control particularly in terms of implementing programs to run for relatively long periods using techniques whose efficacy has been ascertained only in terms of short-term demonstrations.

Drabman, Spitalnik, and O'Leary (1973) extended this research by examining methods to shape matching behavior. After a token economy had been in operation, the children (eight 9- to 10-year-old boys in an adjustment class) were taught matching skills during a 15-minute class. During a 10-day token program, the children recorded the number of points that the teacher had given them. If the children's ratings were within one point of the teacher's ratings, they received the number of points they allotted themselves. If their ratings were more than one point different from the teacher's, they received no points. A perfect match between student and teacher ratings earned the student an additional bonus point and extensive praise from the teacher. A 20-day fading procedure consisted of gradually and systematically reducing the number of children whose ratings were corroborated in the above manner. During a 12-day self-evaluation period, there were no checks with the teacher's ratings. Children were awarded the points they assigned themselves. Throughout the different phases of the study, honesty and the privilege of self-evaluation were stressed, and the children were praised for accurate matching.

Disruptive behavior remained very low and academic output very high during the matching, fading, and self-evaluation parts of the study. These researchers credited the shaping procedure, praise, the climate of honesty, the establishment of self-rating as a privilege, and a less-than-clear specification to the children of exactly what behaviors were being rated by the teacher for the successful results.

Bolstad and Johnson (1972) also were interested in both the different facets of self-control and the use of self-control procedures to promote generalization. Children in this study were from ten combination first- and second-grade classes. Based on the teachers' reports and pre-baseline observations, the four most disruptive children from each class were selected. After baseline, three of these children in each class were placed on an externally regulated system wherein low levels of disruptive behavior were reinforced. The fourth child acted as a control. In the next phase of the study, two of the three children in each class were taught to self-observe their own disruptive behavior following a matching procedure with an in-class observer; this procedure was similar to that used by Drabman et al. (1973). The children received points and reinforcers based on their data. The third child continued on the external reinforcement system. In the fourth phase of the study, the self-regulation children continued their system, but their data were not checked with an independent observer. The other children remained on the external system or acted as controls. In the last phase of the study, all experimental children were placed on extinction; prizes were no longer obtainable. However, half of the self-regulation group continued to self-observe their frequency of disruptive behavior.

During the external reinforcement system, 96% of the children reduced their rate of disruption; 76% reduced their rate to less than one-half of their baseline level. In the next phase, children on either the external or self-regulation system had a much lower rate of disruptive behavior than control children. It was noteworthy that 75% of the children's ratings fell within the permissible range (plus or minus three disruptive behaviors) using an independent observer as the standard.

When children's self-recordings were not checked, both the external and self-regulated children continued to behave at levels similar to the previous phase with no differences between the self-regulation and external groups. Seventy-one percent of the children's self-observations fell within the permissible range, although they were not informed of the observer's recordings or rewarded for matching. During the extinction phase, all groups of children on reinforcement systems displayed lower rates of disruption than the controls; there were no differences between the two self-regulation groups and the external group, nor were there differences between the group that continued to self-record and the self-regulating group that discontinued recordings.

While differences supporting the superiority of self-regulation were not found, these data are encouraging. Together with the Drabman et al. (1973) results, they showed that with some training in accurate self-observation, children as young as first and second graders can learn these skills, and in turn can use self-regulation to modify their own behavior. While initially this training would take a good deal of the teacher's time, some partial checking system (Drabman et al., 1973) could be instituted, thus reducing teacher time while still maintaining self-regulatory effects. One cautionary note with the Bolstad and

Johnson study is that across the different phases, self-regulation procedures were in effect for only 21 sessions (i.e., it was still a short-term demonstration).

After finding that self-recording tied to access to free time successfully maintained high levels of on-task behavior that had been established previously by an external system (Glynn, Thomas, & Shee, 1973), Glynn and Thomas (1974) conducted another study to determine whether self-regulation could be used successfully without prior exposure to an external system. Nine 7- and 8-year-olds who frequently did not attend to their lessons were the participants. Following the baseline, a self-control procedure entailing an audio signal which sounded randomly throughout the lessons was instituted. Children were to record, at the signal, whether they were on or off task. On-task checks were redeemable for free time. Baseline conditions were then reintroduced, followed by a modified self-control condition that included a shortening of the interval between audio cues.

During the two baselines, on-task behavior averaged about 50%. On-task behavior averaged 70% during the first self-control period and 90% during the second self-control condition with much less variability in behavior associated with this second self-control condition.

While Glynn and Thomas (1974) illustrated that external regulation is probably not a prerequisite for self-control procedures, several notes of caution should be identified. The self-control procedures were in effect for only 10 days. Some training and much cueing were apparently essential for the system to be successful. Finally, it might be argued that extensive cueing, including large charts that said, "LOOK AT THE TEACHER—STAY IN YOUR SEAT—BE QUIET" and "WORK AT YOUR PLACE—READ INSTRUCTIONS ON THE BLACKBOARD" (Glynn & Thomas, 1974, p. 302), makes a bit of a travesty of the term "self-control." Demonstration studies are needed in which children decide for themselves, within some guidelines, what is appropriate behavior, are taught how to self-record and match some external criteria, and maintain these skills under gradually faded overt cues. A distinct but currently underdeveloped advantage of self-control procedures is their potential to mitigate partially problems of generalization and to teach children some very worthwhile behaviors applicable under diverse circumstances; for example, self-management and self-reinforcement procedures have been extended recently to composition writing (Ballard & Glynn, 1975). It is expected that future research will extend the applications of self-control methods to new educational targets including prescribed academic and nonacademic skills.

Group and Other Practical Procedures

The purpose of this section is to highlight briefly a number of studies that have investigated procedures to make behavior change programs in schools more practical and less costly. Parallel information also is found in the two previous sections and the section on consultation.

Group Procedures

An intermediate step between the modification of an individual's behavior and that of a school or system is the demonstration of effective change of small groups or whole classrooms. While many behavioral programs (e.g., token economies) have involved entire classrooms or schools, the contingencies usually are individually devised. A large savings of staff time might be incurred if it could be demonstrated that contingencies that focus on the behavior of the group as a whole are as effective in modifying individual behavior as are individual contingencies.

Litow and Pumroy (1975) have developed three categories of group-oriented contingencies: (1) a dependent group-oriented contingency system in which the performance of selected group members determines whether or not the entire group is reinforced—this method has been used primarily to generate peer pressure on classmates deficient in social or academic performance; (2) an independent group-oriented contingency system in which the same contingencies are in effect for all members of the group, but the contingency is applied to each individual based on her/his performance, and each individual's outcomes are independent of other group members—this type of system has been used extensively in special education settings; (3) an interdependent group-oriented contingency system in which the same contingencies are in effect for each group member and also are applied to a specified level of group performance. For example, every student in a class might have to complete a set number of problems for the entire class to have recess. The interdependent group-oriented contingency probably holds the most promise of being an effective and practical method for classroom change. The following studies are examples of this method.

In an early project, Packard (1970), working in four separate elementary classrooms, treated whole classes as "individual organisms." Teachers were trained to discriminate when their classes were attending; they recorded attention by switching on a timer when the class was attentive and stopping the timer when the class was inattentive. In this way it was possible to compute a time-attending percentage score. A light connected to this apparatus provided differential feedback to the class on its attentiveness. Access to play activities was made contingent on the attending score. This group contingency was used successfully in kindergarten, third-, fifth-, and sixth-grade classrooms, and inspection of individual data from a subsample of children indicated fairly uniform effects across different children.

Greenwood, Hops, Delquadri, and Guild (1974) extended Packard's research by examining the effects of rules, feedback, and reinforcement components of the group procedure. A similar timer/clock apparatus was used, and teachers kept track of the percentage of appropriate behavior. Rules were posted in the classroom. Feedback consisted of operating the apparatus during class sessions, explaining the meaning of the light, and calculating a percentage score of appropriate behavior which was announced at the end of the class. Reinforcement (group activities) was contingent on the class meeting a continually increasing criterion of appropriate behavior. Teachers also were instructed to praise individual children as well as the group for appropriate behavior. rules alone had little effect; rules and feedback produced some changes; while the combination of rules, feedback, and reinforcement produced the highest and most uniform levels of appropriate behavior.

Several studies (Barrish, Saunders, & Wolf, 1969; Harris & Sherman, 1973b; Medland & Stachnik, 1972) have investigated what has been called the "good behavior game" in which a class is divided into teams which compete for various group prizes or activities contingent on their good behavior; all teams usually can win if certain criteria are reached. A group's score typically is based on the individual team members' behavior. These studies have shown that the game is simple to operate and reduces disruptive behavior. Initially, consequences are necessary, but after the rules and feedback components of the game have been associated with consequences, they may be used together without consequences and still maintain good behavior.

Two other facets of group procedures are of importance. Comparisons of group and individual contingency procedures (Herman & Tramontana, 1971; Litow & Pumroy, 1975; Long & Williams, 1973) have indicated that group procedures are as effective as individual ones, but group contingencies are somewhat easier to administer. Secondly, Winett, Battersby, and Edwards (1975) found that an interdependent group-oriented contingency in a very disruptive sixth-grade classroom increased the academic performance and improved the social behavior of children who were working at diverse academic ability levels on individualized assignments.

Other Practical Procedures

Because the projects reviewed in this chapter generally are demonstration studies, a major concern involves the applicability of these procedures to "regular" classrooms that are not owned or extensively operated by the experimenters and do not have many resources for reinforcers, observers, and so on. McLaughlin and Malaby (1972a, 1972b) were able to establish a token economy in a normal fifth-grade classroom for an entire year. Data were collected in spelling, language, handwriting, and math. Thus, thousands of assignments (points were awarded for completed assignments) were represented in their data. Features of this project that made it especially practical included the use of natural, cost-free reinforcers such as privileges, games, special projects; point exchanges for back-ups every 4 days rather than every day; student self-correction of work with partial checking by the teacher; and students functioning as "bankers" and observers. A number of studies demonstrated the efficacy of some of the procedures that were used. It was of particular importance that operation of the system required only about 25 minutes per week of the teacher's time. There is a need for similar projects that demonstrate the feasibility and generality of some newly developed techniques (self-control, use of peer change agents) as well as additional research on simple, cost-free procedures such as restructuring academic activities, feedback, and public recognition (Van Houten, Hill & Parsons, 1975; Van Houten & Sullivan, 1975).

Congruent with the themes of practicality and promotion of change in large groups is the development of films that depict alternative ways of behaving. While the use of modeling techniques has gained wide currency in other areas, there have been few studies that have evaluated experimentally the impact of films or other modeling media in classrooms. Unfortunately, a study (O'Connor, 1969) with wide implications for these issues has not received systematic follow-up. Nursery school children who were very socially withdrawn were assigned to experimental and control groups. The former group watched a film that showed increasingly more pronounced social interactions between children who received positive social consequences for their behavior. The audio part of the film stressed the appropriate behavior of the models. Controls saw a film that did not depict social interactions.

Observations indicated that children in the experimental group changed their behavior to the extent that it was similar to the behavior of non-isolates. The control children remained isolated and withdrawn. The comparison of the behavior of isolate children to the normative behavior of non-isolates was a noteworthy aspect of this study that should be incorporated into other projects.

This study suggests that a wide variety of films depicting alternative social and academic behaviors could be developed, evaluated, and disseminated by the use of educational television. Decisions concerning their showing could be determined locally and the immediate and long-term benefits of the films evaluated. Attempts to make procedures more practical so that they can be widely disseminated are a promising yet still limited endeavor. This is an area that clearly needs more attention; a final section of this chapter will discuss the problem.

Generalization

The problem of generalization can be divided into two components—stimulus and response generalization (Kazdin, 1973a). In the first case the concern is whether behavior change will be maintained under different stimulus conditions. In other words, when the contingencies are terminated or the person leaves the treatment environment will her/his behavior deteriorate or return to baseline standards? Unfortunately, the existing data indicate that behavioral persistence is the exception rather than the rule (Atthowe, 1973a; Kazdin & Bootzin, 1972). Kazdin & Bootzin (1972) have characterized many behavioral programs (token economies) as being *prosthetic* rather than *therapeutic*, because change can be demonstrated only within the treatment milieu. However, a number of investigations have been directed at this problem and are beginning to demonstrate behavioral maintenance.

Response generalization refers to the radiating effects of an intervention to other behaviors that were not the initial focus of treatment. Given the movement toward a more systems-ecological perspective (Wahler, 1975; Willems, 1974), the question changes from Does response generalization occur, to How can such effects be measured, for what kinds of classes of responses are radiating effects predictable, and how can therapeutic strategies be organized in light of this phenomenon?

Stimulus Generalization/Maintenance

The examination of maintenance is the next logical step after demonstrations of control of behavior in one situation or under one set of stimulus conditions, although it must be remembered that convincing indications of behavior change in one setting are still relatively recent (O'Leary & O'Leary, 1972). Suggestions to increase generalization are plentiful (O'Leary & Drabman, 1971) and have included:

1)   fading of reinforcement contingencies;
2)   coupling of social reinforcement with tangible reinforcement followed by fading of tangible reinforcement;
3)   training in multiple situations;
4)   treatment in the natural environment;
5)   programming the environment (teachers, peers) to which the person will be returning;
6)   teaching behaviors or skills that are self-reinforcing or that others will readily reinforce; and
7)   teaching self-control strategies that have transituational capacities.

Walker and Buckley (1972) investigated three different methods for programming generalization. Forty-four children were subjects in this 2-year study that entailed special placement in a token economy classroom for a 2-month period followed by a 2-month maintenance program in a regular classroom. Three maintenance strategies were investigated, and one-quarter of the children served as nonmaintenance controls.

A peer-programming procedure involved having the experimental child earn points that could be used for reinforcers (field trips, class parties) for the class. Points were earned in short, bi-weekly sessions that used an experimenter-operated radio-monitor-feedback apparatus. This apparatus provided both the child and the class differential feedback on the appropriateness of the child's behavior. Appropriate behavior earned the class points. In addition, the child had to earn the right to use the apparatus by behaving appropriately between the two sessions. Criteria for acceptable behavior were established by the teacher.

A second maintenance strategy attempted to make the child's environment in the regular classroom as similar as possible to the experimental room. In the experimental room social reinforcement, token reinforcement, response cost, and timeout were used. Teachers in the regular classrooms received instructions on social and token reinforcement; programmed academic materials also were used in the regular classroom. Aversive procedures were not used. Teachers were visited weekly to ensure that the maintenance strategy was being followed, but they did not receive formal training in behavior modification.

Teachers in the third maintenance strategy received direct training and supervision in behavior modification techniques. These teachers observed and worked with the child to be placed in their class while the child was still in the experimental class. These teachers also obtained academic credit for this course and had their tuition paid.

The results indicated that appropriate behavior averaged 45% across all children during baseline, increased to 90% during treatment in the experimental class, and averaged 65% in the regular classrooms. Only the peer reprogramming and equating stimulus conditions maintained behavior at a level significantly different from the control group. Behavior of the children under different treatment conditions did show a good deal of variability, with greatest variability in the teacher training and control conditions. The peer programming required four hours of professional time per child to implement, while seven and nine hours were needed for the equating stimulus conditions and teacher training treatments respectively. Children in the peer reprogramming group maintained 77% of the appropriate behavior produced during treatment; the figures were 74%, 69%, and 67% for equating stimulus conditions, teacher and control conditions, respectively.

It appears that any successful maintenance program will require a good deal of programming. However, in this study, control children maintained program gains almost as well as any of the other groups. It would be important to know what kinds of "maintenance" strategies teachers "naturally" use when accepting a child from a special placement. Such improvised strategies might be more feasible, economical, and effective than the ones used by Walker and Buckley.

Cone (1973) has disputed the findings that teacher training was not an effective maintenance technique, noting that Walker and Buckley's conclusions were based on between-group analyses when there were numerous between-group differences at baseline. Based on scores reflecting mean change from baseline to treatment and loss from treatment to maintenance periods, Cone concluded that the teacher training approach was superior to peer programming but inferior to equating stimulus conditions. More studies are needed to clarify the effectiveness of these strategies. Additional data on the effects of withdrawing maintenance procedures also are needed.

This topic was the focus of a study by Jones and Kazdin (1975), who examined the effects of a maintenance program on the behavior of four educably retarded children whose inappropriate behavior initially was altered by token reinforcement. In the next phase of the study, all children in the special class could earn tokens. Each child who received all possible tokens for the day came to the front of the class and received peer applause and teacher praise; tokens were exchangeable for back-ups on 3 of 5 days per week. Following this phase, token reinforcement was discontinued, and the entire class was reinforced if all four target children behaved well during the day. The teacher continued to use intermittent praise with the four children. Contingent on good behavior, each of the four children could receive peer applause at the end of the morning and afternoon sessions.

Follow-ups were conducted 2 weeks and 9 weeks after all procedures were discontinued. The initial token reinforcement system immediately reduced inappropriate behaviors which were maintained at low levels in the different conditions and during the two follow-up periods when no systematic interventions were used. While the fading techniques were effective and demonstrated that maintenance is possible after the termination of treatment, research should now be directed at evaluating the effective elements in the Jones and Kazdin package.

Walker, Hops, and Johnson (1975) have investigated maintenance of behavior change over time and across settings. In their first study, 10 children who exhibited disruptive behavior and were deficient in basic skills received intensive behavioral treatment and remedial instruction in a special classroom setting. The children were treated separately in two groups of five with one group receiving a maintenance program in the regular classroom. This program involved training and regular consultation with the classroom teacher in behavior modification techniques, regular feedback on the child's behavior, course credit and paid tuition for mastery of a text on behavior modification, an agreement to meet with the consultant and receive feedback, and a course grade based on the behavior maintenance of the child. The other group received no maintenance program.

The results indicated a dramatic change in the behavior of both groups while in the special classroom, and a high level of maintenance for the group receiving the maintenance treatment. The maintenance group averaged 80% appropriate behavior the next school year compared to the nonmaintenance group, which averaged 65%. Caution is warranted since the group receiving the experimental classroom and maintenance program received more and longer treatment than the group receiving only the special class treatment. However, the results suggest that an intensive, relatively short-term maintenance program can lead to long-term maintenance.

Greenwood, Hops, and Walker (1975) discussed the paradoxical nature of single subject designs in which reversal of behavior is required to demonstrate experimental control yet maintenance at some post-treatment point is required to show persistence across time (see also O'Leary & Drabman, 1971). Group designs (Walker & Buckley, 1972) where children are assigned to different maintenance conditions have also been used. A third research strategy to assess maintenance compares children receiving maintenance programs with "normative or representative" peers within the same classroom setting or with peers who are in a regular classroom. Assessments are made on treated and nontreated students before, during, and after treatment in special settings. With this type of design both within- and between-subject comparisons can be made and variables responsible for maintenance effects can be determined.

Greenwood et al. (1975) investigated the effectiveness of a packaged, teacher-directed, group behavior management system that was coupled with a program (PASS) developed at the University of Oregon which focused on academic survival skills (Cobb, 1972). Three different post-treatment conditions were evaluated, as were nontreated control groups. Measures for both experimental and control groups were taken before treatment, after treatment, 1 week after the program's completion, and 5 weeks after the termination of maintenance procedures; a final comparison was made 6 weeks later. Six experimental and four control classrooms were involved in the study. Students were selected who performed poorly in class and on achievement tests. Experimental children (n=36) were matched (based on observational and test data) with control children (n=24) from the same grade; six children from each of the 10 classes participated.

The six experimental teachers were trained to use the PASS program for math and reading in four 2-hour meetings after school. The program stressed group management procedures, and followed a system developed by Greenwood, Hops, et al. (1974). A consultant visited the classroom during program implementation and provided feedback and instruction to the teachers regarding their adherence to the program. This phase of the study lasted for about 30 days. In the maintenance part of the study (15 days), two teachers were assigned to a procedure in which the PASS program was faded, two teachers continued the program, and two teachers terminated the program. Follow-up measures were taken at the end of the school year after all teachers had discontinued the maintenance program.

With the PASS system, the experimental classes showed a 35-40% gain in appropriate math and reading performance. Control classes, which were equivalent to the experimental classes during the baseline, showed an average gain of 15%. During the other phases of the study, experimental classes tended to maintain their treatment level of appropriate behavior but showed only a moderate advantage over the control classes, which also tended to improve across the study. There were no significant differences between the three maintenance strategies in either math or reading. Format changes for experimental and control group classes during the latter phases of the study limited confidence in the results, but this study did indicate maintenance of effects over much of a school year using a repeated-measures, control-group design to assess changes and effective program components across time.

The work on maintenance and self-control, while obviously still in its infancy, offers promise. The studies tend to be methodologically sound and have advanced behavioral evaluative technology toward the goal of developing programs that reliably demonstrate both behavioral change and behavioral persistence (Atthowe, 1973a).

Response Generalization

In a second study by Walker et al. (1975), the five children in the nonmaintenance groups were observed at home to ascertain if children who were deviant in school were also deviant at home and whether any effects of the treatment program in school generalized to the home. Only one of the children exceeded normal limits in the home; none of the families exceeded normative averages of parental negative behavior. There were, however, nonsignificant trends for children's deviant and parents' negative behaviors to increase when the children's school behavior was improved by placement in the special program. While these data suggest a contrast effect, Johnson, Bolstad, and Lobitz (1974) reported no changes in deviant home behaviors that could be attributed to behavior modification programs in the school. As a whole, these results indicate minimal generalization between home and school environments and suggest separate treatment programs need to be conducted in each setting.

This type of data (across settings and responses) is precisely the kind needed to examine important systems-ecological considerations (Willems, 1974). The ecological perspective is predicated on complex interrelationships and interdependencies within organism-behavioral-environmental systems. A number of macro- and micro-level studies have shown, for example, the unexpected, negative "side effects" of insect control (Willems, 1974). Willems also noted several behavior modification studies where the targeted behaviors have decreased but other behaviors have increased, representing unfortunate "side effects."

Two recently reported studies have addressed themselves to the issue of "side effects." Sajwaj, Twardosz, and Burke (1972) found that a teacher's ignoring of a retarded boy's excessive conversation with the teacher during free play decreased his initiation of conversation during this period, increased his social behavior with other children, and decreased his use of "inappropriate girls' toys."[3] However, examination of his behavior in another setting indicated a decrease of appropriate behavior and an increase of disruption during group

---

[3] A pre-liberation study, perhaps.

academics. In a second study the teacher alternately used praise and ignoring for talking with children. While changes in the target behavior were in the expected direction, a higher use of girls' toys, a drop in appropriate behaviors, and an increase in disruptions during group academics also were reported. These covarying effects were not attributable to differential attention contingently directed to performance of these nontargeted behaviors.

Herbert, Pinkston, Hayden, Sajwaj, Pinkston, Cordua, and Jackson (1973) analyzed the effects of differential parental attention in two different environments. Treatments involved a baseline, differential attention, and differential attention plus some other procedure such as timeout or the use of tokens. Training in both settings was in a relatively isolated room and centered around the mothers guiding their children in a structured task. In both settings, as the mothers decreased their rate of responding to the child's deviant behaviors, the child's rate of deviant behavior *increased* and task-oriented behavior *decreased*. Some of the deviant behavior that was observed was new and very dangerous (assault, self-mutilation). Increased disruptions at home also were observed.

These results are particularly distressing in that differential attention is a procedure typically taught to parents and teachers. While the determinants of these outcomes are not yet clear, alternative explanations in terms of a decrease in the absolute amount of maternal attention, an extinction-burst phenomenon, or other changes in reinforcement schedules do not appear to be viable explanations. At the very least, this research suggests that the generality of procedures to different settings and populations cannot be assumed, and that data collection both in research and clinical practice is needed on *nontargeted* behaviors in treatment and nontreatment settings. Another behavioral covariation study involved the observation of two boys in their schools and homes with observations taking place on the same day (Wahler, 1975). A hierarchical cluster analysis was used to examine the covariation of behaviors in the same and different settings over a 3-year period. The major conclusion of the work was that planned interventions in one setting were usually accompanied by unplanned changes in another setting that were neither deviant nor desirable. A suitable explanation could not be found for this phenomenon.

The existing literature suggests that behaviorists need to investigate the system-like quality of behavior/environmental relationships not only in terms of avoiding undesirable "side effects" but for purposefully using ecological considerations to promote therapeutic change. For example, problem behaviors might be modified indirectly through establishing contingencies for their covarying behaviors (Wahler, 1975).

Nontarget Benefits of Contingency Management

One line of research has examined the effects of reinforcing academic products on maladaptive social behavior in the classroom (Ayllon, Layman, &

Burke, 1972; Ayllon & Roberts, 1974; Winett, Battersby, & Edwards, 1975; Winett & Roach, 1973).[4]

Studies examining the relationship of classroom behavior to academic products are important in the light of recent ethical criticisms of behavioral techniques as they are used in schools (Winett & Winkler, 1972). In reviewing earlier behavior modification work (circa 1968-1970), Winett and Winkler suggested that while the primary goal of an educational institution should be the development of academic skills, most studies are concerned with modifying behaviors such as talking, being out of seat, and not following directions. The criteria for successful behavior modification projects should involve increases in learning (variously defined by the type of school the child attends). Further, in many open classrooms, behaviors deemed inappropriate in the typical behavior modification study (walking around the class, talking to other students, singing, and laughing) are the kinds of behaviors inimical to open-setting learning tasks (Winett, 1973). Fortunately, since the appearance of the Winett and Winkler article, a number of studies have been directed at a clarification of these points.

Ayllon et al (1972) discovered that academic structuring (programmed materials, temporal requirements, precise methods of distributing and collecting assignments) was sufficient (without reinforcement) in eliminating much of the disruptive behaviors of special classroom students.

Winett and Roach (1973) worked in an extremely disruptive "educably mentally retarded" classroom; baseline recordings indicated that appropriate behavior averaged 24% in the afternoon period and 50% in the morning. "Appropriate behavior included any behavior in which there was some involvement in work. Therefore, talking to a peer about work, singing and laughing while working, lying on the floor and doing work, sitting and doing work, and requesting teacher aid with work were all scored as appropriate" (Winett & Roach, 1973, p. 393). Inappropriate behavior included only more flagrant behaviors such as fighting, throwing objects, threatening peers or the teacher, and leaving the room without permission; sitting quietly but not working or walking around the room and not working also were considered inappropriate. Thus, by most standards of inappropriate behavior used in behavior modification research, virtually all the appropriate behaviors observed in this study would be defined as inappropriate.

Initially, during the morning and afternoon periods, completed assignments averaged about one per child. These assignments consisted of semi-individualized math and language problems that were made progressively harder throughout the study, although the number of assignments per child remained constant. The intervention program involved making access to a variety of reinforcing activities

---

[4]A study by Ferritor, Buckholdt, Hamblin, and Smith (1972) is inconsistent with the data presented in this section. However, the children in the Ferritor et al. study were behaving and completing academic work at higher levels than the children in the studies discussed here.

contingent on completion of the assignments within a 45-minute period. This program was established in the afternoon with the morning period serving as a control period.

During the afternoon, the children averaged 3.5 assignments completed and their behavior was appropriate about 80% of the time. Completion of assignments increased somewhat in the morning, while appropriate behavior remained about the same. This study strongly suggested that reinforcement of academic assignments would not only increase the children's academic performance but dramatically improve their classroom behavior as well. Further, given the large improvement in academic work while talking, singing, lying on the floor, it is likely that the range of behaviors often considered appropriate in the classroom might well be expanded.

Ayllon and Roberts (1974) have conducted a similar study with five students who were the most disruptive in a class of 38 fifth graders. Academic behavior centered around reading and was defined as the percentage of correct answers in daily performance sessions. Test material consisted of standard, individualized workbook assignments that involved comprehension, vocabulary, and other reading skills. Inappropriate behavior was defined traditionally and consisted of being out of seat, "talking out," and motor behaviors that interfered with other students. A point system was established where points were earned contingent on percentage of assignments correct and were exchangeable for a variety of school-related activities. Substantial increases in the percentage of correct answers on reading assignments and decreases in disruptive behaviors were associated with the reinforcement of academic products for four out of five children. Ayllon and Roberts concluded that educators could focus on academic objectives as a method to increase learning and decrease disruptions but were cautious about applying this strategy to students with less developed academic repertoires. However, Winett and Roach's (1973) study would suggest that this cautionary note might not be essential.

Working in a highly disruptive, normal sixth-grade classroom, Winett, Battersby, and Edwards (1975) demonstrated that an individualized instruction program alone and the program combined with group academic contingencies sharply increased completed assignments and also were associated with significant increases in appropriate social behavior.

Academic reprogramming might be the first intervention in disruptive classrooms or schools followed, if necessary, by other therapeutic programs. The direction of this work also indicated that behavioral psychologists in school settings need to become familiar with curriculum development, or at least collaborate with curriculum experts prior to the design of behavioral interventions.

The following conclusions can be drawn from the research on generalization and maintenance:

1. Maintenance of behavior change is beginning to be demonstrated but
    effective maintenance strategies must be purposefully programmed and
    alternative strategies must be evaluated.
2. There is some evidence for system-level covariations in behavior across
    responses and settings; these correlated changes may or may not be
    desirable, a fact that suggests the need for multiple measurement in
    designing and evaluating clinical and community programs and caution in
    the actual implementation of such programs.
3. The interrelationship of response classes has been demonstrated in the case
    of academic performance and social behavior, and therapeutic strategies
    involving academic programming have been outlined; these data suggest
    that psychologists in schools must have knowledge of curriculum
    development as well as behavioral intervention.

Curriculum Development, Basic Skills, Creativity, and Related Areas

Many of the earlier classroom behavior modification studies have been
criticized for their overemphasis on order and control and the neglect of more
meaningful educational goals such as the development of basic skills (Winett &
Winkler, 1972). However, a good deal of more recent research is investigating
ways to improve academic skills with less emphasis on the control of behaviors
such as sitting and quietness. This development is of great importance because
(1) the inability of the educational system to educate well certain types of
children is well documented (Zax & Cowen, 1972); (2) "basic skills" are the
kinds of abilities and behaviors that should generalize to other settings; (3) as
discussed in the section on response generalization, academic structuring and
reinforcement of academic products are two strategies to improve social
behavior; (4) the development of basic skills is advocated by diverse educational
philosophies (Silberman, 1970; Winett, 1973); and (5) an emphasis on the
"learning environment" will change the framework and focus of behavioral
consultants (Winett, 1976b).

Recent research has displayed a tendency to focus on the development of
basic skills such as writing, reading, and language use. This section will review the
literature in each of these basic skill areas and also discuss a number of other
investigations focusing primarily on academics.

Writing and Creativity

In an early study, Miller and Schneider (1970) developed a token program in
a Head Start project. Tokens were awarded for correct writing responses and
were exchangeable for school-related activities. While a high rate of responding
was maintained with tokens, virtually no responding occurred without them.

Positive side effects of the token program included improvement in vocabulary and following instructions, attitudes toward school, and cooperative play. Salzberg, Wheeler, Devar, and Hopkins (1971) reported that contingent access to play areas could increase the accuracy of kindergarteners' printing, while Hopkins, Schutte, and Garton (1971) confirmed the success of similar contingencies increasing first and second graders' printing rates. Using programmed materials, Brigham, Finfrock, Breunig, and Bushell (1972) demonstrated that token reinforcement will increase the accuracy of writing in kindergarten children.

Working with 13 male children with a combination of behavioral and academic problems, Brigham, Graubard, and Stans (1972) found that simple reinforcement procedures could increase three aspects of composition writing: total number of words, number of different words, and number of new words. Van Houten, Morrison, Jarvis, and McDonald (1974) introduced a simple feedback procedure to normal second- and fifth-grade classrooms in an attempt to increase the number of words each child could write on a specified topic in 10 minutes. In both classrooms, the feedback procedure led to increases in writing rate. Childrens' papers were scored by "blind" raters for several aspects of composition writing (vocabulary, number of ideas, internal consistency of stories) which also improved with the introduction of the feedback procedure.

Creativity

Both Brigham, Graubard, and Stans (1972) and Van Houten et al. (1974) studies are important because the aspects of writing that were influenced were those that most educators would incorporate under the term "creativity." One significant question, then, is whether there is "a reservoir of 'creativity' within children—that if only teachers would leave children alone, original and scintillating stories would soon appear" (Brigham, Graubard, & Stans 1972, p. 429), or whether behaviors termed "creative" are subject to the same kind of environmental influences as other behaviors.

A partial answer to this question rests with studies that have attempted to improve behaviors usually considered to be creative. Maloney and Hopkins (1973), in the context of a voluntary, nonremedial summer class for fourth to sixth graders, used a procedure similar to the "good behavior game" to reinforce different aspects of sentence structure. Dependent measures included grammar, number of letters, and number of different types of words. Children's papers also were rated by two independent judges for creativity.

Specific aspects of writing were correlated with the reinforcement contingencies (action verbs were used more often when reinforced), and the ratings for creativity were lowest during a baseline condition and highest for compositions prepared when writing diversity was reinforced.

Goetz and Baer (1973) demonstrated that children's block-building also might be influenced by the social environment. Prior to the study, it was ascertained that 20 different forms could be constructed with a given set of blocks. Form diversity was defined as the number of forms produced during a session; "new forms" were those which had not appeared previously. The study compared no reinforcement, social reinforcement for production of same forms, and social reinforcement for production of different forms. The production of new forms was restricted largely to those sessions in which the children were socially reinforced for this behavior; children also spent more time block-building during these sessions.

Both these studies are important for demonstrating how attempts by teachers and other school personnel to increase creativity will be bolstered by a more operational definition of the term and the arrangement of both social and physical environments to encourage those behaviors considered to be creative.

Reading

Early reading research (Corey & Shamow, 1972; Gray, Baker, & Stancyk, 1969; Staats & Butterfield, 1965; Staats, Finley, Minke, & Wolf, 1964; Staats, Staats, Schultz, & Wolf, 1972; Whitlock & Bushell, 1967) used operant techniques to increase both the rate and accuracy of reading single words and passages. However, very little research has been concerned with two other important facets of reading ability—retention and comprehension.

Lahey and Drabman (1974) divided 16 second graders into two groups that received token and control treatments in a yoked experimental design. Vocabulary cards (Dolch, 1949) were shown to each child, and individual lists were developed containing words that each child could not identify correctly. During the first acquisition trial, each card was shown to the child, and one second after its presentation the experimenter pronounced the word. On successive trials, the child read the words aloud. In the token group, children were told that they were correct and were given one token for each correct response. If a child gave an incorrect response, (s)he was told "no" and was corrected. Control conditions were identical except that children received noncontingently the same number of tokens as a randomly assigned child from the token condition. Thirty sight words were learned during the three acquisition sessions. Immediately after the third acquisition session, children were shown all 30 cards and asked to identify each one. No feedback or tokens were used. The procedure was repeated 2 days later.

Children in the control group took about twice the number of trials to learn the vocabulary words. Children in the token condition also were able to identify correctly more words on the retention tests. Apparently, procedures that improve acquisition may be able to improve retention as well.

Lahey, McNees, and Brown (1973) investigated comprehension and the discrepancy between high oral reading scores and low comprehension scores. Two sixth graders with this reading pattern and poor performance in other subjects were the participants. Their performance was compared to two children whose oral reading and reading comprehension were not discrepant. The children were brought to an unused classroom two to three times per week for 30-minute sessions and were read short passages from a sixth-grade reader. Depending on each passage's content, they were asked one to four simple factual questions about the reading. The intervention consisted of telling the child "right" and giving a penny for each correct answer.

Social praise and tangible reinforcement led to high levels of correct responses (about 90%) for the two target children. Substantially lower performance levels were associated with a baseline condition. The two children with no discrepancy in their reading skills performed at high levels under both baseline and reinforcement conditions. While the reinforcement condition elevated the performance of the target children to the level of the other children, further research is needed to determine if similar results could be produced with longer, more complex reading passages. In addition, it remains to be established whether such performance increments could be produced in the normal classroom.

Open Classrooms

Haskett and Lanfestey (1974) investigated the effect of multiple interventions on children's reading in an open classroom. They emphasized that:

> The problem for the open classroom would seem to be that of maximizing the number of learning experiences for each child while at the same time maximizing the chances that the pupils will be learning those skills that characterize intellectual development and academic achievement. If that is true, then open-classroom programs like all educational programs must be based on knowledge of the young child. Therefore, how the behavior of pupils can be structured in an open classroom will depend largely on what is known about causes of behavior change. (p. 234)*

Haskett and Lenfestey identified three dimensions of classroom environments that are manipulable and are important in structuring children's behavior: novelty and variety, modeling and material, and social and activity contingencies of reinforcement. The study was conducted in a university preschool attended by eight children of middle- or upper middle-class background. A large area containing 12 different children's books had been designated the reading area. Undergraduates served as "tutors" and engaged in a variety of activities with the children.

Baseline measures of reading were taken for seven consecutive sessions. During each of the next five sessions, a familiar adult would enter the classroom

---

*Haskett, E. J. and Lenfestey, W. Reading—related behavior in an open classroom. *Journal of Applied Behavior Analysis*, 1974, 7, 233-241.

carrying 10 to 15 new books, announce the presence of the new books, and deposit them in the reading area. In the next five sessions, tutors would begin each session by picking up a book in the reading area, going to a separate part of the classroom, settling into a chair, and beginning to read aloud. Tutors did not encourage the children to sit or read with them but did pause briefly to answer children's questions about the reading material. Five sessions were then used to replicate the novel books condition, and three sessions were used to replicate the modeling condition.

The introduction of new books led to moderate reading increases for some of the children while the modeling procedure was effective in substantially increasing reading for all children. During the replications, most of the increases in reading were attributable to the children attending to the tutors' reading. Haskett and Lenfestey (1974) concluded that:

> Free education and the concept of the open classroom do not mean that the child's behavior is freed from *causes*. The larger environment of the open classroom acquires new properties and new meanings when contrasted with that of the traditional school. Both the larger social and physical environment begin to play a more complex, but not unregulated, role in the control of the individual children's behavior in the open classroom. (p. 240)

Language

Behavioral research on language development is not extensive. However, the existing studies are important both in terms of this area and the more general concern of skill development, teaching methods, and school structure. For example, Lahey (1971) showed that for Head Start children modeling without social or tangible reinforcement was an effective procedure for increasing children's use of descriptive adjectives. Hart and Risley (1968) investigated procedures which could modify low rates of adjective-noun combinations present in the everyday speech of Head Start children. A number of procedures (praise, social and intellectual stimulation) were ineffective in increasing the children's low rates of adjective use. A group-teaching method was introduced to increase the children's rates of color- and number-noun combinations. While this procedure was effective in increasing the use of these adjectives in the teaching situation, this effect did not generalize to a free-play situation. In order to increase the children's generalized use of color-noun combinations, it was necessary to work directly in the free-play situation ("incidental teaching") and make access to preschool materials contingent on the use of the targeted adjective-noun combinations.

In a systematic replication of this study, Hart and Risley (1974) demonstrated that reliable increases in children's use of nouns, adjective-noun combinations, and compound sentences were correlated with teacher prompts and the receipt of school materials contingent on the correct use of the particular part of speech. Hart and Risley (1975) also demonstrated that incidental teaching procedures increased the use of compound sentences and stimulated variety in the children's speech.

Most compensatory programs for "disadvantaged" children try to modify language repertoires by using teacher-structured curricula periods; however, the data from these three studies suggest that this is an ineffective strategy. These findings and the style of teaching suggested by the results are also relevant to open classroom teaching and the previous discussion of Haskett and Lenfestey's (1974) reading research.

Future Directions

Two recent papers provide examples of possible future directions that research on academic skills might take—the actual development and evaluation of learning materials and programs.

Quilitch and Risley (1973) studied the effects that different kinds of play materials had on the social play of 7-year-olds. On the basis of pre-testing, some of the toys in the study had been found to be isolate toys (only one child could use them at one time). Under various social conditions, it was discovered that social play was a function of the type of toys available. For example, in one experiment, children engaged in social play about 85% of the time when social toys were available, but only about 10% of the time when isolate toys were used. These results suggest that educational materials should be carefully selected and their effects evaluated to maximize learning opportunities and to facilitate social and cooperative play. Additional research on this topic will be discussed in the section on ecological variables.

Resnick, Wang, and Kaplan (1973) presented preliminary data on an individualized math curriculum that operated on the principle of mastery. The major goal of their research was the development of a procedure to specify and evaluate learning hierarchies so that programs could be designated that would closely match a child's natural sequence of acquisition. The curriculum consisted of a hierarchy of tasks in which lower tasks needed to be mastered before higher ones, and mastery of higher tasks was predictive of mastery of lower ones. The development of the hierarchies involved task analyses in which the specific behavioral components and prerequisite behaviors for each task were identified. In addition, for each analyzed objective, the stimulus situation to be presented and the child's response were described.

The program involves self-paced learning, frequent tests of component behaviors, and tests for mastery. Children can also work on several objectives at one time. Test outcomes can be used as a data base for the evaluation and modification of the program. "The particular form of instruction—group, individual, 'programmed' versus 'discovery' etc.—is not specified. This omission is deliberate. The important question in a mastery curriculum is not how an objective is taught, but whether it is learned by each child. On this view, the school's job is to assure that all children do learn, regardless of time needed or specific teaching method. In this work a carefully sequenced curriculum is one of the essential tools" (Resnick et al., 1973, p. 700). Hopefully, during the next few years more research on classroom and curriculum design will emerge, thereby requiring that the future behavior modifier in school settings will need a knowledge base that exceeds the relatively narrow confines of the behavioral paradigm.

Standard Classroom Procedures

In addition to continuing research on traditional academic subjects (Kirby & Shields, 1972) or vocational training (Clark, Boyd, & Macrae, 1975), a number of studies have investigated other educational techniques intended to facilitate the acquisition of generalized learning skills.

Although homework is a frequently used procedure in schools, there have been few experimental studies of the effectiveness of homework in improving academics and classroom behavior. Harris and Sherman (1974) found that the use of natural reinforcers (e.g., leaving school early) and punishers (no recess for a student until homework was completed at 80% accuracy) resulted in more completed and accurate homework. In addition, in-class quiz scores showed a strong positive relationship to accurate completion of homework.

Knapczyk and Livingston (1974) discussed the importance of question-asking in terms of its double feedback potential—the student receives accurate information and the teacher determines the student's level of understanding. In this study two junior high school students who asked no questions were the participants. The intervention consisted of instructions to the children to raise their hands when they needed academic help, a few prompts by the teacher during the reading period, and quick recognition and answering of student questions by the teacher or aide. In addition to large increases in question asking, there were also increases in on-task behavior and reading performance. This instruction-prompt-reinforcement package is a simple procedure involving little teacher time and no laborious record keeping. However, it does provide valuable reciprocal feedback between the teacher and student which might influence both classroom behavior and academic performance.

Studies of particular importance for classes with heterogeneous ability levels and open classrooms have investigated the nature and duration of teacher-student contacts. Mandelker, Brigham, and Bushell (1970) reported that a teacher's rate of social contact with kindergarten children was higher during the use of contingent tokens than during baseline periods or when tokens were used noncontingently. Sanders and Hanson (1971) found that requiring elementary students to go to a play area when they completed their work resulted in less teacher time being given to better students and more time to poorer students. The number of completed assignments for all students increased during this procedure. In a third-grade classroom Scott and Bushell (1974) demonstrated that instituting lengthy teacher-student contacts led to high levels of off-task behavior, while teacher-student contacts that averaged 40 seconds were associated with lower levels of off-task behavior.

These data converge on the recommendation that classroom procedures emphasize individual student-teacher contacts which give the child feedback and differential attention, are of relatively short duration, and focus on especially troublesome academic material. O'Leary, Kaufman, Kass, and Drabman (1970) describe a "soft" individual reprimand procedure that has these same qualities. Future research should evaluate the extent to which these procedures will require modification to be effective for students of different ages and abilities.

Standard Test Performance

At least two studies have investigated the effects of reinforcement on responses to standard tests. Ayllon and Kelly (1972) showed that the scores of trainable retardates could be raised significantly on the Metropolitan Readiness Test under reinforcement compared to standard testing conditions; similar results were obtained with a group of normal fourth graders. Similarly, children who were in a token program (academic performance was reinforced daily) scored higher under reinforcement and standard testing conditions than a control group. Edlund (1972) matched 11 pairs of young children on various characteristics including revised Stanford-Binet Scale Form-L IQ scores. Each pair then took Form M of the same test, but the experimental group received M&M candy for each plus or correct response. The experimental group scored significantly higher on the second form than the control group. Both these studies seriously question whether testing under "standard conditions" provides an accurate picture of a child's academic performance (Zigler, Abelson, & Seitz, 1973) and indicate the diagnostic utility of conducting ability testing under preplanned incentive conditions.

Hyperactivity—An Instructional Alternative to Drug Control

Recent research by Ayllon, Layman, and Kandel (1975) has demonstrated an alternative to drug control of hyperactivity that emphasizes academic skill development. Ayllon et al.'s (1975) evaluation of their academic reinforcement strategy (Ayllon & Roberts, 1974) as an alternative to medication was motivated by several considerations including ethical concerns about medicating young children and evidence that while drug treatments reduce the frequency of hyperactive behaviors, academic performance may be hindered.

Three children, all diagnosed as clinically hyperactive and taking Ritalin for 1 to 4 years to control this behavior, were the participants. All the children, (8, 9, and 10 years old with IQ scores of 118, 94, and 103) were enrolled in a learning disabilities class. Observations indicated that they were the most hyperactive students in the class. Measures were gathered on math performance, reading, and hyperactive behavior (gross motor behaviors such as running around the room, rocking in chairs and jumping around, being noisy and disturbing others). A multiple baseline design was used because such a strategy "allowed each child to serve as his own control, thereby minimizing the idiosyncratic drug-behavior interactions that have the potential for confounding the interpretations and even the results when comparing one subject with another" (Ayllon et al., 1975, p. 141). Dependent measures were recorded while the children were on medication, off medication (following a 3-day "wash out" period), off medication but with a reinforcement system for math performance, and off medication with reinforcement for both math and reading performance.

The results were very clear. In all three cases with medication, the level of hyperactivity and academic performance was low. Without medication, the frequency of hyperactive behavior increased dramatically and academic performance remained deficient. The introduction of the reinforcement system in each academic area for each child resulted in large reductions in hyperactivity and large increases in academic performance. When the group was on medication, hyperactive behavior occurred in about 25% of the recorded intervals, and academic performance averaged 12% correct. With the reinforcement system and no medication, hyperactive behavior occurred about 20% of the time, while performance in both academic areas averaged 85% correct.

> The present results suggest that the continued use of Ritalin and possibly other drugs to control hyperactivity may result in compliant but academically incompetent students . . .
>
> On the basis of these findings, it would seem appropriate to recommend that hyperactive children under medication periodically be given the opportunity to be drug-free, to minimize drug dependence and to facilitate change through alternative behavioral techniques . . .
>
> This study offers a behavioral and educationally justifiable alternative to the use of medication for hyperactive children. The control of hyperactivity by medication, while effective, may be too costly to the child, in that it may retard his academic and social growth, a human cost that schools and society can ill afford. (Ayllon et al., 1975, pp. 144-145)*

---

*Ayllon, T., Laymen D., and Kandel, H. J. A behavioral-educational alternative to drug control of hyperactive children. *Journal of Applied Behavior Analysis*, 1975, *8*, 137-146.

Interpersonal Relations

Many educational change agents and philosophies have focused attention on the school and classroom for developing a variety of pro-social behaviors. However, most of the behavioral studies reviewed in this chapter have concerned themselves more with increasing academic output, "on-task" behavior, or decreasing instances of aggression. In part this situation reflects the kinds of problems behavior modifiers have chosen or been asked to ameliorate and perhaps also indicates initial preference to establish procedures and methodology by working in areas that are more definable and less controversial. However, a central theme of this book is that a behavioral framework which stresses measurement and evaluation should be capable of delineating alternative approaches to a wide variety of problems whose solutions may, in fact, still be controversial. Racial integration, interpersonal skills, and "self-government" are three such areas.

Racial Integration

The integration of our schools, in some instances by dramatic court actions and equally dramatic community responses, has assured that in many parts of the country white and black children will share the same classrooms. However, this does not mean that social interactions between black and white children will be positive or, for that matter, will occur frequently. It is likely that the environment will have to be programmed to elicit and reinforce pro-social interactions between ethnically different children.

Hauserman, Walen, and Behling (1973) performed the first systematic investigation of this topic. Black and white children in a fifth-grade class were observed rarely interacting despite encouragement by their teacher. In particular, five black children isolated themselves during lunch and other activities. These five children were observed daily for interracial interaction during lunch and immediately following a free-play period.

After a 9-day baseline, a prompting-reinforcement condition (4 days) was introduced. This procedure involved a game in which each black child was paired with a white child, and white children's cliques were broken up. Children were then encouraged to sit with the "new friend." When the children were seated, the teacher praised the children sitting with their assigned mate and gave each child a ticket explaining that it was for sitting with a new friend and could be exchanged for a "goody." At the end of the lunch period, the teacher gave another ticket to children who had remained in their assigned pairs.

In another phase (9 days) experimental procedures were identical to the prompting-reinforcement condition except that the pairing technique was eliminated and children were encouraged only to "sit and eat with a new friend." A second baseline (5 days) followed.

The prompting-reinforcement condition raised the occurrence of interracial interactions to about 80% compared to only 17% during baseline; for the second experimental condition, interactions averaged about 58%. However, it was only during this condition in which more spontaneous interracial activity was reinforced that any significant generalization to behavior during the non-prompted, nonreinforced recess period occurred. The second baseline period revealed that interracial interactions decreased in both settings with the discontinuation of these procedures. Deficiencies in the design of the study precluded data on who initiated social interaction, and whether those children rewarded for eating with a different child also played with that child in recess. Despite these problems, the conclusion of the authors was optimistic:

> this investigation suggests that reinforcement can be a promising tool for dealing with problems of racial integration. The study showed that the global concept of racial integration can be specifically defined and manipulated in order to bring about the desired social integration. Many people assume that racial integration must begin with an attitude change which, hopefully, will then result in some generalized positive behavior change. The present study, however, indicated that positive behavior changes can be brought about directly (Hauserman et al., 1973, p. 200).

Achievement Place

Achievement Place (Phillips, 1968; Phillips, Phillips, Fixsen, & Wolf, 1971) is a small, community-based facility for pre-delinquents which will be highlighted here because of this research's investigations of peer control, self-government, and interpersonal skills. The Achievement Place literature provides a wealth of procedures designed to promote these competencies that may be applicable in the future to normal classrooms. (Additional discussion of Achievement Place research and the juvenile justice system will be provided in Chapter 3.)

Other research (Bronfenbrenner, 1970) has demonstrated that in some countries the peer group is programmed (through differential reinforcement and adult modeling) to reinforce pro-social behavior and to punish anti-social behavior, while the American peer group for the most part serves to reinforce anti-social behavior. Phillips, Phillips, Wolf, and Fixsen (1973) compared the effectiveness of different managerial systems for accomplishing specific tasks at Achievement Place. Four boys participated in this study, which involved the task of cleaning the bathrooms. In one condition, a boy could purchase the job of *peer manager*, assigning specific cleaning tasks to peers each day and providing point penalties or rewards in accordance with work quality. In addition, the peer manager received reward or penalty points contingent on completion or noncompletion of assigned tasks. The peer manager system was compared to (1) a *group assignment-group consequence* condition in which the group as a whole was responsible for the cleanliness of the bathroom, and (2) an *individual assignment-group consequence* condition in which each boy was assigned specific work tasks but received points in the same manner as the group assignment condition (i.e., a group contingency).

The data indicated that with the peer manager system many more bathroom tasks were completed than under the other two conditions. The individual assignment-group consequence condition was superior to the group assignment-group consequence condition.

Another study compared the peer manager system to the individual assignment condition but with individual consequences. Both systems worked equally well, suggesting that specificity in assignments and consequences were the important ingredients of the different plans. Further studies indicated that the peer manager system worked as well when the boys could only give points for completion of tasks. In addition, it was found that the peer manager system worked better when the manager gained or lost points contingent on his group's performance than when he did not participate in such a contingency.

This research is important in terms of the structure of other social and classroom programs. Procedures can be developed and validated that give peers reciprocal control over each other, maintain the program, reduce staff time, and may be preferred by program participants. This work further documents how children's peer groups may be directed so that children are engaged in pro-social educational activities and gain valuable experience in supervisory and supervisee roles.

In a related study, Fixsen, Phillips, and Wolf (1973) observed that persons living in prisons and other institutions (e.g., schools) rarely have a chance to establish the rules by which they would like to live. There is usually an informal type of self-government which is quite severe and is enforced by the peer group through coercion and punishment. Much of the influence of these peer groups is directed at anti-social behavior, although there have been some attempts (Makarenko, 1973; Neill, 1960; cited in Fixsen et al., 1973) to direct children's peer groups toward pro-social behaviors. However, there has been little in the way of experimental analyses of specific training in self-government. The purpose of this study was to examine some of the variables affecting Achievement Place residents' participation in establishing consequences for their peers' rule violations. During the tenure of Achievement Place, a system of conferences had evolved which allowed the boys input into the structure and rules of the program. Through direct teaching and reinforcement, the boys learned how to govern themselves. Conferences gradually became more like group meetings for the discussion and enactment of changes in the program. "Trials," on the other hand, were set up to define and train the boys in self-government and disciplinary skills. This research demonstrated that reinforcing reports of violations and allowing the boys to decide a misbehavior's consequences during a trial led to more reports of misbehaviors and more active participation in trials.

While the "trial" procedures are somewhat similar to some family processes, they do not entirely parallel legal procedures, a problem if the goal of such programs is to teach actual self-government skills. Such techniques should receive further research attention in classroom settings where "variables affecting participation in a government system can be identified and evaluated" (Fixsen et al., 1973, p. 44).

In pilot-level research relevant to the classroom, Kifer, Lewis, Green, and Phillips (1974) taught pre-delinquents and their parents verbal negotiation behaviors. Children often get into trouble with parents, teachers, and peers because deficits in these kinds of verbal skills lead the child to become abusive. In a classroom setting, dyads were trained using an instruction, practice, feedback, and modeling package. Increases were found for negotiation behaviors both within the training sessions and in home observations of the parent-child dyads. While questions remain concerning the durability of these behaviors, and the time for training each dyad was quite high (9-10 hours), the results of future research in this area should be important both for troubled children and perhaps more significantly for the development of methods to teach all children these skills systematically in normal classroom settings.

Ecological Variables

Although some research has examined how the physical structure and social organization of schools directly affect the behavior of students and teachers (Moos & Insel, 1974), very few studies have attempted to modify these structures and observe how they covary with behavior. Research of this nature is vital because (1) the environmental psychology movement (see Chapter 8) has documented psychology's historical neglect of the social and physical context of behavior; (2) a number of educational innovations such as open classrooms stress the importance of classroom designs and organizations that are quite different from traditional classrooms; (3) young children increasingly will be using group (e.g., day-care center) care facilities although little is known about how the physical environment should be designed to facilitate pro-social behaviors, increase safety, enhance adequate supervision, eliminate harmful organizations or structures, and finally how the optimal design for group care environments should correspond to federal and state regulations (Winett, Moffatt, & Fuchs, 1975).

LeLaurin and Risley (1972) investigated two different staffing procedures in a day-care center. In the "Zone" procedure, each teacher was responsible for a particular area and for all the children occupying or passing through it. In the "Man to Man" condition, each teacher was responsible for taking a group of children through different activity areas. The major aim of this study was to compare the time that children lost from planned activities during transitions from lunch, through the bathroom, dressing areas, and to the nap area. A simple observational measure indicated the number of children present in a given area, and the number of these children participating in appropriate area behavior. The Zone procedure was associated with smaller decreases in child participation during the lunch to nap transition.

Doke and Risley (1972) examined the interactive effects of type of activity schedule and quantity of materials on children's participation in preschool activities. The dependent measure involved observing at 3-minute intervals the number of children in an area and the number of children appropriately participating in an activity in that area. The development of such simple, reliable measures is important because it can allow relatively untrained day-care personnel to observe and evaluate systematically their programs.

Doke and Risley discovered that children's participation in preschool activities was as high when children had to adhere to a schedule of sequenced activities (no options) as when they were allowed to choose between several optional activities. The sequenced schedule was effective only when a child could move to a new activity as soon as (s)he was finished with one activity and there was an abundance of materials for each activity. Without a large supply of materials, the level of participation declined unless children were free to choose among a number of activities.

An extensive investigation by Twardosz, Cataldo, and Risley (1974) serves as an excellent example of environmental design research. In Study I, a partitioned environment was compared to an open environment for the number of children visible at different locations and the distance needed to be traveled by an adult to observe a child not readily visible. An additional measure involved having an observer record the distance that a staff person would have to travel to see the child. High reliability was reported for each measure.

Observations indicated that with the open environment 97% of the children were visible compared to 78% in the partitioned environment; the average number of feet traveled per observation was one foot in the open environment and six and one-half feet in the partitioned environment. Study II revealed similar results for the number of staff persons visible to a supervisor and the distance a supervisor would have to travel to see a staff person not readily visible.

Study III investigated whether the open environment which was shown to facilitate supervision would adversely affect infants' sleep. To evaluate this possible problem, the environment of a sleep room was varied. For the "noise and light" condition, the door to the room was left open and activities in progress were audible and visible. In the "quiet and dark" condition, the sleep room's door was closed and the room was darkened. The data consisted of observing whether the children were sleeping, awake, or crying. Under both conditions, there was a good deal of sleeping and very little crying.

Study IV replicated and extended the previous study by showing that infants' sleep was not affected by having the children sleep in the open environment as opposed to the partitioned area. Study V investigated whether toddlers, who are more mobile and possibly more resistant to napping than infants, could sleep in an open environment while other children were engaged in activities or whether a separate and more restricted (dark, closed versus open, separate) room was necessary. There was little overall difference in the amount of sleeping in the different environments.

In a final study, the effects of three environments on the performance of pre-academic activities by small groups of children were examined. Environmental conditions included conducting the activities in a separate room, behind a screen in the open environment, and in the open environment without a screen. Measures included child attention to activity, out-of-seat behavior, number of activities or parts of activities completed, and adult attention to children. In all three environments, attention and completion of activities was high, adults attended to children at a high level (indicating minimal distraction by other children and activities), and children most often remained seated. Finally, other children did not disrupt the activities which were staged in the open environment.

This series of studies demonstrated the advantages of the open environment for supervision, infant and toddler sleeping, and preschool activities. Replications of this work in other group-care environments and schools could determine the advantage of open designs for different settings. Taken together, the studies from Risley's group demonstrate that behavior analytic methods can be applied to the development and evaluation of optimal environments. The range of variables investigated and the goal of establishing optimal educational/care environments suggest that the educational behavior modifier of the future will be an "environmental designer" as well as a contingency manager.

Consultation to Teachers and Teacher Education

Research on behavioral consultation and continuing education programs in behavior modification for teachers is one of the most significant contributions of behavioral community psychology to educational innovation. This conclusion is based on a number of considerations. Systematic data have been collected which examine consultant behaviors affecting teachers' behaviors that in turn influence student behaviors (Kelly, 1971). These studies are in marked contrast to reviews of consultation (Mannino & Shore, 1975) which regularly indicate that much time is committed to consultation despite the absence of data to evaluate such efforts. Educational and consultative efforts with teachers represent potentially powerful and economical methods (Tharp & Wetzel, 1969) to influence current problems in the classroom and to prevent the occurrence of future problems.

Earlier research indicated that teachers could understand and apply various reinforcement procedures to single students and whole classes (Cooper, Thomson, & Baer, 1970; Hall, Cristler, Cranston, & Tucker, 1970; Hall, Panyan, Rabon, & Broden, 1968; Willard, Hall, Fox, Goldsmith, Emerson, Owen, Davis, & Porcia, 1971), that changes in teacher behavior correspond to changes in student behavior (Broden, Bruce, Mitchell, Carter, & Hall, 1970; Pinkston, Reese, LeBlanc, & Baer, 1973), and that teachers could be taught how to observe behaviors and use reversal and multiple baseline designs to evaluate their efforts (Hall et al., 1970; Hall et al., 1971). This research has received some excellent reviews (O'Leary & O'Leary, 1972), but it has lacked (1) a clear delineation of the consultant's behavior and its effect on the teacher and (2) experimental comparisons of different packages to change teacher behavior.

Instruction and Feedback Packages

While differential teacher attention has been shown to change children's behavior, there are few demonstrable procedures for changing a teacher's behavior. For example, although classes in behavior modification have been expanded, many teachers still do not have access to these educational experiences. Cossairt, Hall, and Hopkins (1973) investigated the effects of instructions, feedback, and social praise on teacher's praise and the effects of such praise on children's attention. Three elementary school teachers selected four students who showed minimal attentive behaviors. Throughout the study, the children worked on math problems. Observations were made for teacher praise contingent on student attention, teacher attention to students' non-attentiveness, and student attention itself.

The intervention package consisted of: (1) *instructions*, including an explanation that contingent teacher attention is effective in changing student behavior, details on how to praise students, and a written message which indicated that contingent praise increased attention; (2) *verbal feedback* at the end of each classroom session indicating the frequency of appropriate student attention; and (3) experimenter *social praise* for teacher praise of appropriate student behavior and *feedback* on the number of intervals in which teacher praise was recorded. Initially, social praise and feedback were given after every session; later, they were delivered on an intermittent schedule.

The results revealed that feedback and instruction alone minimally affected teacher and student behavior, while feedback and praise resulted in large increases in teacher praise and in student attention. Contingent social praise by a consultant appeared to be a necessary ingredient in changing teacher behavior. The shift to an intermittent schedule of experimenter praise increased teacher praise. This finding suggests that feedback and praise are inexpensive, powerful methods of change that can be used by school psychologists, principals (Copeland, Brown, & Hall, 1974), and consultants.

In a related experiment intended to evaluate the effects of feedback alone, Parsonson, Baer, and Baer (1974) extended the training package to a larger range of behaviors. This study was conducted in a pre-kindergarten playroom for institutionalized retarded children. The basic intervention consisted of feedback in the form of a note to the teacher after each 15 attention responses to the children. The note informed teachers of the positive and negative attention behaviors they had directed to appropriate and inappropriate child behaviors. With this type of feedback, both teachers markedly increased their positive attention to appropriate child behaviors. After feedback was discontinued, follow-up at 8 weeks for one teacher and 11 weeks for the other indicated that their behavior had been maintained. These findings are even more impressive given the average training time for teachers was only 6½ days (90 minutes per day). This feedback procedure might have been more effective than that employed by Cossairt et al. (1973) because feedback was given frequently in the sessions.

Behavioral Workshops

Similar variables have been investigated in the context of behavior modification workshops (Bowles & Nelson, 1974). Teachers were divided into three groups with two groups first being involved in lecture-discussion workshops and the third group acting as a control. A written test indicated that both workshop groups significantly increased their knowledge of behavior modification principles, but there were no observable differences in actual teacher behavior attributable to the workshop. In the second phase of the study, one workshop group received training using a bug-in-the-ear device with instructions and feedback coming from the experimenters. After discontinuation of the procedure, this group showed changes in classroom behavior such as praise and contingent statements.

These results support the contention that teacher consultation and education should take place in the classroom where teachers can be observed, prompted, instructed, and reinforced in their own setting and style. Purely verbal educational programs will probably result only in changes in the verbal repertoire of teachers. Other potentially effective methods that require empirical investigation include videotape, feedback, graphs of observational data, and various self-monitoring procedures. In addition, different workshop packages (with continuing consultation, take-home assignments, telephone contact) need to be evaluated with measures of cognitive change and in-class behavior.

Clark and Macrae (1976) investigated a training package for interns that included modeling, instruction and feedback, and grades and quizzes. An experienced teacher served as the model, and feedback was given by this teacher and an observer immediately following completion of small teaching segments by the intern. A grade was assigned based on the intern's performance relative to previous performances. Instructions alone had varied effects on intern performance, while the entire package was very effective across different interns and target behaviors. In another part of this research, teachers were allowed to self-select components of the package to be used. The self-selected package method further increased teacher skills. Apparently, while training programs should allow some self-selection, such packages should be constructed around a performance contingency.

The findings of these studies mirror the results of similar work with attendants and mental health technicians (Chapter 7), indicating that informational, verbal workshops do not reliably result in changed work behaviors. This cross-subject, cross-setting generality lends credence to the notion that school consultation efforts will be effective only if contact, feedback, and reinforcement are frequent, *in vivo*, and focused on specific teacher and student behaviors. In addition, Stein (1975), writing in a somewhat different context, has issued a warning about the misapplication of behavior modification principles resulting from short-term workshops and seminars that do not include frequent contact and continual supervision. These same conclusions are applicable to the myriad of formal behavior modification, in-service courses that have been offered (Winett, Deitchman, Woods, & Solernou, 1976). A dilemma exists in that approaches involving extended contacts with teachers may be impractical because "in many, if not most, portions of the country, frequent visits by even a consultant school psychologist is an impossible luxury" (Nelson, 1974, p. 280), but contingent contact seems essential for behavior changes with teachers.

Several alternate and at times overlapping strategies have been proposed to remedy this problem. Tomlinson (1972), working in the Minneapolis public schools, has shown that it is possible to reduce consultant time to 2.4 hours per child referral and 4.2 hours per token economy. These figures were achieved by consulting with small groups of teachers with similar problems, focusing consultation efforts early in intervention programs, making consultation contingent on data collection, minimizing data collection requirements, teaching specific behavioral techniques rather than extensive behavioral principles, having teachers use social and naturalistic reinforcers, and terminating contact with unresponsive teachers. Winett et al. (1976) have demonstrated the feasibility of using paraprofessionals (graduate students) as the differential reinforcer of teacher behavior. In this study, 11 teachers implemented individual change programs in their classrooms; professional contact was limited to about 2.5 hours per week, but the supervised graduate students had frequent telephone and classroom contact with teachers.

It seems likely that the future direction of this work will reflect the prior focus and strategies involved in researching procedures designed to change student behaviors—the development of effective packages, the delineation of key variables in these packages, determination of the most effective but least expensive components, and the investigation of techniques to assure maintenance of changed teacher behavior (Horton, 1975). For example, Van Houten and Sullivan (1975) delivered automated audio signals over the school's public address system as a cue for teachers to praise children engaged in appropriate behavior. This simple, inexpensive procedure resulted in increased praise relative to a contrasted procedure involving the counting and graphing of teacher praise. Jones and Eimers (1975) also are developing a training package for teachers that involves role playing simulated situations. Although the package entails minimal consultation time or expense, it has been shown to be effective in changing targeted student behavior.

Training of Administrators and Support Personnel

Hall and his colleagues (Brown, Copeland, & Hall, 1972; Copeland, Brown, Axelrod, & Hall, 1972; Copeland, Brown, & Hall, 1974) have shown how a principal can prompt and praise parents for their children's attendance at summer school and use a variety of reinforcers to improve school attendance, promptness, and the academic productivity of students. In the Copeland et al. (1974) study, three fifth graders who were working poorly in math and reading were taken to the principal's office for about 1 minute of attention and praise if they surpassed a set of performance criteria. This produced improved academic work. In another demonstration of this technique, a principal went to two third-grade classrooms after a special 5-minute work period on math problems. Students who had improved their performance from the previous day (or the child receiving the highest score) were asked to stand and were praised by the principal. Although the principal did this only twice a week (taking about 3 minutes each time), this intervention led to a 38% increase in problems completed correctly, with 59 of the 74 students showing substantial improvement.

These studies are significant in that the trend for students to have contact with a principal only for negative behavior was reversed, the procedures required few resources, and the measurements necessary for the differential attention procedure could easily be accomplished by the teachers. One promising direction that this research can take would be similar demonstrations involving differential principal attention to teachers contingent on both their own and their students' behavior changes. However, if such procedures are to be widely implemented, they probably will require a role change for the principal—from administrator to "head teacher," similar to the role of the principal in other countries (Weber, 1971).

Additional work has demonstrated the feasibility and effectiveness of training attendance counselors and other mediators in contingency contracting (Cantrell,

Cantrell, Huddleston, & Woolridge, 1969; Tharp & Wetzel, 1969) for school attendance and related problems, instructing a key person per school in behavior modification techniques so as to have available one trainer and resource person in each school (Shimoni, 1973), having parents or other mediators reinforce appropriate school behavior by delivering home reinforcement contingent on good school behavior (Bailey, Wolf, & Phillips, 1970; Tharp & Wetzel, 1969), training children as behavior modifiers, and using a variety of in-service courses for training purposes. In this role, the behavior modifier seeks to expand his/her impact by serving as a trainer/reinforcer of key personnel and providing frequent feedback and reinforcement to these personnel to develop and maintain their therapeutic behaviors.

Summary of Principles and Findings

The purpose of this section is to review briefly the extensive school literature by highlighting key principles and findings. Portions of this summary will be used to evaluate this work and discuss future directions for behavioral school research.

1. Children, even those with severe problems, can be taught to help in the operation of behavioral programs, to modify their peers' and teacher's behavior, and to tutor their peers. The possible benefits to the children themselves, the expansion and individualization of programs, and the savings of teacher time make this an exciting area that presently has received only limited research.

2. An important line of investigation has shown that simple, low-cost procedures can be developed to change the behavior of groups of children or whole classes. This development is important as a midpoint between changing one individual at a time and changing entire schools or school systems.

3. Studies have shown that behavioral programs can be simplified yet remain effective, thereby increasing their practicality.

4. The use of modeling and films for both individual and larger scale changes in educational and social development warrants more extensive study.

5. Self-control in the classroom can be learned by even very young and/or disturbed children if there is shaping and training involved in different self-control components (self-observation, discrimination of acceptable and nonacceptable behavior). Self-control training may be one way to increase generalization from external reinforcement programs, although self-control procedures can be learned without prior participation in external reinforcement programs.

6. The gradual reprogramming of the social environment, the use of fading techniques, and intensive consultation with teachers may be effective strategies to assure generalization of program effects. However, work has just been initiated in this area, and the comparative effectiveness of different strategies

remains unclear. In addition, maintenance of behavior after removal or fading of maintenance programs requires more research attention.

7. While separate treatment programs are probably needed for modification of problem behaviors that occur in different settings, there is some evidence that there are covariations in behaviors across time, settings, and other behaviors. Further, a few studies have shown some harmful side effects—for example, an increase in maladaptive behaviors covarying with changes in target behaviors. These phenomena need much more examination but clearly suggest caution in administering treatment programs as well as the necessity to record multiple measurements of treatment effects.

8. On the other hand, a number of strategies can be developed for the therapeutic exploitation of response generalization. For example, academic reprogramming and reinforcing academic products have been shown to decrease inappropriate classroom behavior.

9. Behavioral methods can be used to increase academic responses and facilitate the acquisition and retention of basic skills. Much more work is needed on the effects of different kinds of materials, models, and classroom patterns on academic behaviors. This research demands that behavioral psychologists in school settings become more familiar with the development and evaluation of curriculum packages.

10. Such "humanistic" areas as creativity and the open classroom can be studied using behavioral methods.

11. Experimental investigation of such common classroom practices as homework, question-asking, and the distribution of teacher-student contacts has been initiated recently. Hopefully, this research will allow a greater specification of more efficient educational techniques.

12. The focus of much behavioral work in the schools has been on academic responses and the modification of disruptive behavior. However, some recent work in schools and other settings has exemplified an important shift to the investigation of racial integration, peer management, self-government, and negotiation behaviors.

13. Although organizational and architectural variables obviously influence behavior, research in this area has been limited. The work of Risley and his colleagues indicates that these kinds of variables can be manipulated systematically and their behavioral effects measured. This research suggests that the behavior modifier of the future might be called an "environmental designer."

14. Work on methods of changing teacher behaviors so as to change student behaviors is a very significant contribution to the consultation literature. The results document that *in vivo* feedback and reinforcement are probably needed to modify teacher behaviors. While this approach is expensive and time consuming, recent research indicates that costs can be reduced by the training of adjunct educational personnel.

Revaluation of the Present Literature and Future Concerns

Behavioral research in school settings is proliferating. In approximately one decade basic processes have been investigated, findings often replicated, and many new areas opened for empirical scrutiny. Problems inherent in some of the procedures (e.g., the expense of *in vivo* interventions, maintenance of outcomes) are being addressed with the prior track record suggesting that the obstacles will not be insurmountable.

At least some of this literature has shifted from the earlier emphasis on severe problems of individuals (Krasner & Ullmann, 1973) to processes affecting many children and educators. Examples include the physical design of classrooms, curriculum development, and the promotion of self-control. This shift is consistent with the emerging emphasis on prevention and system change and the movement away from the "direct service model" (Zax & Specter, 1974). While this research generates numerous prescriptions for the development of optimal educational settings, problems such as severe behavioral and learning problems remain difficult and costly to modify (Lovaas, Koegel, Simmons, & Long, 1973). In our zeal for preventive system-oriented interventions, we should not lose sight of these more extreme, individual problems that have been the traditional focus for behavioral treatments. The field's movement toward prevention has not occurred because such problems have been eliminated.

In the next decade, behavior analysts interested in schools must turn their attention to evaluation and change of some of the broader social and economic conditions affecting educational processes. For example, experiments are being performed on voucher systems (Weiler, 1974) and probably will be conducted on other kinds of financing procedures for schools. If such systems were implemented experimentally on a sequential basis in different school districts, it would be possible to evaluate the effects of these plans using multiple measures on the participating parents, children, teachers, and administrators.

There are at least two encouraging signs to suggest that this scenario for the future is not an illusory one: (1) the development of low-cost, reliable procedures for the efficient behavioral observation of people in different physical settings (Quilitch, 1975; also see Chapter 7) indicates that larger scale intervention projects can still focus on individual human behavior *in situ*; and (2) demonstrations by Schnelle and his colleagues (Schnelle, Kirchner, McNees, & Lawler, 1975; Schnelle & Lee, 1974; Schnelle, Weathers, Hannah, & McNees, 1975) have indicated that quasi-experimental designs (Campbell, 1969) can be used to evaluate changes at institutional and regional levels.

The convergence of these developments should result in a behavior modifier (or "environmental designer") who will be able to provide experimental methodology for the development and evaluation of more optimal educational settings, disseminate positively evaluated practices, and help ameliorate economic and social conditions that limit the adoption and potential utility of worthwhile educational innovations (Winett, 1976b).

Chapter 3
THE JUVENILE JUSTICE SYSTEM

Introduction

During the last 10 years, American society has been the forum for increasing debate and concern for the problems of crime and delinquency. A similar observation led Saleem Shah, Director of the Center for Studies of Crime and Delinquency of the National Institute of Mental Health, to state: "It can be said with little fear of exaggeration that the phenomena of delinquency and crime constitute one of the most critical domestic problems presently facing the country" (1973, p. 12).

The intensity of the debate is a result of the media's continued public illumination of skyrocketing crime rates and campaign rhetoric by aspiring politicians. Although official crime rates have been tapering off some in the last year or two, when recent statistics are compared with 1960 rates, the following compelling results are observed: (1) there has been an increase in the frequency of all crimes of 192%, an increase of 193% in property crimes, and an increase in crimes of violence of 190%; (2) there has been an increase in the rate of all crimes of 151%. Similarly, this figure is reflective of an increase in property crimes of 152% and an increase in the rate of violent crimes of 149% (Federal Bureau of Investigation, 1973). In 1974, official statistics indicated an 18% increase in the overall rate in comparison to the 1973 figures (Federal Bureau of Investigation, 1975).

When the specific area of juvenile crime is examined, it is reported that 34% of all cases cleared by law enforcement agencies involve persons under 18 years of age (Federal Bureau of Investigation, 1973). One-ninth of all youths and one-sixth of all male youths will have formal contact with a juvenile court for law violation by the time they reach their 18th birthday (President's Commission, 1967). Further, in examining delinquency rates in a moderate-sized midwestern city, it was discovered that nearly one-third of all male youths between the ages of 14 and 16 had at least one police contact (Davidson, 1975). Shah (1973) also has noted that the rates of juvenile crime are increasing at a faster rate than general crime figures.

It must be pointed out that official crime and delinquency statistics have come under considerable attack as a valid measure of actual illegal behavior.

Various authors have pointed out the volatile nature of official crime statistics, their susceptibility to alteration by changes in record-keeping procedures, and the political necessity of keeping the crime and delinquency rates high (Milakovich & Weis, 1975). It is often suggested that the success of the last Nixon presidential campaign was due at least in part to the public fear generated by the constant attention to very high crime rates. In short, the actual credibility of official crime rate data is supect at best.

Historically, the phenomenon of juvenile delinquency was created by the initiation of the juvenile courts at the end of the 1800s. Prior to that time, youthful offenders were handled with varying degrees of formality by the adult justice system. The initial thrust for the creation of the separate system for juvenile law violators came from the socially altruistic desire to protect children from mistreatment while at the same time providing a vehicle for safeguarding society. The failure of refuge homes, used for wayward youth in the 19th century, had resulted in children being severely treated and used as cheap manual labor. The court was to provide an alternative to this undesirable situation. The mandate was to provide for the care of children in a manner that would ideally approximate that provided by "responsible" parents. Another central issue was that the court per se would provide a highly flexible procedural format amenable to individualized justice and treatment. The rationale for the procedural informality was that juveniles would exchange their access to constitutionally specified rights, usually guaranteed by procedural formality, in return for the benevolent and parent-like concern of the court. When necessary, the court was to assume the role of the interested parent; such court processing was thought to require minimum formal safeguards (Mennel, 1972; Schultz, 1973).

The court had been created with all the fervor of a publicly supported social movement and its influence quickly expanded. For example, the Illinois Juvenile Courts, usually cited as indicative of early juvenile court development, were created by the 1899 Juvenile Court Act and given jurisdiction over any youth who had violated the criminal code of the state. Its operation was based on the work of appointed, unpaid probation officers. By 1901, legislative change expanded the legal definition of juvenile delinquency to include uniquely juvenile offenses. These "status offenses"—offenses for which a youth could not be prosecuted if (s)he were an adult—came to comprise nearly half of the caseload of the juvenile justice system in modern times (Schur, 1973). In 1905, the court's mandate was further expanded. In addition to the adjudication and disposition of cases, it was to supervise directly the treatment services provided pursuant to its orders. In 1907, legislation further expanded the Illinois Juvenile Court's arena by providing for professional probation officers and adjunct staff.

After the fervor of the first decade of this century, the juvenile courts conducted their mission in a rather dormant fashion. Most other states had followed Illinois in creating separate courts for juveniles by the 1920s.

Procedural informality, individualized justice and treatment, and provision of services approximating those of the natural home were held as the basic operating principles. Juvenile courts proceeded in relative quiet until the middle 1960s. The juvenile justice system, like many other social institutions, became the target of a variety of attacks, both from those within and outside its ranks.

The first line of criticism attacked the juvenile court's justification for acting with procedural informality while at the same time holding the fate of individual youth in its hands. Characterized by the Supreme Court decision in the case of Gault (1967), it was suggested that the entire juvenile court movement had been a fiasco. In its majority opinion the Supreme Court stated that regardless of the good intentions of procedural informality and the desire to act in a parental fashion, "the condition of being a boy does not justify a kangaroo court." The failure of the juvenile court to provide either sound, effective treatment or procedural safeguards insuring constitutional rights left the youth with the worst of both worlds. Such criticisms struck at the very basis of the rationale for the principles of individualized juvenile justice (Renn, 1973). Some evidence concerning these contentions has been forthcoming. For example, Scarpitti and Stephenson (1969), in surveying 1,200 juvenile court decisions in the last 1960s, found that rather than individualized justice, the severity of disposition handed down by judges was related inversely to the socioeconomic standing of the youth. Susman (1973) examined the effects of a juvenile judge's experience on his dispositional decisions and found that to some degree case outcome was related more to the individual judge than to the circumstances surrounding a particular youth. Further, Langley, Graves, & Norris (1972), in surveying the cases of 229 youth in a state training school, found that an important factor in a judge's decision to order institutionalization was the judge's perception of the community demand to remove a youth.

A second set of criticisms of the juvenile justice system was focused on its mistreatment of youth in malignant correctional institutions. This line of attack was quiet similar to the arguments which had provided the impetus and rationale for the creation of a separate justice system for juveniles (Schultz, 1973). Recidivism rates for juvenile correctional institutions usually ran as high as 50% and above (Stephenson & Scarpitti, 1969). In addition, Pulitizer Prize-winning reporter Howard James, in his book *Children in Trouble* (1969), outlined the deplorable conditions which existed in juvenile detention and correctional facilities across the country. A national moratorium in the construction of all correctional facilities has been called for (Nagel, 1973). Irwin (1974) has further argued that the current system is so malignant that any serious attempts at innovation can only be thwarted. Other authors have characterized the juvenile court as part of America's process of throwing away undesirable citizens (Richette, 1969), ignoring social problems, providing a forum to regiment the poor (Polier, 1973), isolating undersocialized youth (Feldman, Wodarski, Flax, & Goodman, 1972), and punishing youth who are reacting to social inequality

(Jordan, 1974). Even those less critical see little hope in the future for the nation's juvenile correctional institutions (Luger, 1973).

A third and somewhat more pervasive flaw attributed to the juvenile justice system was its insistence on viewing the problems of delinquency as unique to only apprehended and convicted youth. The deductions from this assumption usually led to the conclusion that delinquency was centered among lower class groups. However, several self-report studies of youth inquiring about involvement in various illegal behaviors indicated that there was widespread commission of unlawful acts quite unrelated to social standing (Erickson, 1973; Williams & Gold, 1972). Thus, officially labeled delinquent youth may have been more representative of the actions of the juvenile justice system than the behavior of the youth apprehended. A similar position has been presented by Polk and Schafer (1972), who observed that delinquency in relation to schools must be viewed from an interactionist position rather than only looking to youth in trouble. More recently, Elliot and Voss (1974) have reported the outcome of an extensive longitudinal study of delinquency. Their results seem to indicate that official delinquency is intricately related to a multitude of social variables usually quite unrelated to illegal behavior per se.

The area of juvenile delinquency theory, practice, and policy has been in a state of considerable turmoil. This situation has led to several sets of events related to the application of behaviorally based approaches to the juvenile crime problem. The next section of this chapter will detail the development of three major policy level responses to the problem and their theoretical underpinnings. These developments, while more general in nature than the specific technical and scientific events which led to the current widespread use of behavioral techniques with delinquent populations, provide a framework for understanding how the behavioral approaches fit into related innovations in the field. It is therefore necessary to provide a brief description of (1) the policy moves toward community-based/preventive interventions, (2) the use of nonprofessional and volunteer staff, and (3) diversion or alternatives to justice system processing as being intricately related to and providing the scenario for the use of behaviorally based approaches.

Community-Based Intervention Policy Recommendations

One change in policy for the juvenile justice system which began to gain prominence by the mid-1960s was the proposing of increased use of community-based remedies. As was pointed out earlier, this response was in part a result of the increasing evidence that traditional, institutionally based correctional approaches for youthful offenders were ineffective, expensive, and inappropriate in their focus (Empey, 1967). In addition, the juvenile justice system was influenced by the more pervasive moves toward community-based interventions prevalent in the other social service fields (Cowen, Gardner, & Zax, 1967; Spergel, 1973).

An apparent critical development in the early implementation of the community-based intervention policy innovation was the report of the President's Commission on Law Enforcement and the Administration of Justice (1967) with its heavy reliance on environmentalist, sociological thought. A prevalent position among criminologists at the time stemmed from the earlier work of Robert Merton (1957) and his general conception of human deviance. Heavy emphasis was placed on the importance of the social milieu. Using official delinquency rates as a data base, earlier classic studies such as those by Shaw and McKay (1942) had demonstrated disproportional distributions of various social and physical problems among socioeconomic and geographic groups. Combining such information with the propositions of anomie theory led to the conclusion that juvenile delinquency was a result of differential access to legitimate and illegitimate means to attainment of societally defined personal and material goals (Cloward & Ohlin, 1960). Varieties of youthful crime were explained by several available modes of coping with blocked opportunity structure including criminal, conflict, and disorganized subcultures. Similar explanations led to theories of gang delinquency (Short, 1968), the importance of exposure to deviance by peers and family members (Severy, 1973), citing the schools as a primary source of blocked opportunity (Gold & Mann, 1972; Harry, 1974; Kelly, 1974; Polk, Frease, & Richmond, 1974; Polk & Schafer, 1972), pointing to the juvenile justice system itself as a perpetuator of continued delinquency (Goldenberg, 1971), and highlighting population density as an etiological factor (Beasley & Antunes, 1974). As part of these developments, "environmentalism" was given a considerable boost in acceptability as an explanation for delinquent behavior. It was a short jump from social structural and conflict theory to recommendations for the importance of making modifications in the environments of delinquent youth.

A related development gave increased credibility to the changeability of delinquent behavior which was to become so central to the behavior modification approach to delinquent youth. Ironically, this indirect support was to come from the individual differences ideology. The classic work in the area had been carried out in the 1940s by the Gluecks. In comparing 500 institutionalized delinquent youth with 500 demographically matched nondelinquents on over 400 physical, psychological, and social variables, the Gluecks sought to identify dimensions which would discriminate delinquents in early elementary school for predictive and preventive interventions. A large number of statistically reliable differences were identified in all domains in the initial *post hoc* study (Glueck & Glueck, 1951). After several further analyses of the data, the Gluecks concluded that five social factors, essentially descriptive of differential levels of parenting mode, best distinguished delinquents early in elementary school, were most amenable to application by school personnel, and were most descriptive of different types of delinquent youth (Glueck & Glueck, 1970).

The highly influential work of the Gluecks is representative of a large body of work focusing on the individual differences between delinquents and non-delinquents from a multitude of theoretical perspectives. A review of that literature has indicated that the research since 1950 shows consistent differences between delinquents and nondelinquents on a variety of objective personality tests, performance measures, and projective techniques (Waldo & Dinitz, 1967). The criterion group research model, exemplified by the work of the Gluecks, has led to a myriad of "individual difference" explanations for delinquency. Recent representative work found delinquents to be less socialized (Smith & Austrin, 1974), psychologically abnormal (K. Adams, 1974), morally immature (Prentice, 1972), and the product of dysfunctional upbringing (Alexander, 1973).

The results of this work were the propositions that if the products of psychologically and socially harmful environments could be identified early in life, interventions could be applied in a preventive fashion. The services which were proposed for identified future delinquents included intensive casework (Tait & Hodges, 1971), community day-care centers (Grossman, 1972), the "Big Brother" projects (Davis, 1957), corrective foster homes (*Columbia Journal of Law and Social Problems*, 1972), detached workers for youthful gang members (Klein, 1971), child guidance services (Craig & Furst, 1965), mental health services for vulnerable children (Cowen, Dorr, Trost, & Izzo, 1972), educational enrichment for likely delinquents (Wenk, 1974), and increased services to disadvantaged families (Epstein & Shainline, 1974).

These developments, although theoretically and technically divergent from the behavioral approach per se, provided tangential support for the argument that delinquency was functionally related to social phenomena and potentially amenable to modification. In the context of the history of delinquency theory and intervention, these were landmark breaks with the past and added to the juvenile justice system's amenability to innovative approaches.

Nonprofessional and Volunteer Staffing Policy Recommendations.

A second set of policy recommendations which coincided with the advent of the behavioral approaches in the field of juvenile delinquency was suggestions for the widespread use of nonprofessional and volunteer staffing. Such proposals were the result of several factors which centered primarily around the ineffectiveness of the juvenile courts in preventing or correcting delinquency and the projected lack of additional personnel resources.

One of the main contributors to the staff shortage rationale, George Albee (1968), suggested that the mental health field's traditional view of human problems as intra-individual in locus had and would lead to massive shortages in professional personnel to provide the required therapeutic services. This argument led Gruver (1971) to conclude:

Albee's continuing investigation of professional manpower resources in the mental health fields had made apparent the severe current shortages, and further, has suggested the probability of even greater future shortages.

A second aspect of the mental health manpower dilemma is that even if there were sufficient numbers of professional personnel, present mental health ideology would prevent many of those needing help from receiving it ... groups such as drug abusers, alcoholics, and juvenile delinquents have also been neglected by the mental health professionals primarily because professional contact with them has been for the most part fruitless. (p. 111)

More provocative is the evidence that nonprofessionals are more effective than their professional counterparts in working with some populations which are presently receiving professional focus. (p. 112)

In fact, the evidence had been mounting for some time that traditional one-to-one counseling and therapeutic techniques with delinquents produced less than desired results. The classic Cambridge-Sommerville Youth Study cast serious doubt on the value of one-to-one counseling approaches to troubled youth. Multiple follow-ups of 325 male pre-delinquents, who had received individual counseling from model adults, and a matched control group indicated no impact on crime rates, type of offense committed, incarceration rates, or post-institutional adjustment (McCord & McCord, 1959). Further, it appeared that traditional casework methods and psychotherapeutic techniques were similarly quite ineffective (Grey & Dermody, 1972; Levitt, 1971). Levitt concluded that in general "conventional psychotherapy methods appear to be least effective with delinquents. The reported improvement rate is more than a standard deviation below the mean for all treated cases" (p. 484).

The questionable effectiveness of traditional approaches to juvenile delinquency *and* the current and projected shortages of professional personnel led to recommendations for the use of nonprofessional and volunteer services in the juvenile justice system (Joint Commission on Correctional Manpower and Training, 1970; Joint Commission on Mental Health of Children, 1973; Tomaino, 1968). Again, these developments added credence to suggestions for the use of behavioral approaches with delinquent populations. The behaviorists were suggesting that their methods could and must be employed by on-line correctional staff. In fact, it was the behavioral position that the individuals in the immediate day-to-day, social environment of the delinquent youth were the very individuals who must be engaged in the rehabilitation effort. They were also suggesting that behavioral techniques could be taught to relevant staff and family members in a relatively brief time and without the acquisition of a doctoral degree (Cohen & Filipczak, 1971; Tharp & Wetzel, 1969; Thorne, Tharp, & Wetzel, 1967).

Diversion Policy Recommendations.

A third set of policy recommendations also was tied closely to the report of the President's Commission on Law Enforcement (1967). The recommendation for diversion specified that delinquent youth should be handled through alternatives to juvenile court processing and institutionalization whenever possible. The general argument was that the court's functioning and institutional rehabilitation had become so malignant that alternatives for social control and rehabilitation had to be provided. Proponents of the diversion alternatives found instant allies among social labeling theorists. Further, early propositions concerning the use of behavioral approaches to human problems drew heavily on the social labeling conceptualization of deviance (see, for example, the introduction to Ullmann & Krasner, 1965).

Prominent authors had suggested that deviance was a characteristic conferred upon various acts by an influential audience. In addition, society used deviance labels to specify the limits of acceptable behavior by selecting certain groups as deviant, formally identifying them in a variety of social ceremonies, and relegating them to inferior social standing (Becker, 1963; Garfinkel, 1956). From this point of view, deviance—i.e., juvenile delinquency—was not seen as a characteristic of the individual violator or his pathological/deprived environment, rather deviance was said to be the result of intricate social processes. In fact, this chain of thought led to a definition of power as the ability to socially label (Matza, 1969).

Social labeling theory, in combination with self-report studies of delinquency reporting the widespread incidence of unreported youthful crime was highly inconsistent with traditional views of the delinquency problem. Essentially, if most youth drifted in and out of illegal behavior patterns until either apprehended or left unnoticed, and if the conferring of a negative social label of delinquency had adverse effects on the future incidence of illegal performance, the overuse of a juvenile court or institutional remedy seemed contraindicated (Faust, 1973; Lemert, 1974; Matza, 1964; Schur, 1969, 1973).

Again, recommendations for diversion and the theoretical underpinnings of social labeling theory provided the behavioral position with adjunct support. The behavioral approaches also were suggesting that delinquency was not an intraindividual or intrinsic characteristic of apprehended youth amenable to remedy by traditional therapeutic interventions or institutional punishment. Rather, the importance of the social environment in maintaining the illegal performances and in failing to provide support for alternative acceptable behaviors was the central thesis of the behavioral position as it entered the realm of juvenile corrections.

The Advent of Behavioral Procedures in the Juvenile Justice System.

As we will see in the more formal review section of this chapter, the systematic use of behavioral procedures with delinquent groups has occurred within the last 15 years. Yates (1970) recalled that a conference convened in the early 1960s to discuss the application of social learning theory to the problems of delinquency involved almost entirely theoretical discussions. While the principles of behavior modification had demonstrated a considerable degree of effectiveness with a variety of human problems, they had not been used in any systematic fashion with adolescent law violators prior to the early '60s.

The suggestions for the use of behavioral procedures with delinquents came at a time when the juvenile justice system and its supportive political and theoretical undergirding were under considerable duress. These attacks and suggested remedies coincided well with the optimistic recommendations for the use of behavioral principles. The door had been opened for considering relatively "radical" alternatives. The suggestions for community-based intervention, the importance of nonprofessional personnel, and diversionary alternatives were all directly supportive of the advent of the behavioral corrective technology. The importance of the social environment and the contingencies it imparted, the potency of interpersonal contingencies on a day-to-day basis rather than only during the therapy hour, and the ineffectiveness of the traditional juvenile justice system were all critical issues for the behavioral movement in juvenile corrections.

More specific events occurred within the behavioral movement per se which enhanced its palatability for juvenile corrections. First, early writings tended to outline the general principles and strategies of behavior modification and suggest their conceptual and technical appropriateness for use in correctional settings. The concerns for specifiable behavioral acts, overt as opposed to internal events, and the importance of consequation were quite consistent with the judicial tradition and required a minimal amount of "translation." This convergence between the language of the behavioral approach and legalistic thinking was an important contributing factor. The juvenile justice system had always placed heavy emphasis on its close relationship with social and clinical practitioners. However, the apparent marriage was always suspected as illegitimate (Steketee, 1973). The clinical "nosology" of probation officers, case workers, and court psychologists made little sense to juvenile judges or correctional program administrators. In one sense, then, the behavioral movement had considerably more in common with the juvenile justice system than had prior attempts at therapeutic innovation.

Second, the behavior modification approach to juvenile delinquents was quick to point out that on-line staff, parents, teachers, case workers, etc. were the very individuals who were most likely to be in a position to alter the behavior of the youth and should therefore become the focus of the innovations. Juvenile courts and their related agencies and institutions had always struggled with the unavailability of professional therapeutic personnel to work with adjudicated delinquents. In fact, juvenile court casework was often considered low on the totem pole of social service professionals. The suggestion of the behavioral movement that many years of graduate and clinical training were nonessential for becoming a highly effective change agent fit nicely with the times. Court and correctional staff could be provided relatively short-term instruction and supervision. Efficiency as well as effectiveness issues provided strong arguments.

Third, behavior modification held some promise of providing a strategy for dealing with previously unreachable youth. Traditional therapeutic approaches had always experienced difficulty in getting "unsocialized, lower class, and incorrigible" delinquent youth to even attend, let alone meaningfully participate in therapy sessions. The early work of Slack (1960) had demonstrated that it was possible to induce unreachable delinquents into intensive psychotherapy. One of the initiators of behavioral work with delinquents, Schwitzgebel (1964) proposed that Slack's work provided the basis for a new conception and treatment of juvenile delinquency—namely, delinquency could be viewed as youth who had been exposed to contingency systems functionally related to illegal performances. Therapeutic approaches, then, required the rearrangement of environmental contingencies (Schwitzgebel, 1967).

The fourth component of the behavioral movement was the suggestion that in order for rehabilitation to be successful and durable it had to involve increases in desired behavior rather than only the reduction or elimination of undesired behavior. Earlier writers pointed out that the behavioral approach provided the probation or parole officer with techniques for increasing desired performances rather than targeting only the removal of undesired behavior (Shah, 1966; Thorne, Tharp, & Wetzel, 1967). Cohen (1968) in presenting the principles and procedures of the CASE I program at the National Training School for Boys, outlined a general model for behavioral interventions with delinquents that drew heavily on these propositions. The importance of scheduling and arranging consequences in programming success for an educational environment was stressed. Cohen's closing comments reflected the positive and educational focus of behavior modification with delinquent youth. "Learning, putting in new successful behaviors, not unlearning, is the program for successful rehabilitation. The unlearning part is done by the individual differentiating his own behaviors by the newly learned set of values which are imprintable and discoverable through the educational process." Although the building of alternative positive behaviors was a relatively new conception for the juvenile justice system in the early and mid-1960s, the other events described earlier had added sufficient flexibility to the system allowing for the addition of the positive focus of the behavioral approach. In addition, suggesting that the juvenile justice system must concern itself with positive as well as illegal behavior meshed nicely with more general concerns for rehabilitation.

A fifth component of the entry of behavioral approaches to the area of juvenile delinquency is an issue which pervades many of the specific social and human problems where behavioral approaches have played a major role. In many ways, behavior modifiers gained access to delinquent groups somewhat by default. The behavioral movement was gaining momentum at exactly the time when juvenile corrections were under considerable attack. Juvenile corrections had not attracted the best therapists and program directors in the social service fields. In fact, relative to the prevalence of the problem, delinquency had attracted relatively little attention from the social service profession. This situation was due in large measure to the conceptions of the early and mid-1900s, which saw delinquency and criminality as relatively intractable conditions. Also, it was quite evident experientially and empirically that delinquents as a group did not appear amenable to traditional therapeutic interventions. In short, the area of juvenile delinquency theory and practice was ripe for the innovations offered by behavior modification.

The next section will provide a review of representative programs and research. For organizational purposes, the review will be divided into sections dependent on the setting in which the intervention and research took place. These sections will be determined by whether the program took place in an institutional setting, a residential community-based setting, or a nonresidential community setting. Each of these sections will be further subdivided according to the type of research methodology employed: case studies, pre-post single-group studies, control-group studies, and A-B-A studies.

Review

Institutional Programs.

A good deal of the research on behavioral approaches to delinquent populations has been carried out in correctional or detention facilities. The overriding concern has been the upgrading of institutional programs and the training and involvement of institutional personnel in the change procedures. The ultimate goal was to enhance the effectiveness of juvenile correctional programs.

Case studies. Early implementation of behavioral principles with delinquent populations tended to focus on individual youth. Staats and Butterfield (1965) designed procedures which focused on the academic deficiencies of a 14-year-old institutionalized delinquent male. The program called for earning extra privileges by completing units from programmed reading materials. These procedures produced an increase in the amount of time spent reading and in comprehension of assigned reading material. This individual program was instituted over a 4½-month time period and included 40 hours of instruction. Follow-up testing indicated a 2½-year gain in reading level as well as a reduction in errors made in the programmed instruction. In addition, the in-house schoolteacher reported that the youth had reduced the amount of misbehavior displayed in the classroom.

Tyler (1967) followed similar procedures in focusing on the school performance of a 16-year-old delinquent in a state training school. Again, the youth was allowed to earn privileges contingent upon academic performance. Daily report card grades were given in each class attended. Tokens were administered on the basis of the grade level earned. Tokens were exchangeable for somewhat more "basic" items such as a mattress to sleep on and civilian clothes. In addition, the youth could obtain general canteen items for his earnings. The results of these procedures indicated that the youth improved the report card grades over the half year covered in the study.

Other studies in institutional settings have been concerned with the elimination of undesired behavior. Burchard and Tyler (1965) designed a program consisting of a brief timeout period and a token economy for reduction of aggressive behavior in a 9-year-old institutionalized delinquent. Each instance of aggressive behavior by the youth was met with a brief isolation period, while privileges could be earned for nonaggressive performance. Gradually, the disruptions decreased in occurrence and finally disappeared. An additional case study was aimed at the reduction of stealing in a 10-year-old institutionalized youth. The approach involved making home visits, which were apparently very important to the youth, contingent on the absence of theft for weekly intervals. This contingency system resulted in the elimination of the stealing over a 3-month time period and at 1-month follow-up (Wetzel, 1966).

Several years later Brown and Tyler (1968) sought to eliminate the intimidating-aggressive actions of a 16-year-old delinquent youth in an institutional setting. They also designed a brief isolation procedure to be used contingent upon the undesired actions. These procedures were followed for the 10-month time period covered by their study. A check of staff records showed that the behavior of the youth had improved and that the incidence of intimidation had decreased considerably.

Single-group designs. Fineman (1968) described a program involving the use of contingent rewards over a 6-month time period in a juvenile detention facility. Although the contingency system was based on individualized contingencies, the token economy allowed for exchangeable points for the "top point earner." The system concentrated on staff-defined desirable behaviors. Undesirable behavior resulted in point penalties. Assessment of the program consisted of staff interviews at the end of the 6-month exploratory period. The interviews indicated that staff rated the program as generally positive in producing the desired behaviors from the youth. A nearly identical program, with parallel results and measures, was presented as part of a discussion of token economy programs in a particular state training school system (Rice, 1970).

The use of isolation or timeout procedures for the elimination of undesired behavior in institutional settings was a major focus of early work in this area. Somewhat more recently, Burchard and Barrera (1972) examined the specific effectiveness of such procedures. They began by identifying the impact of varying timeout and response cost procedures in reducing undesired behaviors such as swearing, fighting, destroying property, and disobedience to staff instructions. Alternating conditions of a 5-token penalty, a 5-minute period of isolation, a 30-token penalty, and a 30-minute period of isolation were applied to 11 institutionalized delinquent youth. Each of the four conditions lasted 12 consecutive days. The results indicated that a relatively severe penalty was required to reduce the undesired behavior below baseline levels—only the two conditions with the larger penalties were successful in reducing the undesired behavior.

Fodor (1972) presented a somewhat less detailed description of attempts to remove undesired actions in an institutional setting. The behavior change strategy consisted of group discussion sessions with eight training school inmates. The group training sessions focused on the runaway behavior of the girls and consisted of negative verbal feedback from the staff whenever the girls talked of running away. In comparing the runaway rates of this group of females prior to and following the group discussion project, it was reported that the rate of runaway behavior was reduced considerably.

Comparison group designs. An early issue which needed to be examined in behavioral programs in institutional settings was to what extent the positive results which had been observed were attributable to the initiation of "positive" procedures. In other words, given the state of most juvenile correctional programs, wouldn't any positive reinforcement, systematic or not, be expected to produce desired results? Tyler and Brown (1968) examined this question directly. Fifteen institutionalized males were randomly assigned to one of two intervention groups. Each intervention group was exposed to both experimental conditions. The first group earned privileges for correct answers to daily news quizzes for the first 17 days of the study. This procedure was followed by 12 days of noncontingent privileges for the first group. The second group received the noncontingent reinforcement (privileges for the first 17 days followed by a 12-day period during which they had to earn their privileges by correct answers to the news quizzes. In other words, the two groups of youth were exposed to the same two procedures, except in reverse order. The results of this study indicated that both groups performed better on the news quizzes when privileges were contingent upon performance. Further, the group which was exposed to the contingent reinforcement condition first showed less of a decrement in performance when exposed to the noncontingent condition.

An expanded criterion of school behavior was the focus of Meichenbaum,

Bowers, and Ross (1968) who designed a set of procedures to increase the appropriate classroom behavior rates of 10 institutionalized female delinquents. At baseline, the appropriate classroom behavior rate of this group was half the rate of similar nondelinquent peers. The criterion for this study consisted of a dichotomous behavioral observation system which provided a tabulation of appropriate versus inappropriate behavior. Tasks set forth in the classroom by the teacher formed the boundary conditions of appropriate behavior. The girls in this study attended both morning and afternoon classrooms. This study involved four sequential intervention conditions. The first condition lasted for 5 days and involved the usual classroom procedures. The second condition lasted for 7 days, during which the girls earned up to $2.00 in the afternoon classroom only. Their earnings were based on the proportion of appropriate behavior exhibited. The third condition lasted for 3 days and expanded the previous earning opportunities to the morning classroom. In this condition, the girls could earn up to $3.50 based on the proportion of appropriate behavior displayed in both the morning and afternoon classroom. In addition, the verbal feedback to the girls was provided in terms of dollars and cents in this condition rather than in terms of percent-of-desired-behavior as had been the case in the second condition. The fourth condition included the addition of fines for inappropriate classroom behavior and a reduction in the reinforcement available to $1.50. This final condition lasted for 3 days. The results of this study demonstrated that the appropriate behavior levels of the delinquent females could be raised to the same level as those of nondelinquent peers (80%). However, the differential effectiveness of the three experimental conditions was not explicitly demonstrated.

A somewhat different approach to examining the effectiveness of behavioral procedures in the educational realm was reported by Bednar, Zelhart, Greathouse, and Weinberg (1970). Thirty-two institutionalized male delinquents were randomly assigned to one of two procedures. The first group attended 18 weekly evening study sessions, they earned monetary reinforcement for 5-minute intervals of "attending, cooperating, and persisting" on their assigned work. During the remainder of the sessions, they were paid on a prorated scale on the basis of their level of performance on proficiency tests. The second group also attended the weekly study sessions except that they were not paid either for their attention to the assigned work or for their performance on tests. Several assessments of both groups were accomplished on a pre-post basis. First, on the SPA achievement tests, both groups showed significant increases in their reading achievement, while the experimental group made significantly greater gains in terms of word comprehension. On the Gaites-MacGinitie Achievement Test series, the experimental group also showed significantly greater improvement in both reading achievement and word comprehension. Both groups had also been given an attitude survey to assess their attitudes toward reading. Neither group exhibited any change in their attitudes toward reading. Teacher ratings indicated significantly more improvement for the experimental youth in terms of persistence, attention, liking school, sociability, and cooperation.

Coleman (1974) further examined the effective conditions for the use of behavioral principles with institutionalized delinquent populations. Nineteen youth were randomly assigned to one of two conditions. During the initial baseline period, both groups participated in work-study sessions consisting of 30-minute study periods followed by noncontingent 15-minute breaks. The baseline sessions exposed the youth to usual classroom educational materials. During the next phase of the project, both groups were put on programmed instructional materials. The first group was paid points, exchangeable for a variety of privileges, for on-task behavior in the study sessions. The second group could earn points contingent on the accuracy of work completed during this segment. The results indicated that programmed instruction alone failed to enhance the performance of either group. The contingencies, however, did increase the academic performance of both groups with the group who had been reinforced on the basis of the accuracy of work completed showing the higher rates of improvement. Post-testing of the two groups on standard achievement tests did not reveal any differential effects.

Other applications of behavioral principles in institutional settings have been concerned with more general behavior within the residential setting. A study by Pavlott (1971) investigated the effectiveness of behavioral procedures in producing general rule compliance. Sixty female delinquents were placed randomly in either a special token economy program or the traditional institutional regimen. The token economy system in this particular project employed contingencies for a variety of self-care and social behaviors. The criteria for success in this project were staff ratings of the behavior on a problem behavior checklist. After 3 months of operating the experimental program, the group that had participated in the token economy was rated as exhibiting significantly less problem behaviors—i.e., greater improvement.

Buehler, Patterson, and Furness (1966) highlighted the importance of peer reinforcement systems in correctional programs and their potential contribution to the juvenile "schools for crime." A project designed and executed by Krueger (1971) examined the relative impact of differential sources of reinforcement. Eighteen institutionalized male offenders were randomly assigned to attend one of three different group sessions. The first two groups were designed to provide reinforcement to the youth contingent upon positive verbal statements about themselves or others. In the first group, the dispensers of the reinforcement were peer members. In the second group, the institutional staff dispensed the reinforcement. The third group received reinforcement randomly throughout the sessions from the staff members. The criteria for this study included behavioral observations of the rates of positive comments about self or others within the group and in other day-to-day settings throughout the institutional program. The group which had been exposed to the peer reinforcement in the group sessions displayed a significantly higher rate of positive comments in the sessions themselves. In addition, these rates were more resistant to extinction once the formal system had been terminated and showed greater generalization to other institutional settings.

Cohen and Filipczak (1971) reported the outcome of a 2-year contingency management program at the former National Training School for Boys. The token economy program which was developed focused to a large extent on educational achievement and accomplishments. The 41 boys who participated in the program over the 2 years of its experimental operation demonstrated highly significant gains in academic achievement. The students from this program were compared later with a similar group of youth who had completed the regular training school program. In addition, the youth who were released from the case project directly were compared with those who first were sent to another institutional setting prior to release. Those youth who could be located at 3 years of follow-up (less than half) displayed a continued high level of achievement as measured by standard achievement tests. However, by the end of the 3-year follow-up, the rates of recidivism for the experimental group were highly similar to those of the matched control group.

Sloan and Ralph (1973) present a description of the implementation of a behavioral program in one dormitory at a state training school. This project involved retraining the regular institutional staff to use a point system to make institutional contingencies specific. The point system involved contingencies for both educational behaviors and accomplishments and social performances. A daily record-keeping system was established to provide the youth with immediate feedback. The point system in this program involved both immediate daily payoffs as well as point-earning goals in order to be considered for parole. This experimental dormitory was compared to another similar dormitory in the same training school system. In the area of academic achievement, the experimental dormitory group showed greater gains. Recidivism rates for both dormitories dropped during the period covered by the study.

Jesness (1974) reports an extensive evaluation of two California Youth Authority programs in institutional settings. The aim of the evaluation was a direct comparison of two innovative approaches to institutional treatment for delinquent youth. Nearly 1,000 youth were assigned to either the experimental behavior modification units or to the experimental transactional analysis units. Both experimental programs involved institution-wide innovations and may represent the most comprehensive reported in institutional settings to date. In addition to examining the relative efficacy of the two innovative approaches, the study also included an examination of the differential impact of the two approaches on various types of youth as categorized by the interpersonal maturity dimension used by the California Youth Authority. One important finding of the study was that the two programs generated rather specific treatment effects. The behavior modification program showed greater gains in behavioral observational data while the transactional analysis units demonstrated greater gains on attitudinal and self-report scales. The results of the two programs in reducing recidivism are somewhat less promising—namely, there did not appear to be differential impact on recidivism rates between the two experimental programs. Both programs showed a reduction in illegal behavior when the follow-up time period was compared to the time before the subjects had entered the program. In addition, both experimental programs showed lower recidivism rates than those exhibited by the regular state training school rates. However, after 2 years (24-month follow-up) over half of the youth who had attended both programs had recidivated.

A-B-A designs. While some investigators have chosen to use control-group designs to examine the effectiveness of their innovative procedures, others have used single-subject reversal procedures. An early study of this type by Tyler and Brown (1967) was aimed at the reduction of rule violations by 15 male delinquents in an institutional setting. The investigators concerned themselves with the elimination of these undesired behaviors during the "pool-playing" recreation period. During the first 6 weeks of the project, rule violations resulted in the youth being immediately placed in isolation for 15 minutes. During the next 14 weeks, rule violations resulted in only the usual staff verbal reprimands. The final 15 weeks of the study involved a return to the initial isolation methods. Recordings of the incidence of rule violations throughout the study indicated that the swift isolation procedures were effective in suppressing undesired behavior.

Burchard (1967) employed a similar methodology to determine the effectiveness of a combined positive token economy and penalty system. Twelve institutionalized retarded delinquent males were exposed alternately to contingent and noncontingent reward and penalty conditions for both their school and workshop performances. It was demonstrated that such procedures were successful in bringing both the classroom and workshop behavior to desired levels.

Horton (1970) examined the extent to which the aggressive behavior of delinquent boys would generalize from a situation in which it was directly reinforced to a similar situation in which it was not. Aggressive actions and behavior were observed in two settings. The first situation consisted of pairs of youth playing the card game "war." In this situation, the youth were exposed to five separate conditions. In the baseline and two reversal conditions, the youth earned money on the basis of the number of cards they won in the game. During the two intermittent experimental conditions, the six male youth were reinforced for aggressive behaviors. In the second situation, the pairs of youth played the game "steal-the-bacon." There were no formal contingencies in effect during the "steal-the-bacon" situations. The results indicated that the youth were more aggressive when reinforced for being so. Further, when the youth were more aggressive in the card game situation, it tended to generalize to the second situation.

Jesness and DeRisi (1973) reported interim results of the efficacy of the behavior modification procedures which were utilized in the program (Jesness, 1974) mentioned earlier. Of concern in this particular investigation was the relative impact of immediate versus delayed reinforcement for desired educational behaviors. An average of 15 institutionalized male delinquents were the students in this classroom. During the baseline and reversal conditions, which lasted 39 days and 30 days respectively, points earned for the completion of academic assignments were exchangeable only in the institution-wide token economy program. The experimental manipulation established a separate contingency payoff system within the classroom and was in effect for 62 days. Classroom payoffs could be exchanged immediately for better working materials, breaks, cigarettes, and free time. Undesired behavior resulted in penalties within either system. During the time that reinforcers were available in the classroom, the rate of penalties for undesired behavior was less than half the rate when only the general token program was in effect. This pattern indicated a substantial improvement in classroom performance.

The reader can see that the majority of attempts to demonstrate the efficacy of behavioral approaches to delinquent youth have occurred in institutional settings. In most instances, the studies and procedures reported have focused on only single behaviors or single domains of behavior. These reports have detailed a set of positive results which is without exception in its demonstration of improvement in specific behavioral performances. The broader outcome studies, particularly in the area of recidivism, have produced neutral or negative results.

Community-Based Residential Programs.

The major contributions in this area have come from the Achievement Place Project operated in conjunction with the Department of Human Development of the University of Kansas. Consequently, this section will consist primarily of summaries of representative studies from that project (see also Chapter 2).

A-B-A designs. The first study on the Achievement Place program (Phillips, 1968) was concerned with examining the efficacy of the total contingency system which was set up in the home-style residential setting for delinquent boys. Three of the youth participated in five experiments designed to check the effectiveness of various contingency procedures in enhancing different behaviors. One concern in generating the family-like program was the elimination of aggressive verbal statements from the youth. The conditions included the observation of naturally occurring rates, verbal correction by the house parents, penalties within the program's token economy, and verbal threats of penalties. It was clear that only the actual penalty conditions were successful in eliminating the aggressive statements, and further it took the higher of the two penalty conditions to completely eliminate the aggressive statements.

A second concern was getting the youth to keep their rooms clean. This study represented one of the first attempts by the Achievement Place program to involve the youth themselves in the management of contingencies, a procedure which was to become an integral part of the operation of the program over the years. The different procedures attempted in this study included baseline, auctioning the right to manage the room-cleaning contingencies among the students in the program, fining the entire group of students if the rooms were not kept clean, the house parents appointing a manager of the contingencies for room cleaning, and having the group elect a manager. The resulting study indicated that the appointed and elected manager conditions were most effective in producing the highest rates of room cleaning. A third experiment was aimed at getting the youth to do a variety of tasks on time. This study indicated that fines within the general token economy were the most effective in getting the youth to return on time from school, return from errands on time, and getting to bed on time.

Another early issue was finding an effective procedure for getting the youth to complete their assigned schoolwork in homework sessions. The conditions in this study included a baseline, monetary payoff for completion of homework, earning time out of the house on a weekly basis for completion of homework, earning time out of the house on a daily basis, and earning points within the general token economy. In this instance, the earning of points within the general token economy was found to be most effective in getting the youth to complete their homework.

A final study in this initial set focused on the elimination of the word "ain't" from the conversation of the Achievement Place youth. The procedures tried in this experiment included baseline, verbal correction by the staff for using the word "ain't," and verbal correction plus point penalties within the general contingency system. Only the correction-plus-penalty condition was successful in eliminating "ain't" from students' conversation. A post-check indicated that the experimental effects had been maintained.

An early series of three studies from the Achievement Place project is presented by Bailey et al. (1970). Achievement Place youth live in a small group (6-8 youth) home organized to reflect a natural family situation. Those youth attending Achievement Place attend the community schools to continue their educational careers. An initial concern of the project was developing procedures which would effectively modify the school performance of the youth. This early series of three studies demonstrated the effectiveness of a reinforcement system administered from the home in effecting change in the youth's school performance. A system was set up whereby the youth received additional privileges at Achievement Place contingent on performance in school, as rated by teachers on daily report cards. In a series of conditions including positive contingencies, negative contingencies, and report cards only, it was demonstrated that when home privileges were earned for classroom accomplishments and lost for failure to do daily classwork, significant improvement in teacher ratings occurred. Further, it was shown that when the formal contingencies and daily report cards were gradually faded out, the improvements in classroom behavior were maintained.

Another series of studies at the Achievement Place project was reported by Phillips et al. (1971). This report included four separate experiments. The first was concerned with getting the youth to attend meals promptly. In this situation, the loss of points within the general contingency system was found to be more effective than threats by the house parents. The second experiment was concerned with getting the youth to clean their rooms, as had been the focus of an earlier study. During this study, a variety of positive and negative contingency procedures was tried. It was found that a combined payoff and fine condition was more effective than verbal demands from the house parents, verbal threats, feedback about performance, or specific verbal instructions about how the task was to be completed. The third study in this set was aimed at getting the youth to place a proportion of their earnings in a savings account. This study demonstrated that the youth could be induced to engage in saving if their rate of saving was matched with earnings within the general contingency system. The fourth behavior targeted for change in this report was correct answers by the youth to daily news quizzes covering material presented in the nightly news. Again, a system involving point earnings for correct answers and point loss for incorrect answers was demonstrated superior to a number of other options. In addition, the youth were much more likely to watch the news in that condition.

Another innovation attempted by the Achievement Place project was the use of the youth themselves as reliable reporters of their own and others' behavior. The general result of several procedures and conditions was that the youth would accurately report when they could earn points for it and when the situations for reporting were combined with specific instructions and supervision by the house parents. However, it was also demonstrated that the accurate reporting by the youth did not generalize to reporting on performance not under close supervision by the house parents or any of the performances after the close supervision was terminated (Fixsen, Phillips, & Wolf, 1972).

Related work on the efficacy of the Achievement Place model has included the modification of articulation errors (Bailey, Timbers, Phillips, & Wolf, 1971), training in interviewing skills (Braukmann, Maloney, Fixsen, Phillips, & Wolf, 1971), the importance of self-government in the total program (Fixsen et al., 1973; Kifer, Ayala, Fixsen, Phillips, & Wolf, 1975), further work on the use of home-based reinforcement and academic performance (Kirigin, Phillips, Fixsen, & Wolf, 1971), and modification of the verbal interactions of the youth (Timbers, Phillips, Fixsen, & Wolf, 1971).

Control-group designs. Preliminary results from outcome studies concerning the effectiveness of the total Achievement Place approach have been reported by Kirigin, Phillips, Fixsen, Atwater, Taubman, and Wolf (1974). Comparison of institutionalization rates of eight Achievement Place youth with 18 control youth, who were randomly rejected from the program due to lack of space, indicated that Achievement Place was serving as an alternative to institutionalization. Over half of the rejected youth had been institutionalized within 2 years. Follow-up comparisons of the Achievement Place youth are only available for a matched comparison group that had been institutionalized in the state school. One- and 2-year follow-up comparisons with this matched group indicate that the Achievement Place youth are much less likely to be reinstitutionalized, have further police contact, or be school dropouts.

A somewhat similar follow-up study was recently completed by Davidson and Wolfred (in press). Fifty-four youth were followed for 9 months following release from a community-based residential behavior modification program. This project consisted of a residential token economy including individualized as well as group contingencies for desired social and self-care performances. In addition, the program involved an in-house classroom run according to the principles of individualized instruction and contingency management. Descriptive as well as empirical examination of the residential program indicated its effectiveness in bringing the academic, social, and self-care behaviors of the youth to highly desirable levels prior to release. The youth from this program were compared with a matched group, from the state child-care agency in a neighboring community, not participating in such a program. The two groups were matched in terms of age, race, sex, presenting problem, and length of time the youth had been a ward of the state. Pre-post comparisons were accomplished on school attendance and grades, police contacts, institutionalization rates, foster home placement rates, and school suspensions. While analyses of the pre-data indicated that the groups were essentially equivalent on the dependent variables for 1 year prior to the project, the group that participated in the experimental program was more likely to have been institutionalized and have police contacts by 9 months following the program.

Again, in community-based residential settings, behavioral procedures with delinquent youth have produced universally positive results in terms of eliciting specific positive behavioral changes and eliminating undesired behaviors. The results of the follow-up studies are mixed. Neither of the two studies reviewed are based on true experimental designs, making definitive conclusions difficult.

Community-Based Nonresidential Programs.

Another strategy in applying behavioral techniques to delinquent populations has been to employ procedures in naturalistic and open community settings.

Case studies. Stuart (1971) presented the procedures for the behavioral contracting method of altering interpersonal contingencies. The contracting method consists of explicit written agreements concerning the interpersonal exchanges which will take place between two parties. It is necessary to identify and specifically detail what each party expects changed in the interpersonal situation. In the case of delinquent youth, such exchanges are usually negotiated between the youth and the parents or teachers. A case study is presented of a female delinquent who had a history of incorrigibility, alleged sexual offenses, and school-related difficulty. Behaviors such as curfew, free time, household chores, and schoolwork were included in the contract, which was negotiated between the girl and her parents. The data regarding the performance of contracted behaviors indicated a high rate of contract compliance by both parties, court wardship was terminated, and there was no indication of further delinquency.

Single-group designs. The Behavioral Research Project (Tharp & Wetzel, 1969) worked from the assumption that naturally occurring mediators of reinforcement in the lives of delinquent youth were the key to successful intervention. A program was designed whereby parents and teachers were provided consultation from bachelor's level behavior analysts. The behavioral analysts met on a regular basis for supervision with doctoral level professionals who had expertise in the use of behavioral methods. Individualized programs and contingency systems were devised. A number of individual cases are presented from this project as representative of typical increases in desired performances. Three follow-up assessments of up to 18 months were performed on the group of youth who completed this project. Those assessments indicated that the youth who participated showed considerable decreases in their delinquency rates, increases in grades, and improvements in behavior problem ratings.

A similar program is described by Rose, Sundel, Delange, Corwin, and Palumbo (1970). This project used a detached caseworker model for providing behavioral consultation and community resource development. Descriptions of several cases in the report indicate that the youth who participated in this project were likely to stay out of trouble and improve their school performance.

A related strategy was outlined by Alvord (1971) who emphasized the importance of involving parents in the change procedure. Twenty-eight families of incorrigible children were trained in the operation of contingency management systems. Considerable attention was paid in the training sessions to the use of contracting procedures and the importance of reciprocity. On post-assessment questionnaires, 24 of the 28 families indicated that they considered the interventions a success.

Davidson and Robinson (1975) reported the development of a daytime program for hard-core delinquent males as an alternative to state training school commitment. The program consisted of half-day work projects in the local community and half-day intensive educational sessions in a neighborhood center. The entire program included various individual and group contingencies for work-task completion and academic achievement gains. Using a modified, multiple baseline design, one specific study carried out within the half-day classroom demonstrated the dependence of the high rates of desired behavior on the contingency system. The program also included behaviorally oriented group sessions twice a week for the purpose of having the youth make decisions about desired changes in the contingency system, discuss their progress in the program, discuss their advancement through the three hierarchical program levels, and make plans for graduation. Pre- to post-standard achievement testing indicated significant improvement in the academic levels of the youth in the project. Further, 18-month follow-up of the first 125 youth in the program indicated a dramatic reduction in their delinquent activities.

Control-group designs. One of the first programs to use behavioral procedures with delinquent youth was carried out in a street corner project (Schwitzgebel, 1964; Schwitzgebel & Kolb, 1964). The project consisted of hiring youth, recruited from local pool halls, clubs, hang-outs, etc., to tell their stories into tape recorders. In order to participate, the youth had to provide proof of previous official delinquent status. Twenty male delinquents, averaging 17 years of age and eight previous arrests, served as experimental subjects. For purposes of follow-up, they were matched with 20 control youth on demographic characteristics and previous offenses. Those youth who were hired to participate in the interviews were gradually shaped into prompt attendance and talking about positive life events. The contingencies in this project consisted of monetary wages, food, and other individualized privileges. One part of the investigation demonstrated that prompt attendance and interview content improved over the course of the year. Follow-up checks of justice system records indicated that at 1-, 2-, and 3-year intervals, the experimental youth were arrested significantly less and had spent significantly less time incarcerated. The methodology and procedures developed in this pioneering study provided the basis for replication and expansion in subsequent work (Schwitzgebel, 1967, 1969).

In one of the few comparative investigations in this area, Alexander and Parsons (1973) examined the relative effectiveness of short-term family-based behavioral intervention, client-centered group therapy, psychodynamic group therapy, and a control condition. Forty-six families who had been referred to the project from the juvenile court were randomly assigned to the behavioral intervention. The intervention sessions were aimed at the negotiation of interpersonal contracts, systematic feedback, and instruction from the therapists concerning the patterns of family communication, studying family training manuals, and setting up home-based token economies. Nineteen families were assigned to the client-centered group therapy sessions. Eleven families were assigned to a church-sponsored family group, and an additional 10 families were released from the court with no additional formal contact. A 20-minute test-discussion session was set up to assess the specific effects of the interventions on the interaction patterns. The test sessions consisted of having each family discuss the changes that they wanted in each other's behavior. Systematic observations of the discussion sessions indicated that families who had received the behavioral interventions were significantly more balanced in their discussion, talked significantly more during the 20-minute discussions, and interrupted each other for clarification significantly more often. This study also examined the relationships between the family interaction patterns and subsequent recidivism, which was assessed in 6- to 18-month follow-up assessment. It was demonstrated that the interaction patterns demonstrated by the behavioral group were highly predictive of lack of further delinquency. When the recidivism rates were analyzed directly, the behavioral group showed only a 26% recidivism rate while the other three groups recidivated approximately 50% of the time. The difference was highly significant. When further criminal offenses were examined, there was no significant difference between the groups.

A recent examination of a diversion project is reported by Davidson, Rappaport, Seidman, Berck, and Herring (1975). In this project, adolescent delinquents were assigned to the diversion project by the juvenile divisions of two metropolitan police departments in lieu of juvenile court processing. Following pre-assessment, the youth were randomly assigned to a college student interventionist or a control condition. The experimental intervention in this project consisted of a conglomerate behavioral approach including family contracting, contracting with school teachers, recreational activities, job recruitment, and parent training. One-year follow-up of both groups indicated a highly significant difference favoring the experimental group in terms of further offenses, the seriousness of those offenses, and further referral to the juvenile court.

The applications of behavioral principles in nonresidential community settings have also met with considerable success. The techniques have demonstrated the ability to produce specific behavioral changes *and* positive outcome results. Each program described in this section included both the specific application of behavioral procedures and the creation of alternatives to traditional juvenile justice system handling.

Critical Issues and a Systems Perspective

The results of the research and program descriptions presented in the preceding section reflect an array of innovative programs. The research to date has indicated a pattern of positive results in terms of improvements in specific targeted behaviors. Additionally, these positive results have shown some generalization to socially defined criteria such as recidivism, particularly when the interventions were accomplished in community settings. In order to highlight areas for further innovation in both program design and research methodology, this area of work needs to be scrutinized according to several additional criteria. This section will examine the methodological adequacy of the research to date and needed future empirical directions, the theoretical adequacy of the behavioral explanation of delinquency and the resultant intervention programs, and the ethical and political issues involved in future work in the juvenile justice system.

Methodological Evaluations.

An initial set of questions which must be raised about this area of intervention and research surround the issues of the credibility of the results. In short, how sound are the grounds for belief in the effectiveness of behavior modification procedures with delinquent populations. Another way of approaching these issues is to ask to what extent alternative explanations have been ruled out. Table 3-1 provides a summary of the research issues to be addressed and denotes whether or not each study provides the relevant control.

Attribution to effect to procedures under investigation. The first concern which must be addressed is whether or not the observed changes in the behavior of the delinquent youth would have occurred without the specific procedures used. Potential confounding of experimental effects is always a central concern when examining the efficacy of interventions with human populations. However, these concerns are magnified when adolescent youth are under study. They are at a developmental and social era when maturation, social role alteration, etc. also produce dramatic behavioral changes. Some authors have gone as far as to suggest that the most therapeutic intervention for delinquents would be to leave them alone (Schur, 1973). In general, two strategies are suggested to control for such confounding. The group-design tradition (Underwood, 1957) suggests that random assignment of individuals to the experimental condition and a concomitant control condition is called for. The single-subject design or functional analysis tradition (Sidman, 1960) proposes the use of reversal conditions or multiple baseline designs. In the studies and programs reviewed in the preceding section only 26% included an equivalent no-treatment control group, while only 28% of the investigations reported reversal data. These figures

TABLE 3-1

Research Issues in Behavioral Approaches to Delinquent Youth

Author	N	Target Behavior	Control Group (Randomized)	Baseline	Reversal	Systematic Variation of Treatment	Multiple Measures	Unbiased Data Collector	Follow-Up
			Institutional Programs						
Staats & Butterfield, 1965	1	Programmed instruction	No	Yes	No	No	Yes	No	No
Tyler, 1967	1	Grades	No	No	No	No	No	No	No
Burchard & Tyler, 1965	1	Disruptive behavior	No	No	No	No	No	No	No
Wetzel, 1966	1	Stealing	No	No	No	No	No	No	Yes
Brown & Tyler, 1968	1	Intimidation	No	No	No	No	No	No	No
Fineman, 1968	20	Rule compliance	No	No	No	No	No	No	No
Rice, 1970	10	Rule compliance	No	No	No	No	No	No	No
Buchard & Barrera, 1972	11	Aggressive behavior	No	Yes	No	Yes	No	No	No
Fodor, 1972	8	Runaway	No	Yes	No	No	No	No	No
Tyler & Brown, 1968	15	Answers to news quiz	Yes	No	—	Yes	No	No	No

Study	N	Behavior							
Meichenbaum et al., 1968	10	Appropriate class behavior	No	Yes	No	Yes	No	Yes	No
Bednar et al., 1970	32	Academic achievement	Yes	No	—	No	Yes	No	No
Coleman, 1974	19	Academic achievement	Yes	Yes	—	Yes	Yes	Yes	No
Pavlott, 1971	60	Self-care	Yes	No	—	No	No	No	No
Krueger, 1971	18	Positive comments	Yes	No	No	Yes	No	No	No
Cohen & Filipczak, 1971	41	Academic achievement	No	Yes	No	No	Yes	No	Yes
Sloan & Ralph, 1973	?	Social and educational	No	No	No	No	No	No	Yes
Jesness, 1974	904	Social and educational	Yes	Yes	—	Yes	Yes	No	Yes
Tyler & Brown, 1967	15	Rule violation	—	No	Yes	No	Yes	No	No
Burchard, 1967	12	Sitting in seat	—	No	Yes	No	No	No	No
Horton, 1970	6	Aggressive	—	Yes	Yes	No	No	No	No
Jesness & DeRisi, 1973	15	Classroom behavior	—	Yes	Yes	No	No	No	No

Table 3 (Continued)

Author	N	Target Behavior	Control Group (Randomized)	Baseline	Reversal	Systematic Variation of Treatment	Multiple Measures	Unbiased Data Collector	Follow-Up
Community-Based Residential Programs									
Phillips, 1968	3	Aggressive statements	—	Yes	Yes	Yes	No	No	No
Bailey et al., 1970	5	Daily teacher ratings	—	Yes	Yes	Yes	No	No	No
Phillips et al., 1971	4	Promptness	—	Yes	Yes	Yes	No	No	No
Fixsen et al., 1972	8	Accurate observation	—	Yes	Yes	Yes	No	No	No
Kirigin et al., 1974	26	Institutionalization	No	Yes	No	No	No	No	Yes
Davidson & Wolfred, in press	86	Social and educational	No	Yes	No	Yes	Yes	No	Yes
Community-Based Nonresidential Programs									
Stuart, 1971	1	Curfew, chores, runaway	No	Yes	No	No	No	No	No
Tharp & Wetzel, 1969	89	Desired performances	No	Yes	No	No	Yes	No	Yes
Rose, et al., 1970	?	Desired performances	No	No	No	No	No	No	No

Study	N	Measure							
Alvord, 1971	28	Child management	No	No	No	No	No	No	No
Davidson & Robinson, 1975	125	Educational and work performances	No	Yes	Yes	Yes	No	No	Yes
Schwitzgebel, 1964	20	Recidivism	No	Yes	No	No	Yes	No	Yes
Schwitzgebel & Kolb, 1964	20	Interview attendance	No	Yes	—	No	Yes	No	Yes
Schwitzgebel, 1967	48	Interview content	No	Yes	—	Yes	Yes	No	No
Schwitzgebel, 1969	18	Interview attendance	No	Yes	No	Yes	No	No	No
Alexander & Parsons, 1973	86	Family interaction	Yes	No	—	Yes	Yes	No	Yes
Davidson, et al., 1975	36	Recidivism	Yes	Yes	—	No	Yes	Yes	Yes
Percentage of Studies Controlling for Each Specific Issue			8/31	23/39	9/32	15/39	13/39	3/39	12/39
			26%	59%	28%	38%	33%	8%	31%

have the impact of considerably restricting the confidence which can be placed in the positive results reported.

Credibility of the assessments of observed changes. The second concern which must be assessed encapsulates two specific research problems. Within the Sidman (1960) single-subject paradigm, a critical tactic for the demonstration of behavioral control is the notion of stable states of behavior. In short, if inference is going to be made from the changes in behavioral rates, the initial rate has to demonstrate sufficient stability to make accurate interpretations of the changes observed. The establishment of a stable rate during baseline conditions is a necessary condition for initiating the particular procedure or manipulation under investigation. Similarly, the rate resulting from the manipulation must demonstrate sufficient stability before the reversal condition can be initiated. The question of stable state occurrence is not difficult in the abstract or absolute sense. However, difficulties arise when highly variable human performances are under study. This is particularly true when infrequent actions are being examined. Short of the criteria of the highly subjective "inter-occular t-test," adequate interpretations of observed changes in "rates of appropriate behavior" are difficult. None of the studies reviewed in the above section include such basic checks of the stability of behavior rates as the analysis of variance and time series analyses models suggested recently by several authors (Gentile, Roden, & Klein, 1972; Gottman, 1973). These procedures will not make interpretations any more clear-cut in an absolute sense. They will provide a beginning estimate of the stability of effects over time and the concomitant rate variability during baseline, manipulation, and reversal conditions.

A related component of this issue addresses more general assessment and research design issues. When single-performance criteria or standardized assessment devices are given as pre- and post-measures in combination with a single-group design, practice and regression artifacts become viable alternative explanations for observed changes. These concerns are particularly salient when the levels of performance are at the extreme ends of the natural distribution, as is often the case with adolescent delinquents. Although 59% of the studies reported pre- or baseline data, few ruled out the inherent effects of multiple assessment prior to the initiation of the intervention. Of those which presented only a single pre-assessment measure with a single-group design, all are open to the regression or practice counterargument. Future research must include safeguards against such confounding. Also at issue here is the potential for interaction between the assessment instruments and the intervention procedures. Often it is clear to subjects in experimental conditions what changes are desired by the experimenter or the program director (Lana, 1969). The same may not be true for control subjects or to the experimental youth during reversal phases. To what extent such factors affect observed changes must be examined by further work in the field.

Important components of the intervention. A third methodological issue is concerned with the relative potency of the components of the intervention procedures or program. In most of the studies reviewed, the procedure investigated actually involved a composite of contingencies, instructions, additional community resources, etc. These concerns are critical for maximum routinization of procedures, replicating experimental effects, and removing unnecessary components from innovative programs. In the work reviewed, 62% of the studies included no such manipulation.

Convergence of observed results. When focusing on a social problem with the complexity of juvenile delinquency, credibility is added to the observed results when multiple methods of measurement are used. Less credibility exists when the results are dependent on the behavior rates observed by a single coder, on the behavior rates reflected by a single observation scheme, on the reports of the interventionist, on the attitudinal changes reflected by a single attitudinal measure, etc. No single assessment procedure, including behavioral observations, is inherently valid. Convergence with other methods must be demonstrated to enhance the credibility of the results reported. Although these issues have been most eloquently described in areas of more traditional intra-individual assessment (see, e.g., Campbell & Fiske, 1959), they are also of considerable importance when examining the efficacy of social intervention procedures. The complexity of the phenomena of delinquency dictates that assessment of effects be taken from the perspective of the youth, parents, significant others, independent observers, as well as the interventionist. It is then incumbent on the investigator to examine the covariation of the several measurement procedures. For example, the multi-trait, multi-method paradigm provides one scheme for beginning this undertaking. Even though 33% of the research in this area included the collection of data from multiple perspectives and the data generally exhibited general agreement within groups across measures, it is necessary to examine the extent to which the multiple methods covary across individuals both within and between targeted variables.

Unbiased collection of data. A fifth issue concerning methodological adequacy has to do with the potential effects of the experimenter's expectations of the data collected and the artifactual performance of the participants (Rosenthal & Rosnow, 1969). Given that only three of the studies reviewed here included purposefully naive observers and data collectors, that many took place in applied correctional settings at a time when positive evaluation of the procedures was crucial to their acceptance, and that contemporary publication practices are biased toward positive results, an additional note of caution must be added to the positive pattern of results reported.

Durability of effects. In an area such as delinquency intervention, it is important to examine not only the immediate impact of the behavioral procedures but the durability and generalizability of the effects in follow-up situations. For behavioral interventions particularly, there is an inherent dilemma in these concerns. On the one hand, if there is a functional relationship between the environmental manipulations which were part of the intervention and the positive behavior changes, it would be anticipated that improvements would terminate at the same time the interventions conclude. This is particularly true if the intervention did not involve programming of the follow-up situation. The behavioral movement does not posit the existence or importance of traditional intra-individual therapeutic changes and is therefore unable to rely on such assumptions for expectations of therapeutic durability. It could also be argued that durable effects are not the focus of strict research efforts aimed at demonstrating the operation of behavioral procedures with delinquent groups. Yet, if the intervention is initiated under the guise of mandatory or court-ordered treatment or rehabilitation, the responsibility to assess and insure carryover to the follow-up situation is critical. In addition, the professional and scientific role advocated by this book argues for both social responsibility and action. The fact that only 31% of the studies reviewed here report follow-up data is far less than desirable.

Systematic monitoring of intervention processes. Without exception, the programs and procedures reviewed in the preceding section consisted of a complex intervention program or took place in the context of a complex social program. Inferences about their effectiveness would be very difficult even if the above-mentioned methodological shortcomings did not exist. The issue here is that no data are presented relevant to the independent variables operating to produce the effects observed; the relationship of the effects to other events in the lives of the youth, the initial characteristics of the youth, or the characteristics of the interventionist; or the relationship of the sequences of events within the intervention project or procedures. It seems imperative that the behavioral movement keep in mind its beginnings with heavy emphasis on systematic investigation, serendipitous findings, open investigations, and specificity. Unfortunately, the pseudo-control of laboratory methods transferred to field research settings cannot be realized. Conceptual narrowness, monolithic approaches to assessment, and assumptions about control over independent variables have precluded the field from adding to the understanding of the functional relationships between the behavior of delinquent youth, the social environment, the juvenile justice system, and resultant outcomes. Future research must assume this perspective in its approaches to data collection and project implementation.

Although the review of the research and programs using behavioral techniques with delinquent youth have indicated the success of the approach, careful scrutiny of the research methods employed has indicated that there is considerable work remaining to be done. This conclusion should not indicate unrealistic pessimism about the field, for a similar scrutiny of most therapeutic and social interventions would have an identical outcome. It would also appear that if progress is to be achieved, considerable "opening" of the research process will have to be undertaken.

Theoretical and Conceptual Adequacy.

It is obvious that the methods and procedures of behavior modification have had considerable impact on the practices of the juvenile justice system. Although recently the intensity of the behavior mod movement has waned slightly (London, 1972), the break it represents with past correctional practices is of landmark proportions. It clearly represented a paradigm shift at a time when existing paradigms were being strained. This section will argue that since that initial breakthrough, the field has returned to science and practice as usual.

Initial conception. In its early phase of involvement, the behavior modification movement and its participant practitioners and researchers operated in almost total isolation in a few institutional settings. Their conception of delinquency was little different than their operant conception of all human behavior—namely, delinquency was a result of environmental contingencies which had systematically reinforced illegal behavior and failed to reinforce socially appropriate behavior. The recommended course of action was the rearrangement of the environmental contingencies to produce behavior patterns more like those exhibited by nondelinquent groups. These propositions were extensions of information and data from the experimental laboratories and, as we have seen, the early work in this area was concerned solely with direct replication of learning experiments with delinquent youth as subjects. Having demonstrated that when delinquent youth received reinforcement for some desired action they were more likely to perform that act, the behavioral group made a "conceptual leap of faith." Stuart (1971) delineated the behavioral position concerning the etiology of delinquency that included the following three propositions: first, the parents of delinquent youth disproportionately displayed and reinforced anti-social actions and failed to reinforce pro-social actions; second, the peers of delinquent youth disproportionately displayed and reinforced delinquent activities and under-reinforced pro-social activities; and third, the teachers of delinquent youth disproportionately reinforced the undesirable actions of the youth and failed to reinforce the desirable actions. At least one of these propositions was empirically examined in two studies. Stuart (1971) and Alexander and Parsons (1973) used criterion group designs to compare groups of delinquents and nondelinquents and groups of recidivists and nonrecidivists, respectively. Both studies demonstrated the disproportionate amount of negative interactions displayed between delinquent youth and their parents. From this work and the earlier demonstrations of the responsiveness of delinquent youth to positive contingencies in institutional settings, the movement expanded considerably.

Conceptual closure and implications for intervention strategies. Following the success of early efforts in the field, it would appear that considerably less attention was paid to conceptual and technical expansion. While the settings in which the techniques were applied were expanded to some extent, programs using behavioral approaches were introduced relatively late in the juvenile justice system. In other words, most remained in institutional settings or, as in the case of Achievement Place, provided an alternative to institutional placement for adjudicated youth. This and other factors have contributed to what could be viewed as conceptual backsliding. The environmentalist position could at this point have been extended into preventive efforts earlier in the justice system or into programs for social change involving marginal youth likely to be apprehended. However, the environmentalist position was gradually transferred into the intra-individual learning-history explanation of delinquent youth. Delinquents began being described in introductions to journal articles and program reports as individuals with "learning deficits" and "behavioral excesses." They had "deficits" in their histories of pro-social behaviors and possessed excess anti-social repertoires. Further attention was paid to technical sophistication and innovation for the purpose of building pro-social repertoires and eradicating or replacing anti-social performances. This position was most explicitly stated by Braukman et al. (1975): "The educational model suggests that the deviant youth has a behavioral deficiency in that he has not learned socially appropriate behaviors that will allow him to successfully interact with others in an appropriate way" (p. 6). An extreme statement of this position is contained in a report of the necessity for implementing a behavior modification program in a private institution as it began to take delinquent youth. This program had traditionally serviced orphans and neglected youth. The delinquent youth were described as "children from families with long histories of maladjustment, from abusing and incestuous families, from drug usage, years of school failure, with learning disabilities, and perhaps with constitutionally difficult personalities" (Meyer, Odom, & Wax, 1973). Just how close the behaviorists concerned with delinquent youth have come to a "learning-lingo medical model" is difficult to discern. However, many of the negative side effects of the medical model which had been so adamantly opposed by behaviorists' initial work with delinquent youth have again come to the fore. The apparent result has been an increased focus on refinement of existing techniques in situations to which the behaviorists had already gained access. The danger is that negative expectations, subprofessionalization, and business as usual will now be promoted by the behavioral movement.

These developments have contributed in many ways to technical, methodological, and theoretical stagnation. The literature reviewed earlier reveals the conceptual status of behavioral explanations of delinquency to be highly questionable. As indicated in the methodological evaluation, the research cannot be viewed as confirmatory of the original propositions of the behavioral explanation of delinquency due to methodological shortcomings. In addition, the work to this point has not been exploratory in any real sense. Investigators in the area have been lured into ideologically based inattention to multiple methods of measurement and omission of critically important variables. Most important has been the acceptance of unwarranted assumptions about the operation of functional relationships between the social environment and the youth in the justice system. All too often the variables to be examined have been selected before the fact while others have been left out. The result of these developments has been a reduction in innovation and the institutionalization of behavioral procedures for delinquent youth.

The current conceptual strain. It is apparent that the current developments in this area should be exerting considerable conceptual strain on the behavioral movement in the juvenile justice system. The effects observed in the review section indicate a differential effectiveness between the institutionally based programs which demonstrated little if any positive outcomes in follow-up, the community-based residential programs which showed considerably more positive outcomes in follow-up, and the community-based nonresidential programs which showed exclusively positive outcomes in follow-up. It would seem plausible that other processes are operating here than just the particular manipulation of contingencies described as the intervention. Unfortunately, the proposed operation of other variables in affecting delinquent youth must be left as conjecture at this point given the lack of relevant data within the area. The field is also experiencing considerable ambiguity about how it will respond to this strain. That ambiguity exists is reflected in the recent article by Reppucci and Saunders (1974) in their description of attempts to introduce a behavioral program in an institution for delinquent youth. They suggest very clearly that organizational factors and processes can play an important role. However, they appear to be suggesting that such variables are conditions which the good behaviorist will have to learn to put up with and work around so that he or she can get down to the business of instituting the necessary contingency management system. The choice appears clear. The conceptions of delinquency can be reopened by those working on behavioral approaches to delinquent youth, or the behavioral conception can consummate closure and the field will have to await another impetus for theoretical and practical innovation.

Several serious issues concerning the conceptual and theoretical adequacy of the behavioral position in this area have been raised. It appears that early innovation and the struggle for acceptance and the successes it brought have placed the movement in danger of stagnation.

Ethical and Political Issues.

Behavior modification with delinquent populations involves major ethical and political entanglements. The events of the last 5 years in the public and legal arenas have given considerable political overtones to any attempts at changing and studying human behavior. The cessation of funds for behavior modification programs by the Law Enforcement Assistance Administration, increasingly stringent Department of Health, Education, and Welfare requirements for safeguards in research with human subjects, and increasing advocacy of the rights of juveniles (Silbert & Sussman, 1975) have all contributed heavily to this situation. Ironically, the assumed right of the state to formally punish those convicted of crimes has not come under similar scrutiny. The right to treatment, right to be different, and right to be left alone are currently meeting in an unparalleled clash. It is imperative to first understand how behavior modification efforts with delinquents came under attack for overlooking and ultimately violating ethical standards and supporting the status quo. The concluding section will outline the steps which must be taken in dealings with juveniles to guarantee their rights while continuing innovation.

Professional and scientific oversights. Much of the early work involving behavior modification with delinquent youth, intentionally or otherwise, had the effect of making behavior modifiers appear to be concerned with retraining wayward youth to the norm, being unconcerned with their future well-being, and siding with "establishment-oriented" forces in the juvenile justice system. Rehabilitation meant increasing pro-social behavior and removing or decreasing anti-social behavior. (Lest the reader think that stones are being thrown at a glass house from the outside, this sentence is nearly a direct quote from a report written by the fourth author in 1970.) Further, the most visible efforts were accomplished in highly removed juvenile correctional institutions. In the middle to late 1960s and early 1970s, the predominant position of behavior modifiers was that they were politically neutral scientists interested in demonstrating the empirical validity of their principles and procedures. The position of those in the movement at the time was that they recognized the potential political use of their techniques, but that such concerns were both outside their professional domain and professional responsibility. Some even went so far as to suggest that we should use behavioral techniques in intense doses to completely retrain, reshape, and "brainwash" convicted criminals, or, further, that "we should reshape our society so that we all would be trained from birth to do what society wants us to do" (McConnell, 1970).

An additional factor was the laboratory-based history of the behavior modification movement. Environmental control became the synonym for experimental excellence. Hence, the behavior modifiers who entered the field of juvenile delinquency searched for situations where they would have control. They entered the field laboratory of the juvenile correctional institution by siding with the institution's administration, thereby gaining access to experimental subjects and settings.

The controversy became not so much what techniques were being used but how they were being administered and, more importantly, for what purposes. At some abstract level, the programming of increments in pro-social behavior and educational achievement seemed like universally acceptable goals for the use of behavioral procedures. Token economy programs, contracting procedures, timeout rooms, and staff training sessions were all instituted toward those ends. Yet, the question is "toward what ends?" Who was to decide what constituted pro-social behavior or academic achievement? It appeared that this new technology might be used for the more effective and efficient attainment of old ends. The staff had less trouble with institutionalized delinquent youth under the token economy system than under the nonprogram which existed previously. An additional tool for control had been added to the armamentarium of staff who made up a generally damaging juvenile justice system. Holland (1974) recently outlined these concerns in rather succinct fashion: "Simply put, today's token economies support established power structures" (p. 10). Another related issue was the apparent monolithic focus of most residential behavior modification programs for delinquents. It appeared that the techniques were being used for shaping all adjudicated youth in the direction of passive attention to programmed materials, coming to the evening meal on time, and serving their sentences more appropriately. Again, Holland (1974) captures this issue in one of the beatitudes according to T. Economy: "Blessed are the meek for they shall be promoted to level two" (p. 8).

Part of the attack may have been due to the form of the reports of most behavior modification work with delinquent groups. In many research reports there was seldom sufficient detail to discern to what extent there was voluntary agreement by the youth for participation in the study, selection of the target behaviors and desired rates, etc. In most cases participative democracy procedures did not appear to be part of the programs. A second contributing factor to the problems was the delay by the behavior modifiers in responding to the queries. They held to the scientific-neutrality position for considerable time. A third factor was the conceptual closure which had taken place in the field by the time the attacks were in full swing. Earlier concern with potent institutional, social, and organizational factors which contributed to the phenomena of delinquency would have put the behavior modifiers in a better position to respond professionally as well as scientifically. The issues which must be addressed go well beyond the ethical treatment of human subjects in scientific experimentation. Attention to the systemic and political factors which lead to official delinquency must determine future strategy.

Future directions and ethical-political options. It is necessary for the behavior modification movement to consider some new directions in its work with delinquent populations. These new directions must stem from two basic assumptions about the work which needs to be done. First, as practitioners and scientists we should take on the position of advocates for youth. This is necessary both as a basic value position and a practical policy in order to balance the scales a small step toward equality in the power position of adjudicated and pre-delinquent youth. Second, as practitioners and scientists, we should take on a systemic view of the issues related to delinquency: the designs of interventions, the analysis of outcomes, and the dissemination of results for use in future social policy decisions.

The final form of the ethical and political safeguards necessary for all future interventions and investigations involving delinquent youth must await the formation of ethical codes by the field. Preliminary suggestions have been offered by Braun (1975) and should prompt further professional activity and debate. It seems imperative that the field engage in self-regulation before further outside legislating takes place (Halleck, 1974). The remainder of this section will detail the apparent choice points in the intervention-research process and the preferred safeguards and options available at each. This section draws heavily on input from the writing of Stuart (1974) and Davison and Stuart (1975).

1. *Selection of therapeutic or program goals.* Each intervention or empirical investigation, explicitly or implicitly, begins with the selection of goals to be accomplished. These may involve both the behaviors to be changed as well as the ultimate behavioral pattern to be established. The options at this point involve those ranging from selection by the investigator, joint selection by the investigator and an administrator or staff member from the juvenile justice system, to solitary selection by the participant in the project (e.g., youth). It seems desirable at this point that program decisions involve all concerned parties as well as an outside person or group in the form of a review board. This procedure also has the benefit of providing the investigator access to information about the workings of the system and the participants' perspective from the very beginning.

2. *Selection of intervention method and entry point.* The next step has been the focus of much of the recent debate. Table 3-2 outlines the potential options and likely level of political and ethical ramifications. This table highlights the conditions under which the interventionist and researcher must directly confront ethical issues. It can be seen that within the framework presented here, whenever someone other than the program participants selects the intervention goals, the need for ethical safeguards is high. Also the use of aversive procedures generally indicates the need for intense concern. The use of positive approaches to behavior change in the situation where the youth participate in goal selection reduces, but never eliminates, the need for stringent safeguards. Again, the openness of a democratic group which includes participants is the recommended course of action. The overriding concern is that as the potential seriousness of

TABLE 3-2

Level of Ethical Implications and Intervention Strategy

	Type of Intervention				
	Aversive		Positive		
Level of Intervention	Others Select Goals	Youth Selects Goal	Others Select Goals	Youth Selects Goals	
Institutional	High	High	High	Moderate	
Community-based residential	High	Moderate	High	Low	
Open community	High	Moderate	High	Low	

the ethical problems increases, the power of the participants in influencing the decision to implement must be increased to veto power in the "high" conditions.

3. *Research design and assessment procedures.* At the decision point of selecting a research design, there is also a range of options for protecting the interests of the various people involved in an innovative research effort. Decisions concerning the use of random assignment, control groups, reversal conditions, etc. are of considerable concern in terms of human rights as well as interpretability of the results. Outside review is essential, with the investigator being given the most influence concerning this particular point. The denial of service to controls is not an issue in the juvenile justice system which currently provides most participants with little treatment. However, the next step, enlisting participant agreement, must include an explanation to each subject of the research design as part of the voluntary agreement.

4. *Subject participation.* The range of options at this point includes physically forced participation, aversively manipulated participation, seduced participation, and completely voluntary participation. Without getting into the philosophical debate of determinism versus free will, it would appear that the realistic ideal which must be sought in investigations with identified delinquent youth is seduced participation with all the formal safeguards of voluntary participation. This step should involve a complete disclosure of the procedures, design, and measures to the youth and his or her verbal and written consent to participate. Obviously, the youth has veto power at this juncture.

Reporting of outcome. Traditionally, scientific investigation has ended with the publication of a scholarly work in a professional journal. Responsibility for dissemination or preparation of results in an understandable format has not often been part of the scientific enterprise. In addition to the urgency of having subjects participate in the research process fully, current ineffectiveness of the juvenile justice system demands that new avenues be explored for the dissemination of results to consumer groups and policy making bodies. Further, it is incumbent on the applied social scientist to take an active role in seeing that empirically sound innovations are diffused and that efforts are undertaken to influence the quality of disseminated programs and procedures. Innovative work highlighting the importance of such concerns has recently been reported by Fairweather et al. (1974) and by Braukman et al. (1975).

This section has been particularly stringent in its call for change in the process of undertaking behavioral innovations and research in the juvenile justice system. However, the urgency of empirically based innovation in the juvenile justice system dictates that anything less is shortsighted. The position of youth cannot be compromised. Open discussion of assumptions, techniques, results, and ultimate goals will reopen the potential for innovation.

Chapter 4
ADULT CORRECTIONS

Crime is a social problem of compelling magnitude. Since the 1920s, virtually every indicator of adult crime has increased to the point where lawlessness has been proclaimed as one of our most serious domestic ills (Harris, 1968). Approximately six million nontraffic crimes are reported to the police each year; probably five to ten times this many have actually occurred. Over the past 11 years, the year-to-year increase in Federal Bureau of Investigation "index crimes"[1] has totaled 110%—see Fig. 4.1 (Federal Bureau of Investigation, *Federal Crime Reporting*, 1965-1975). While FBI crime statistics have been subjected to numerous criticisms (Morris & Hawkins, 1970; Waldo, 1971; Zeisel, 1973), they are the principal data by which the public monitors crime trends. Even though there may be no fully acceptable procedure for measuring the "true" extent of crime, both unobtrusive and official measures reflect consistent increases (Nettler, 1974).

The total cost of this increasing crime is not easily determined. The cost to the public must include the financing of justice system functions on the local, state, and federal level. In the late 1960s the cost of the collective services from these agencies was estimated at more than four billion dollars per year (President's Commission, 1967). Both the offender and the public are faced with the financial hardships of enforced unemployment (which itself has become a recent target of behavioral community psychology—see Chapter 10), and the resultant decrements in earning power following incarceration. Moreover, the victims of crime have been a neglected population. Recent development of victim compensation (Schafer, 1968) and restitution (Laster, 1970) programs has directed attention to the very real personal and economic adversities encountered by the victim of either property or violent crime.

As crime has increased, so have the institutions and the interventions intended to rehabilitate its perpetrators. Official figures place the number of adults in our more than 4,000 jails and prisons or on supervised release at over 1.3 million (Fox, 1973; President's Commission, 1967); approximately 2.5

---

[1]The seven FBI index crimes are murder, forcible rape, robbery, aggravated assault, burglary, theft, and motor vehicle theft.

98   BEHAVIORAL APPROACHES TO COMMUNITY PSYCHOLOGY

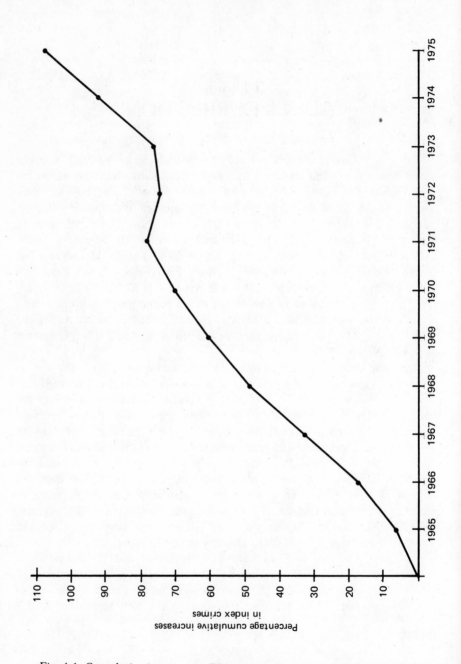

Fig. 4-1. Cumulative increases in FBI index crimes over the past 11 years

million offenders are processed through the correctional system in the course of a given year (President's Commission, 1967). Not included in this figure are the thousands of offenders in hospitals, short-term detention centers, clinics, and special treatment programs. The annual budget for corrections is over one billion dollars, the largest percentage of which is used to guard, feed, and clothe inmates (Morris & Hawkins, 1970). Torok (1971) has estimated that the cost of maintaining one inmate in a state correctional facility is approximately $6,000 for a single year.

The control of crime has become one of the critical political issues of the times. The last three Presidential elections have had a deliberate emphasis on the "law and order" theme. Recently, the Ford Administration proposed that "flat time" or mandatory minimum sentences be required for certain categories of offenders as a means of furthering "domestic tranquility." Federal legislative programs have proliferated: the Omnibus Crime Control and Safe Streets Act (1968), the Juvenile Delinquency Control Act (1968), the Law Enforcement and Assistance Act (1965), the Model Cities Program (1967), and several seemingly uncoordinated efforts from the Department of Labor, Federal Bureau of Prisons, and the Department of Health, Education, and Welfare provide a few examples. Proponents of numerous other pieces of social legislation have attempted to justify their programs on the basis of potential crime prevention and constraint.

One of the few phenomena which has kept pace with the burgeoning statistics of criminality is the plethora of unconfirmed (often unconfirmable) theories that attempt to explain proscribed behavior (Nettler, 1974; Shore, 1971). Property crime has been most prone to a rich variety of sociological explanations that includes class theory (W. Miller, 1958), anomie (Merton, 1957), differential association theory (Sutherland & Cressey, 1960), labeling or stigmatization hypotheses (Becker, 1963; Lemert, 1967), and opportunity-structure theory (Cloward & Ohlin, 1960). Biophysical explanations are most likely to be invoked when accounting for episodic or repetitive violence. Prominent on the roster of biophysical theories are chromosomal abnormalities (Amir & Berman, 1970; Jarvik, Klodin, & Matsuyama, 1973), genetic transmission (Rosenthal, 1973), and morphological features (Lombroso, 1911). An ample range of deviant conduct has received the attention of psychological interpretations such as conditioning (Eysenck, 1964), social-learning (Bandura, 1973; Shah, 1966), psychodynamics (Freud, 1933), stimulus seeking (Quay, 1965), and inadequate socialization (Bender, 1946). Unfortunately, the collective impact of this rich theoretical array on questions concerning criminal correction has been minimal. The practical implications that are suggested are often conflictual. The result is that the field of criminology is still awaiting a well-articulated, empirically supported theory that could direct correctional efforts (Peterson & Thomas, 1973).

Correctional outcome data are disconcertingly consistent. Present-day corrections do not correct, rehabilitate, or deter the adult offender. Baily

(1961), in a review of over 100 outcome studies, concluded that there was little evidence for rehabilitative efficacy and that the most rigorously designed investigations were the most likely to discover harmful or no effects for the evaluated correctional effort. Robison and Smith's judgment (1971) is equally direct: "While considerable evidence exists that some types of offenders have relatively more or less likelihood of recidivism than others, there is, as yet, almost no evidence that available correctional alternatives have any impact on these likelihoods" (p. 67). Similar assessments have been made by Hindelang (1970), Meehl (1970), Schwitzgebel (1974b), Shireman, Mann, Larsen, & Young (1972), Shuman (1973), the President's Commission (1967), and Clark (1970). The most optimistic of views is reflected by S. Adam's (1974) conclusion that "if one takes only controlled experimental designs in selected areas of corrections, at least half of the studies will show either statistically significant effects associated with treatment or benefit/cost ratios higher than unity" (p. 15). The recidivism rate for adult offenders is commonly placed at anywhere from a third (President's Commission, 1967), to 75%[2] (Clark, 1970). To compound matters, recidivist crimes tend to become increasingly more violent, deliberate, and felonious (President's Commission, 1967). Even if one were to assume a degree of treatment success, the cost-effectivensss of modern corrections is not at all apparent. It may be the case that the dual criteria of efficacy and economy would be satisfied best by "outmoded" alternatives such as punishment, restraint, banishment, and retribution (see Leeke and Clements, 1973, for a brief historical review of correctional objectives).

An impressive quality of behavior modification has been its success with problems characteristically known for their intractableness—for example, retardation (Gardner, 1971), chronic psychoses (Ullmann & Krasner, 1975), autism (Lovaas et al., 1973), and life-jeopardizing habits such as smoking (Bernstein, 1969). In this regard, the recent but increasing application of behavioral principles to criminal conduct is understandable. Few categories of behavior appear as refractory to alteration as does criminal comportment. The introduction of behavior modification to the domain of offender correction was promoted by the expectation that it could provide a viable, ameliorative technology with a determinable impact on unlawful conduct. A review of the

---

[2]Glaser (1964) has argued that the "legend" of the two-third's recidivism rate is the result of methodological confusion. The fact that two-thirds of the inmates in a prison may have been in prison before is not equivalent to the conclusion that prison has approximately a 70% failure rate. Morris and Hawkins (1970) observe that, "one of the principal conclusions of Glaser's study is that 'in the first two to five years after their release, only about a third of the men released from an entire prison system are returned to prison.' In view of the fact that many studies have shown that a three-year follow-up provides about 90 percent of the probable future returns to prison, Glaser's finding suggests that it is unwise to dismiss prisons as complete failures" (p. 117).

extent to which this promise has been fulfilled will be the goal of the present chapter.

Since the early to mid-1960s, there have been approximately 30 descriptions of behaviorally oriented interventions with adult offenders. The review of these reports will be organized according to the correctional setting in which they have occurred.

Institutional Programs

While behavior modification procedures for identified criminals have been applied in a diversity of settings, they have most frequently been conducted in penal institutions. For the most part, the target behaviors of these applications have been components of a larger, extant rehabilitory effort. Typical of such programs have been those aimed at increasing inmate participation in educational or vocational training.

McKee (1964) and his associates (Clements & McKee, 1968) have used programmed instruction for several years at the Draper Correctional Center in Alabama. While programmed materials offer advantages over traditional educational modes, they have not proven successful in sustaining learning in inmate populations. In an effort to increase the learning productivity of 16 inmates, Clements and McKee (1968) employed a combination of performance contracts and contingency management procedures. Following a 3-week baseline during which subjects completed programmed materials at their own pace, a 4-week "experimenter management" phase was introduced. For each week during this period, the experimenter assigned an amount of work which was approximately 20% greater than the average for the immediately previous week. Successful completion of the specified materials was followed by short reinforcement periods (15 minutes) that allowed the subject to choose preferred activities from a "reinforcement menu." In the final phase of the study inmates themselves specified the amount of materials to be completed. The one restriction was that output had to be at least as great as the baseline average. The same reinforcement schedule was in effect as during Phase 2.

The results indicated that educational output during the two contingency periods was significantly greater than the baseline level. The experimenter and self-management phases did not differ significantly in output. Level of performance during the last week of the "experimenter management" phase was maintained for both weeks of Phase 3. These changes were accompanied by greater work efficiency and improvements on periodic achievement tests.

The absence of a reversal-to-baseline condition in this study makes it difficult to attribute unambiguously the effects to the procedures during the second and third phases. In addition, the design confounds the effects of the performance contracts with those of the contingency procedure.

In an effort to increase participation in educational programs, Milan (1972) examined the influences of a "license" procedure in which inmates could exchange tokens for back-up reinforcers only if they possessed an exchange license. While the tokens were earned by successful participation in a broad-scale token economy, licenses could be obtained only by completing specified amounts of educational material. The effect of the license procedure was substantial. During the token only phase, 17.4% of the inmates were involved in the program for an average of 37.3 minutes per day. Participation during the license phase increased to 41.9% of the inmates devoting an average of 161.8 minutes per day to the program. Milan and McKee (1974) report other variations on the basic model such as the use of "regular performance" charts and financial payment for educational achievement.

Contingency-managed programmed instruction has yielded some impressive outcomes. Reviewing the Draper project, Milan, Wood, Williams, Rogers, Hampton, and McKee (1974) report that "offenders enrolled in the projects averaged gains of 1.4 grades per 208 hours of programmed instruction. High school equivalencies were earned by 95% of those who qualified for and took the GED, and nine former students entered college after leaving prison" (p. 11). It is not possible to determine how those figures compare to the performance of nonprogram inmates, because such data have not appeared in published form.

Bassett, Blanchard, Harrison, and Wood (1973) report a program at an adult prison farm in which expanded access to phone privileges was made contingent on attendance at a remedial educational center. The results indicated that during a 17-day contingency period, man-hours utilization of the educational center was almost tripled over baseline levels. Reinstatement of baseline conditions resulted in a return to baseline use levels. The man-hour increase associated with the contingency period was significantly related to grade-level improvement on a monthly achievement test. Methodologically, this study was an advance over the earlier work of Clements and McKee (1968), which found academic achievement to be substantially related to the introduction of a contingency program but did not include either a control group or an attempt to reverse behavior to baseline levels.

A second prevalent, behavioral target of correctional facilities is increasing compliance with institutional rules of conduct. Published reports of such programs are rare, possible because their implementations are quite uneven and unsystematized. Opton (1974) cites estimates that more than 20 states have some variant of a prison token economy in operation. As an example of these programs, one study (Von Holden, 1969; cited by Brodsky, 1973a) reported increasing inmate compliance with military prison rules via a contingency program that utilized a variety of reinforcers (e.g., snacks, release from segregation). Maintenance of these changes was evidenced at a 60-day follow-up. Four additional prison token economies are described in more detail in the following sections.

The Walter Reed Project

A special ward program for soldiers classified as "character or behavior disorders" was established at Walter Reed Hospital in 1967 (Boren & Colman, 1970; Colman & Baker, 1969; Colman & Boren, 1969). The program was intended for soldiers who had had a civilian history of minor arrests, been AWOL repeatedly, made suicidal gestures, and evidenced difficulty with adjustment requirements presented by military life. The program was not open to homosexuals, alcoholics, or drug addicts. Soldiers transferred to this unit for treatment were conceptualized as having behavioral deficiencies in educational, occupational, and social areas of functioning.

During its first year of operation, 48 men participated in the program. The mean age was 20 years; 83% of the men were white, the remainder were black; three-fourths were in a low socioeconomic class category; half had civilian police records. A token economy was instituted as the preferred method of behavior change. Points were provided for soldier performance in each of the following areas: military assignments, educational classes, work duty, and ward operation (e.g., meeting attendance, appropriate attire). Points could then be exchanged for the usual assortment of privileges—semi-private rooms, free coffee, passes, and access to recreational activities. Deliberate efforts were directed at individualization of the behavioral skills to be emphasized, and the men were to some degree responsible for their own treatment programming.

The program had two phases. During the initial 10 weeks, each man had to purchase all reinforcers with the token points. After 10 weeks of satisfactory performance, participants moved to Phase II, in which program rewards were contingent on positive weekly performance reviews. Phase II soldiers also were expected to take an active leadership role in the therapeutic management of new assignees to the ward. The duration of treatment was 16 weeks.

A comparison was made between 46 program participants who had been released for at least 3 months and 48 "control" subjects who had apparently received either general disciplinary or psychiatric attention. Of those men who had been in the token economy, 69.5% were functioning in a regular military unit ("successes") and 30.5% had received either an administrative discharge from duty or were AWOL ("failures"). In contrast, 71.7% of the control subjects were discharged from duty or in the stockade ("failures"), while 28.3% were regarded as "successes."

Methodologically, these limited data are difficult to evaluate. First, it is not clear from the published version of the program what constituted the standard treatments to which the control subjects were exposed. Also it is not clear that program and control subjects were similar on demographic characteristics, length of treatment, or interval between treatment and follow-up. While some components of the program were anlayzed with a reversal design (Boren & Colman, 1970), behavioral functioning in the four targeted areas was assessed neither at baseline nor following any reversal of program contingencies.

The Cellblock Token Economy

The major work of the Experimental Manpower Laboratory for Corrections at the Draper Correctional Center in Elmore, Alabama, is described by Milan and McKee (1974) and Milan et al. (1974). The Cellblock Token Economy, as this project is known, represents the most thoroughly researched behaviorally oriented prison program to date. Three representative Draper experiments are reviewed below (for additional examples, see Milan et al., 1974).

Experiment 1. The characteristic mode of inmate control is the punishment model in which prisoners either lose initially available resources and privileges contingent on "bad behavior" or receive direct disciplinary punishment (verbal harassment, isolation, etc.). The systematic and swift application of punishment is routinized in our prisons despite numerous suggestions of limited effectiveness and adverse side effects. The first study examined the effects of the usual institutional control procedures upon prisoner conduct.

The study took place in a 40-bed cellblock of the Draper Correctional Center. Impact of the punishment model was assessed by the following three measures: percentage of self-management skills performed (e.g., bed-making, area maintenance, personal appearance), percentage of voluntarily performed maintenance tasks completed (e.g., cell upkeep, mopping, cleaning), and behavioral incidents (e.g., fighting, property destruction, insubordination).

An A-B-A design was employed. Stage A (baseline) involved verbal instructions to perform the self-management and maintenance tasks, but no contingencies were applied for noncompliance. In Stage B ("officer corrects"), the correctional officer for the cellblock applied the usual methods of institutional control (e.g., isolation, loss of good time) to increase performance of self-management duties. Maintenance tasks were not targeted during this phase. Phase C involved reinstitution of the baseline procedures.

Median level of self-maintanance skills during baseline (32%) was almost doubled during the "officer corrects" conditions (62%), but slowly declined following introduction of the second baseline. Baseline levels of cell maintenance tasks (35%) were relatively unaffected by subsequent phases.

While the effects of punishment-based procedures did not generalize to nontargeted areas, they were quite effective with respect to the targeted behavior of self-maintenance. As expected, however, introduction of aversive control was coincidental with marked increase in behavioral incidents. The percentage of days during baseline 1 in which at least one behavioral incident occurred was only 11.8%, while incidents occurred on 47.8% of "officer corrects" days. Behavioral incidents were recorded on 28.6% of baseline -2 days (Milan & McKee, 1974). These data are consistent with laboratory evidence that aversive control provides immediate effects at the expense of increased undesirable side effects (Azrin & Holz, 1966).

Experiment 2. The first EMLC token economy examined the potential of an alternative management regime based on principles of positive reinforcement. The project was in operation only during inmates' off-work hours (approximately 7 hours per week day and 15 hours per holiday and weekend day) for a 420-day period. "The token economy focused primarily upon those aspects of inmate performance of concern to custodial personnel: arising at the appointed hour, making the bed, cleaning the general living area, and maintaining a presentable personal appearance. A secondary objective was to motivate participation and performance in a voluntary remedial education program in operation evenings and weekends" (Milan & McKee, 1974, pp. 32-33).

Token points were credited to inmate checking accounts and could be exchanged for a variety of incentives by simply writing a check for the desired item. Accounts were individualized and balanced daily. Observations of critical behaviors were recorded by a correctional officer. Independently acquired reliability checks by project staff revealed interrater reliabilities that typically exceeded .90.

The design of the study was complex, involving a sequence of 13 experimental manipulations in which differential levels of token points were presented contingently or noncontingently (see Milan et al., 1974, pp. 33-37). The results justify the conclusion that "Performance-contingent token reinforcement was shown to be considerably more effective in motivating the performance of routine chores of concern to the institution administration than either the social reinforcement conditions of the *baseline* phases or the coercive procedures of the *officer treats* phase" (Milan et al., 1974, p. 54). Percentage of satisfactory performance of targeted behaviors surpassed 90% when the contingency phases were in effect as opposed to pre-contingency levels of 40% (maintenance tasks) and 60% (self-management skills). Participation in the remedial education program increased from .2% of inmates participating to 20%.

Introduction of a final baseline condition resulted in an expected and significant decrease in level of completed activities. Performance during the initial days of this phase was higher than that recorded during the pre-token economy baseline. However, there was no significant difference in completed activities between the initial baseline and the second half of the final baseline. These data were interpreted as suggesting a steady decline in performance over the course of the baseline condition.

Experiment 3. The general success of this project resulted in introduction of an expanded token economy involving inmate performance across the entire day. In addition to being more comprehensive in scope, this program (in effect for 390 days) substituted a punch card system for the simulated banking system of the previous economy.

The reinforcers, contingencies, and operation of this token economy were quite similar to that of the first one. Its administrators stated that the results were "as promising as those of the first. Inmate performance improved in each of the three areas under study and was maintained at high levels throughout the duration of the token economy. In addition, these changes in performance occurred without the concomitant increase in behavioral incidents witnessed during examination of the punishment model" (Milan & McKee, 1974, p. 34).

The EMCL token economies produced impressive results on almost all of the "in-house" criteria employed. Their effect on extra-institutional indices of success is less convincing. Saunders (1974) cites 15-month follow-up data that indicated no differences in recidivism rates for token economy graduates from two types of vocational training programs. In neither of the major summaries of the Draper program was there reference to post-release criteria such as recidivism or employment status. Indeed, the objective of the first token economy explicitly was described as "motivating the performance of activities that administrators consider important for the orderly operation of their institutions" (Milan et al., 1974, p. 15). Justification of this goal is based apparently on the contention that until administrators develop more effective, less tempestuous means of institution management, "it is unlikely that they will have either the time or the inclination to turn their fuller attention to the more general problems involved in preparing the offender for his eventual return to community life" (Milan et al., 1974, p. 15). This logic is hardly compelling, especially in light of the failure to collect any data which would bear upon the point. One might just as easily suggest that implementation of an efficacious managerial system would result in a level of prisoner passivity and compliance that would be dysfunctional for present-day societal demands.

The START Tier Program

The most notorious of prison token economies was the now inoperative Special Treatment and Rehabilitative Training Program (START) developed in 1972 at the Medical Center for Federal Prisoners in Springfield, Missouri. The program was created as a means of more effectively dealing with the most hard-to-manage residents of federal prisons. Prisoners for whom a START placement was deemed appropriate were male inmates who were already in a prison's segregation unit because of repetitive assault, destruction, or violation of regulations. The major intention of START was to help the participant gain sufficient control over his aggressive behavior to allow a return to an institution for "training programs designed to help him make a more successful community adjustment" (Levinson, 1974, p. 5).

During the 16 months of program operation, 99 offenders were considered for START placement. Twenty-six met the program's admission requirements (see Levinson, 1974); of these, 19 individuals participated. The average program population at any one time was 12. Selected START residents have been defined by program opponents as "the few who had managed to maintain the individuality, leadership, self-interest, and independence often felt to be important behaviors outside of institutions, but somehow intolerable within their walls" (Holland, 1974; cited by Levinson, 1974, p. 6) and by program proponents as "destructive" and "physically assaultive" (Levinson, 1975, p. 5). Levinson also indicates that 11 of these men had received additional sentences for offenses committed in other prisons (murder, n=6; assault, n=4; possession of weapon, n=1) in addition to an average of 12 major disciplinary "incidents" (e.g., arson, bombing, and stabbing fellow inmates).

START was an eight-level program with each level having certain behavioral requirements that, when successfully completed, were consequated by institutional privileges. The levels were progressive, with each succeeding level demanding more behavioral control than the previous one while at the same time increasing the range of available privileges. Promotion through the eight stages was expected in 8 to 9 months.

Of the 19 participants, Levinson (1974) classified 10 as successes defined by progression through the eight levels and transfer back to an "open" institution setting. Six months after termination of START, six of the successes "continue to show positive behavior, including three who were released to the community" (Levinson, 1974, p. 8). Of the nine failures, eight remain in an institutional segregation unit of some kind.

It is unlikely that a totally noncoercive treatment environment for START-suitable prisoners will be developed. Notwithstanding the claims of the ACLU, it might be argued that START was less coercive than the segregation units by which it has been replaced. Unfortunately, outcome data comparing START with other procedures for handling troublesome inmates are not available. It is questionable that a large enough difference would exist to justify START's per capita cost of $39.18 as compared to the Federal Bureau of Prison's average of $14.50 (Levinson, 1974). It appears that if START was not an expensive failure neither was it an economic success.

Virginia's Contingency Management Program

Similar in intent to START, the LEAA-funded Contingency Management Program (CMP) in Virginia was initiated in June 1973 and halted early in 1975 when state officials refused to renew the project. According to an early CMP operations manual, the program intended to (1) "receive inmates who are particularly troublesome to themselves, to other inmates, and thus to the smooth administration of correctional programs and (2) to modify the actions of such inmates so that they may be returned to the beneficial influence of correctional programs in the general population of another institution until their sentences are fulfilled" (Johnson & Geller, 1973, p. 5). START and the CMP have been compared frequently, even though the program differences were numerous. For example, in contrast to START, inmate participation in CMP was completely voluntary. Table 4-1 presents a fine-point comparison of other START-CMP differences.

As an alternative to the segregation units at the Richmond State Penitentiary and the Goochland County State Farm, the CMP was designed as a four-tier token economy (Oliver, 1974). Inmates entered the CMP merely by requesting a credit card upon which credits for designated behaviors were punched and later exchanged for commissary and recreational items. Reinforced behavior during Stage I, conducted at the Richmond Penitentiary, included educational involvement, cell maintenance, and improved personal appearance. Satisfactory performance in these areas warranted promotion to Stage II, at the State Farm, where inmates encountered both more freedom and performance requirements.

The major additions at Stage II were job training (emphasis was placed on learning rudimentary skills for data-processing operations—e.g., typing) and social skill training. At this stage, contingencies were applied systematically for the acquisition of "appropriate interpersonal strategies."

Stages III and IV of the "progressive living plan" were located at the St. Bride's Correctional Unit in Chesapeake, Virginia. Stage III was distinguished by "direct training on data processing machinery" and an increasing focus on the development of social repertoires that would permit the harmonious group living that was expected during Stage IV. Beginning in Stage III, there was a gradual fading of the CMP credit economy. By Stage IV, the credit economy was discontinued completely, and CMP residents were paid money for their work on data-processing jobs. Stage IV living was virtually indistinguishable from life in the general prison population; available services and privileges were greatly increased over Stage I levels.

Aversive control was minimized in the operation of the CMP. "Counterfeiting" of CMP credit cards was the only punishable behavior in the program. Punishment consisted of a 1-week restriction on the spending (not earning) of credits. Inmates who failed to perform satisfactorily at any level could be reassigned to a lower level. While such a demotion involved a loss of available privileges, it was a mild form of punishment since cessation of program participation remained an inmate prerogative.

Evaluation of the Contingency Management Program is limited to preliminary data on a small number of graduates. Apparently, the level of inmate participation exceeded that of START. Geller (1974) estimated the number of Stage I and II residents to be about 90 each week; approximately 30 inmates progressed to Stages III and IV. After 14 months of operation, 12 inmates graduated from the program. Placement of these men was varied but indicative of positive changes. "Three will remain in Stage IV as inmate-CMP staff, five will be transferred to a field unit or pre-work release center where they will hopefully continue their education and vocational training compatible with their interests and skills, three were recommended for parole, and one was released to

Table 4-1

Contrasts Between START and CMP*

START (Special Treatment and Rehabilitative Training)	CMP (Contingency Management Program)
1. Eight stages in one building (maximum capacity = 30 inmates). Medical Center for Federal Prisoners, Springfield, Mo. Four levels of privileges: orientation, Level 1, Levels 2-6, Levels 7 and 8.	1. Four stages, each in separate facilities (maximum capacity in each unit is 70 inmates). Stage 1—Richmond Penitentiary, Stage 2—Virginia State Farm, Stages 3 and 4—St. Bridges Correctional Unit Chesapeake, Va. Each successive stage added privileges and reduced environmental restrictions.
2. One-week orientation (relative deprivation) = no personal property, no commisary, 1 hr. recreation.	2. No orientation stage: inmate assigned to segregation received CMP information and could join at any time.
3. Involuntary participation. Revision provided for nonparticipation status; inmate lives in first deprivation stage (i.e., same as orientation).	3. An inmate could enter or drop CMP at any time. Nonparticipants were dealt with by the institution as regular segregated inmates.
4. Full-time staff (besides security officers): 2 managers, 2 industrial specialists, 2 counselors, 1 recreation-education specialist = total of 7.	4. Full-time staff (besides security officers): 3 counselors per building, 1 data analyst per building, a vocational instructor for Stage 3 and 4 = total of 18.
5. Part-time staff = one each of the following: chaplain, education specialist, doctor, caseworker, physician's assistant, occupational therapist = total of 6.	5. Part-time staff: four PhD psychologists, one nurse per building, one teacher per building = total of 12.

(Table 4-1 continued)

6. Muslim religious services and/or discussions were allegedly prevented.

6. No implications for religious practices.

7. Two graduates after 17 months.

7. Twelve graduates after 14 months.

8. Graduates returned to the general population of a high-security prison.

8. Relocation units compatible with inmates' vocational interests; e.g., general population with reduced custody-level, pre-work release facility, or work release unit.

9. Vocational training = broom production.

9. Vocational training = typing computer card key-punching.

10. Privileges existing in prior segregation status were allegedly removed during initial levels (e.g., home-town newspapers and magazines).

10. All privileges existing in segregation status continued.

11. Less than 30 inmates involved.

11. One hundred to 200 inmates were participating at any particular time.

12. Direct input from one PhD psychologist during program development and refinement.

12. Direct input from four PhD psychologists throughout program development and refinement.

13. Reduction of regular, expected privileges during orientation stage.

13. No reduction in the regular, expected privileges.

14. No immediate and tangible behavior-contingent reinforcers administered, apart from advancement to levels with more privileges.

14. A "credit-economy" nested within the first two stages of a four-stage, progressive living plan. Tangible credits absent in the latter two stages.

(Table 4-1 continued)

15. Educational activities not expected in the orientation stage, and not directly reinforced at any level.

15. Educational activities expected and directly reinforced at all stages.

16. No personally owned property allowed during orientation and in nonparticipation status. Some property permitted in levels 1 thru 8, upon approval.

16. All personal property normally allowed in the general prison population allowed at each stage.

17. Recreation severely limited at orientation and nonparticipation levels (i.e., 1 hr. per week); Levels 1-6 = 1 hr. daily; Levels 7 and 8 = more than 1 hr. daily.

17. At least three hrs. daily recreation was available at each stage except the first stage (i.e., padlock status = 2 days of 3 hrs. each per week).

18. No commissary spending during orientation status and nonparticipation status

18. Commissary privileges at all levels. Inmates at each stage could earn credits for commissary spending (1 credit = 1 cent).

19. Frequent use of aversive consequences; e.g., removal of status, or Good Time.

19. Minimal use of punishment; i.e., one inmate lost his CMP card for one week (timeout from credit spending) following a detection of counterfeited punches on his CMP card.

---

*From Geller (1975). Reprinted by permission

the street" (Geller & Johnson, 1974, p. 17).

The first stages of the CMP still are maintained by Virginia prison officials. Its purposes apparently no longer include the systematic preparation of inmates either for group living or job training. Trotter (1975) quotes prison officials' intentions as "modify(ing) the behavior of inmates who 'disrupt institutional routine by venting aggression, cowering or simply refusing to obey rules and regulations' " (p. 10). It is clear that START and CMP have met somewhat parallel fates. An especially ironic outcome for both programs is that successful or threatened legel action has resulted in the departure of the professional, supervisory staff while the custodial staff remains. Both programs continue in either truncated and disguised forms or have been replaced by previously existing methods of securing inmate compliance.

Aversion Therapy in Institutions (Atascadero and Vacaville)

Aversion therapies are used most often in correctional institutions for the control of aggressive, sexually deviant, or uncooperative behaviors. It is not certain how widespread their use is in prisons; published accounts of aversion programs are quite uncommon. The number of court cases challenging the legality of these treatments makes it clear that the incidence of aversive techniques is substantially greater than that reflected by the existing professional literature. In addition to the programs described in this section, the systematic use of aversion procedures has occurred at the California Institute for Women (Spece, 1972), the Wisconsin State Penitentiary (Sage, 1974), the Iowa Security Medical Facility (*Knecht v. Gillman*, 1973), and the Connecticut State Prison (Opton, 1974). The present section will examine two widely discussed aversion programs that were implemented at two California facilities—Atascadero State Hospital and the Vacaville Rehabilitation Center.

Atascadero. Remringer, Morgan, and Bramwell (1970) report a chemically based aversion technique for the elimination of "persistent physical or verbal violence, deviant sexual behavior, and lack of cooperation and involvement with the individual treatment program prescribed by the patient's ward team" (pp. 28-29). A total of 90 male patients received the procedure apparently in lieu of the facility's traditional responses (restraint, isolation, and tranquilization) to unacceptable behavior.

The technique was procedurally simple. Following a predetermined schedule, the staff administered to the patient an intravenous, 20 mg dose of succinyl-choline, a neuromuscular blocking agent that produces rapid (34-40 seconds after administration) but brief paralysis of the diaphragm and suppression of breathing. Inmates were conscious during the period of apnea. Subjectively, the experience was defined as an intensely terrifying one. Upon suppression of breathing, the "talking phase" of the technique began. This involved verbal admonishments to discontinue unacceptable behaviors along with suggestions to increase positive "constructive socialization." Suggestions were repeated until the inmate was able to respond verbally to the attending staff.

Frequency of acting-out behavior was the outcome measure. Sixty-eight percent of the patients were classified as improved (no incidents for more than 3 months), 18% were listed as temporarily improved (no incidents for up to 3 months), and 13% were placed in a "no-change" category. One inmate (1%) increased his violent episodes over the course of the treatment. Evaluation of these data is difficult. The criteria for reported incidents were not specified, and it is doubtful that raters were blind to the experimental status of those receiving aversion trials. No reliability data were provided nor were there any comparisons made to suitable controls.

Conceptually, this demonstration is difficult to classify. At times it appeared to follow a punishment paradigm; at least some of the time succinylcholine was delivered contingent on the occurrence of some objectionable behavior. In other instances the procedure was described as a kind of chemically assisted sensitization technique. As a third alternative, Dirks (1974) suggests that the drug actually was not used as an aversive UCS but as a means of introducing "a state of heightened suggestibility" (p. 1328).

Regardless of its theoretical paradigm, the Atascadero experiment has evoked much professional criticism. At best it represented a rather corrupted treatment. At worst, its failure to obtain informed consent from the inmates may have made it both unethical and illegal (Spece, 1972). Intolerance for the program resulted in its termination and in some efforts to replace it with more innovative treatments. One such effort is the Sexual Reorientation Program for homosexual pedophiles, a population to which succinylcholine often was administered.

The goal of this program is to teach homosexual inmates the skills necessary for adult homosexual behavior (Keith, 1974; Serber & Keith, 1974). Its methods involve a wide range of group-based behavior theory techniques including modeling, role-playing, behavioral rehearsal, and feedback. The program has been broadened by its incorporation of consciousness-raising meetings and rational-emotive therapy. One of the most noteworthy features of the project is its utilization of gay community volunteers as models who teach and role-play appropriate adult, homosexual behaviors (e.g., conversational skills, "cruising," seduction). In addition, this involvement has increased the amount of positive support which the gay community extends to inmates upon their release.

To date, 25 inmates have received the project's services. Formal evaluation has not occurred. Apparently there are no recidivism figures for program graduates. Subjective assessments (Keith, 1974) of the project's impact have included the following observations: (a) the program has not been effective in reducing the arousal that many patients experience in relation to male children; (b) some patients have "outgrown" the program and now require assistance with the problems that accompany intense, long-term relationships; (c) the project has been well-received by the gay community, the patients, and an unusually responsive administration; and (d) the overall consequences of the program have been positive with patients learning new gay and "straight" skills and establishing their own self-help organization. A final benefit of the program has been the opportunity it has afforded professionals to reexamine their traditional prescriptions for the treatment of homosexuals.

Vacaville. The California Medical Facility at Vacaville is a medical correctional institution for "convicted felons who either develop mental illness during their incarceration in prison or are found by the staff of the Department of Corrections to have personality or psychological problems even though they were held responsible for their crimes" (Spece, 1972, p. 634). Sixty-four inmates were included in an experimental, 11-month succinylcholine aversion program intended for inmates who were unamenable to other treatments by reason of their extreme aggressive or withdrawn behaviors (Mattocks & Jew, 1970; cited by Spece, 1972).

The Vacaville program can be distinguished from Atascadero's on two points. First, most of the participating prisoners signed a pre-treatment contract which specified that succinylcholine would be administered contingent on the occurrence of proscribed behaviors (interpersonal violence, property damage, suicide attempts). It appears that at least five inmates were treated without consent while many were treated only with the consent of a relative (Spece, 1972). In any case, this contrasts with the Atascadero experiment in which no attempt to obtain informed consent was evidenced. A second difference is that Vacaville officials intended their program to follow a punishment paradigm; "the actual administration of the succinylcholine injection followed as temporally close as possible to the subsequent (sic) commission of one of the designated behaviors by the patient" (Mattocks & Jew, 1970; cited by Spece, 1972, p. 635). Procedurally, punishment took many forms; some inmates received threats but no injections, others received injections without warning. Vacaville prisoners also received verbal admonishments similar in kind to those used at Atascadero. This "counseling" was seen as strengthening the association between the behavior and its consequences.

Treatment evaluation involved comparison of the incidence of proscribed acts, rule infractions, and number of patients made accessible to other treatments before, during, and after the aversion program. Of the inmates evaluated, 61% did not commit a proscribed act during the program, while 11% committed only one such act. There was also a 27% decrease in rule infractions by participants during this time. Twenty prisoners were made amenable to other forms of treatment.

As Spece indicates, these data are not sufficient to justify a conclusion of program effectiveness. A major methodological problem was attrition. Data was supplied for only 35 of the original 64 participants; more than 50% of the subjects were never evaluated. Of the 35 evaluated subjects, only 15 actually received an injection; apparently the other 20 subjects were threatened only with its use. There was no control group of any kind.

On a theoretical level, the program was as perplexingly eclectic as its Atascadero counterpart. Spece's review of the project identifies operational components of operant conditioning, classical conditioning, pseudo-hypnosis, and threats of punishment. Dissatisfaction with the program appears to have been widespread. Spece (1972) reports that it was terminated sometime in 1970 because of a lack of both staff and consenting patients.

Nonresidential Behavior Therapy

There have been several experimental and case-study descriptions of successful behavior therapy with adult offenders. Most often the targeted behavior has been some repetitive, illegal sexual practice such as exhibitionism, pedophilia, or rape. A diversity of techniques including faradic aversion, covert sensitization, sexual retraining, and desensitization have been applied in outpatient contexts. Table 4-2 summarizes the methods, offender characteristics, and outcomes for a range of sexual and nonsexual criminal activities that have been treated by behavioral techniques.

As with many other approaches to "isolated" (e.g., sexual) deviations, behavioral interventions provide generally successful treatment outcomes (Coleman, 1972). Maintenance and generalizability of change exceeds that obtained with other disturbances, but the methodological inadequacies of case studies (Paul, 1969a) preclude any conclusions concerning factors responsible for the alleged durability. Given the social undesirability of these behaviors, it is doubtful that the minimum components of experimental designs (e.g., reversal, sequential application to multiple behaviors, no-treatment controls) required to demonstrate causality will be attempted. These limitations should not obscure either the apparent clinical utility of these procedures or their potential for generating hypotheses that can be examined later with rigorous, factorial designs.

Shah (1970) has utilized what many therapists would recognize as "broad spectrum" behavior therapy with an "outpatient" offender population. Shah's (1966) conceptualization of illegal conduct is based on a combination of operant and respondent principles. The process of shaping is seen as crucial in the early, inadequate development of self-control, conscience, and frustration tolerance—a set of complex behaviors which are hypothesized to be salient to socialized conduct. Contributing to deficits in these areas is a developmental history with a surfeit of punishment as a disciplinary technique and the resulting impairment of parents as effective models or sources of positive influence (Bandura & Walters, 1964). With parental influence thus diminished, it is expected that patterns of peer reinforcement will emerge as potent determinants of behavior. Citing research by Patterson and Anderson (1964), Shah (1966) concludes, "at least part of the learning of delinquent behaviors seem to result from reinforcements fairly typically provided by the adolescent culture for nonconformism to adult and other middle class behaviors" (p. 22). Drawing from the work of Eysenck (1964), Shah further suggests that deficits in moral development may be attributed to the generally low conditionability of extraverted personalities.

The immediate goal of Shah's behavioral treatment is "cessation of the antisocial activities." Attainment of this goal is related to therapeutic activity in three treatment areas.

1. *Elimination of behavioral deficits.* The offender is seen as lacking

Table 4-2

Examples of Behavior Therapy with Noninstitutionalized Offenders

Author	Sex	Age	Arrest History	Target Behavior	Treatment Procedures and Outcomes	Follow-Up
	Subject					
Mees, 1966	Male (n = 1)	19	Committment to state hospital for sexual assault	Sadistic fantasies	Electrical aversive conditioning, group therapy, and fantasy substitution. reduction of sadistic fantasies was accompanied by increases in "normal" fantasizing and sexual intercourse.	Six months; infrequent sadistic fantasies unaccompanied by masturbation. Continuation of heterosexual relationships
Jackson, 1969	Male (n = 1)	20	None reported	Voyeurism	Orgasmic reconditioning to heterosexual fantasies. Rapid reduction of voyeurism and increase in heterosexual contacts.	Nine months; treatment effects were maintained.
Kellam, 1969	Female (n = 1)	48	10 prior arrests	Shoplifting	Electrical aversion was unsuccessful. Symbolic (film) presentation of social disapproval in an aversion paradigm resulted in cessation of stealing.	Three months; continued urge to steal when in shops but no occurrence of actual theft. "Booster sessions" were instituted.
Kushner, 1965	Male (n = 1)	21	2 prior convictions	Fetishistic behavior	Electrical aversion; desensitization to heterosexual stimuli. Isolated relapse of fetish was treated by booster session.	Informal reports; occasional occurrence of fetishistic fantasies during intercourse.
Kohlenberg, 1974	Male (n = 1)	34	2 prior arrests for child molestation	Reduction of child contacts, increase in sexual responsiveness to adult males	Electrical aversion, "Masters & Johnson" sexual reprogramming. Elimination of child attacks, increase in sexual attractiveness and contacts with adult males.	Six months; no sexual contact with children reported.

Callahan & Leitenberg, 1973	Male (n = 6)	(15, 19, 22, 29, 30, 38)	Exhibition (n = 2) transvestite-transexual (n = 1), homosexual (n = 2), pedophilic homosexual (n = 1)	Court commitment (n = 1), arrest without charges (n = 1), suspended sentence (n = 1)	Comparison of counterbalanced, within-subject presentations of contingent shock versus covert sensitization. General effectiveness of both procedures was found, subjective reports favored covert sensitization.	4-18 months; continued suppression of target behavior was evidenced. Deterioration of effects was reported by one of the exhibitionists.
Marshall, 1973	Male (n = 12)	(range = 19-38)	Homosexuality (n = 3), fetishism (n = 2), rape (n = 2), pedophilia (n = 5)	Penitentiary referred (n = 5), court referral (n = 1), private referral (n = 6)	Combination of electrical aversion and orgasmic reconditioning for reduction of deviant fantasies. Eleven of 12 patients report modification of fantasies and disappearance of problem behavior.	3-16 months; 75% reported success was maintained.
Epstein & Peterson, 1973	Male (n = 1)	college age	Reduction of stealing	One prior felony conviction for theft	Self-control procedures involving self-initiated positive contingencies and response costs, in vivo graduated exposure to high-rise situations, no stealing evidenced at treatment termination.	None
Raymond, 1956	Male (n = 1)	33	Elimination of perambulator/handbag fetish	Numerous charges involving malicious damage to perambulators	Chemical aversion therapy	19 months; reduction of deviant behaviors and fantasies, improved sexual relations with wife, positive reports from probation and police officials.

appropriate educational, vocational, sexual, and interpersonal skills. The lack of adequate repertoires in these areas may result in the selection of alternative behaviors that are periodically consequated by positive outcomes but are nonetheless legally proscribed. Interventions such as assertion training, job training, and therapist modeling of social skills are frequently directed at the acquisition of critical responses.

2. *Discrimination training.* Certain behaviors (e.g., sexual offenses) are socially disturbing because "they occur at the wrong time, with the wrong people, or in socially inappropriate situations." The treatment goal in this case is to bring the behaviors under adequate stimulus control. Techniques such as desensitization, aversive conditioning, and cognitive restructuring are often employed.

3. *Development of self-control.* Related to deficits in stimulus control is inept self-control of certain responses. Often behavior is offensive because of its inappropriate frequency, duration, or intensity. Acquisition of self-control over these parameters may be facilitated via modeling, contingency contracting, role-playing, or aversive methods.

Community Settings

Probation

Among available correctional dispositions, probation represents the preferred settlement for most first-time offenders, some misdemeanants, and offenders who present little hazard for community disruption. Together with parole, probation provides for the bulk of community treatment available in our criminal justice system. Probation offers the advantages of community placement and regular supervision of the offender but does not require any period of incarceration as does parole.

Although the theory of probation is widely endorsed, its actual practice is broadly criticized. Probation caseloads are unmanageably large; the recommended ratio is 35 offenders per officer, yet over two-thirds of probated adults are seen by an officer with a caseload in excess of 100 (President's Commission, 1967). Because of this caseload, community supervision is often only nominal; many periods of probation are really unsupervised suspended sentences. Goals for the probationer are either vague or concerned only with identifying behaviors that should not occur. In lieu of adequate case management probation officers must rely on aversive control of their clients' behavior.

Augmentation of adult probation services with behavior therapy techniques is an innovative development in correctional behavior modification. It represents a welcomed demonstration of behavioral techniques' utility in a noninstitutional setting. To date, the most comprehensive examination of a behavioral approach to probation is a well-controlled study by Polakow and Doctor (1974a; see also

Doctor and Polakow, 1973, for an abbreviated description of this research). Subjects were 26 adults (11 males, 15 females) who had served a mean of 12.5 months probation prior to the initiation of the study. They had been transferred to the program because previous probation officers, using traditional case management procedures had found them too difficult to work with. The vast majority of the crimes for which the subjects had been convicted were drug-related.

The probation period consisted of three graduated contingency phases. In phase 1, the probationer received a credit for weekly meetings with his probation officer. Accumulation of eight points allowed an advance to stage 2, where points were earned for attendance at a group meeting with other probationers. These meetings were devoted to "experience sharing within a social context, discussion of problems, and support for positive self-correction of deviant behavior." Phase 2 was a minimum of 10 weeks in duration.

Phase 3 required subjects to execute a written, individualized contract with their officer that specified new behaviors which the probationer felt (s)he needed to develop (e.g., obtaining employment, new social activities). Successful completion of contracted behaviors resulted in predetermined reductions in remaining probation time. Aversive control was deliberately minimized. The only "punishment" was demotion to phase 1 for violation of written probation conditions.

Using an own-control design, the authors compared participants' performance on traditional probation to that achieved with the contingency management format. Program evaluation focused on four outcomes: number of probation violations, number of new arrests, proportion of probation time the subject was employed, and attendance at scheduled probation meetings. The results for the first three measures are presented in Table 4-3 and clearly indicate the superior effectiveness of contingency-based probation. Attendance at meetings was also increased significantly during the contingency program. The rearrest data are especially impressive in light of the fact that no systematic contingencies were applied to the occurrence of illegal conduct including drug usage.

Behaviorally based probation has been successfully extended to other targets. Polakow and Peabody (1975) report the treatment of a 30-year-old woman placed on probation for child abuse involving her young son. Therapy was multifaceted, involving (a) negotiation of a behavioral contract between mother and son that set limits on the permissible behavior for both parties (satisfactory performance of their contract resulted in reduction in total probation time); (b) discrimination training to improve the mother's control of the son's aggressive behavior; and (c) assertion training designed to develop a more effective interpersonal repertoire for the mother. Follow-up at 18 months revealed sustained improvement for both mother and son. Child abuse had not reoccurred in this interval.

Polakow (1975) treated a 24-year-old female barbiturate addict who was on

Table 4-3

Mean Scores and Associated t Tests for Number of Probation Violations, Arrests, and Months Employed While on Intensive Probation and Contingency Management†

Dependent variable	Type of probation	Sex		Total	t_{diff}
		M	F		
Mean number of probation viola- tions/year	Regular	1.43	2.05	1.75	5.05*
	Contingency	0.00	.26	.15	
Mean number of arrests while on probation	Regular	2.64	1.53	200	4.22*
	Contingency	.18	.13	.15	
Percentage of months em- ployed while on probation	Regular	51.9	38.6	44.6	3.30*
	Contingency	74.7	78.9	76.9	

*$p<.001$.

†From Doctor, R. M. and Polakow, R. L. Copyright (1973) by the American Psychological Association. Reprinted by permission.

3-year probation with a record that included felonious drug possession, sale of drugs, and robbery. Contingency contracting for pro-social behavior was combined with covert sensitization for barbiturate use. Treatment was continued over a 15-month period and was supplemented by *in vivo* practice of the sensitization technique. The subject was employed and had experienced neither rearrest nor resumption of drug use at an 18-month follow-up.

Future efforts in this area might examine the extent to which behavioral techniques could permit a redefinition of many probation functions. Table 4-4 contrasts several activities as they would be implemented with behavioral or probation methods. As yet, we do not have empirical support for the usefulness of all such behavioral redefinitions. The preliminary data which have compared probation counseling with contingency contracting would seem to warrant further investigations of the efficacy of acquainting probation officers with the behavioral alternatives described in Table 4-4.

Table 4-4

A Comparison of Standard and Behavioral Approaches to Probation Practice*

Institutional Activity	Probation Method	Behavioral Method
Record keeping	Enter descriptive information about client, what he says about what he is doing.	Definition and charting of target behavior. Identify goals in behavioral terms. Enter objective information as well as impressions about the client. Objective sources of information would involve proof of activities, visits to client in natural environment, visits or calls to significant others in environment. Changes in behavior would be monitored.
Plans for work with client	Develop generalized nonbehavioral goals that have good social value such as reduce acting-out behavior, improve self-image, and ability to get along with others.	Develop organized sequential plan to work with client. Define your goals in objective behavioral terms and secondary steps toward goals. Behavioral plan as an educational function.
Structure of contact with client	Be open, responsive, inactive listener. The client is responsible for making self-corrections, you provide warm atmosphere and reflection. Probation officer is positive and client is acting appropriately for contingent verbal response upon appropriate client verbal behavior.	Consequation rules are clearly defined as well as behavioral expectations within each sequential step. Client controls reinforcements. Behavior outside of office is reinforced regardless of relationship with probation officer.
Accountability	Report psychological status of client on how hard you are working with him. Try not to get pinned down to specifics. Focus on terminal goals and deficits.	Keep accurate records of target behaviors. Baseline and continual recording provide evidence and speed of change.
Incentives	Use aversive control via threats, punishment by incarceration, fines, or continued probation if behavioral demands are not made.	Use of natural reinforcers in the system such as time off probation, sequence of behavioral expectations show probability of successful responses.

*From Polakow, R. M. and Doctor, R. L. (1974b). Reprinted by permission

PORT

PORT (an acronym for Probationed Offenders Rehabilitation and Training) is a residential, community-based program for offenders who require a correctional alternative with more structure than that of traditional probation but with less restriction than institutional confinement. Originated in 1969 in Rochester, Minnesota, PORT is distinguished by two innovative elements (Keve, 1974; Schoen, 1972).

First, the program represents a combination of group therapy and behavior modification procedures. Progress through the five levels of the program is determined jointly by group (i.e., residents) staff decisions and the accumulation of points for performance in such areas as budget management, educational achievement, social activities, and work completion. The emphasis on group decision-making in a token economy framework is reminiscent of Fairweather's very successful work with chronic psychiatric patients (Fairweather, Sanders, Tornatzky, 1974). This programmatic affirmation of self-direction and social responsibility differentiates PORT from many prison token economies.

Another unusual variation of PORT is that it simultaneously serves juvenile and adult offenders (age range, 13-47). Such an integration is virogously avoided in most institutions because of the suspected danger of criminalizing younger residents. In the case of PORT, the direction of influence is intended to be reversed in that older residents benefit from the decriminalizing efforts extended to juveniles. An additional attempt to make a PORT placement less stigmatic is provided by the use of a staff consisting largely of live-in college students.

Available descriptions of PORT suggest that it closely approximates an optimal alliance of community corrections with behavior modification techniques. Confirmatory outcome research is minimal at this time however. A recent review of the program (Schoen, 1972) revealed that of the first 60 residents, 34 have been discharged successfully to full probation.

Evaluation

The efficacious application of behavior modification procedures for the alteration, control, and prevention of adult criminal behavior is a promise that is currently unfulfilled. This discrepancy between current status and potential promise is attributable to a failure of the behaviorally inclined professionals in the area to confront effectively five major limitations or constraints on their craft. The remaining sections of this chapter involve an evaluation of the ecological, conceptual, methodological, legal, and ethical status of correctional behavior modification.

Before examining each of these in more detail, it is important to attend to their interrelationships. The first three criteria (ecological, conceptual, and methodological) converge on the question, "Can the promise be fulfilled?" The last two (legal and ethical) ask essentially, "Should it be?" Despite the obvious importance of the second question, it may be premature unless one is interested in the morality or legality of unverified, often ill-conceived procedures.

Ecological Conventionality

Despite its relatively recent history, the community-based corrections movement has exerted a momentous impact on the American criminal justice system. It has been heralded consensually as the single most important innovation in prisoner rehabilitation. While the initial panacean proclamations have now become somewhat muted, the concept of community corrections still enjoys as high a status as its psychological sibling—the community psychology movement. Both orientations share many conceptual components: an emphasis on environmental-sociological explanations of conduct, creation of non-institutional modes of helping, increased employment of nonprofessionals, a preference for prevention rather than reparation of social dysfunction, and attempts at system rather than individual change (Cowen, 1973). These diverse principles have been operationalized into the following three general strategies for effective offender programming via community corrections: deinstitutionalization, decriminalization, and diversion. Each of these efforts will be discussed briefly below.

Deinstitutionalization as a correctional goal rests on the dual assumptions that offender restoration will be maximized to the extent that institutional confinement is minimized, and that the preferred correctional setting is one which possesses the greatest similarity to the social milieu in which adjustment should occur. Alternatives to institutionalization are numerous and historically recognized. Work-release programs in which offenders obtain or retain jobs in the community while serving their sentences have been in existence since Wisconsin's passage of the Huber Act in 1913. In the United States the concept of parole as an alternative to continued incarceration dates to the so-called "good-time" laws of the 19th century (Clegg, 1964). Newer partial or noninstitutional alternatives include halfway houses (Killinger & Cromwell, 1974), educational release (Leeke & Clements, 1973), and furlough. At the judicial level, probation (with origins in Massachusetts in the late 1800s) and sentence suspension are dispositions most frequently utilized with first-time offenders. Unfortunately, the lack of systematic supervision associated with these procedures has reduced their correctional potential.

Decriminalization involves strategies intended to reverse the stigmatization process that accompanies the criminal justice system's processing of the accused and the convicted. The movement of an accused through the justice system reveals few available "exit points" from the law enforcement bureaucracy. Following arrest, there are only five procedures by which an individual can interrupt or terminate his contact with the criminal justice system: release on bail, dismissal of charges, acquittal, reversal by a reviewing court, and completion of correctional disposition after a finding or plea of guilt. At a conceptually simple level, decriminalization can be thought of as a collection of procedures for increasing the alternatives to existing "exit points" from the system. Special emphasis has been placed on the development of exits during the early stages of processing the accused.

A recently popular proposal designed to minimize the legal system's tendency to create deviance is the dismantling of portions of the substantive criminal law. From this perspective, decriminalization would occur at the statutory level. Statutes against drunkenness, acquisition and possession of drugs, gambling, and varieties of sexual behavior between consenting adults are generally recognized as ineffective controls of socially unpopular conduct because they attempt to enforce a morality to which many people do not adhere. It has been suggested that this flowering of moral prohibitions is a reflection of a "too ready notion that the way to deal with any kind of reprehensible conduct is to make it criminal" (President's Commission, 1967). Whatever their origins, the so-called "victimless crimes" (Schur, 1965) create a multitude of difficulties. They represent over one-half of all nontraffic arrests and impose an unworkable burden on administrative and judicial agencies. Decisions to regard these behaviors as "unlawful" result in the association of those engaged in such activities with more violent and skillful offenders. Such associations are among the most powerful sources of criminalization. They divert law enforcement resources from the control of more dangerous crime and at the same time provide unusually fertile grounds for bribery and corruption. Decriminalization of victimless crime need not be construed as a sanction of such behavior. A search for alternative procedures to control or discourage such conduct, coupled with a systematic reexamination of the appropriateness of many of our criminal statutes, might reduce objectionable behavior as well as objectionable means of regulating it.

A second point at which decriminalization efforts have been concentrated is the interval between arrest and final case disposition. The predominant instrument by which persons charged with crime secure their release during this time is through financial bail. Failure to gain release has been associated with numerous deleterious effects for those detained, including loss of job, restrictions on the preparation of an adequate defense, and lengthy imprisonment. More pertinent to the issue of criminalization is the ubiquitous finding that a person who is living in the community at the time of adjudication has a better chance of acquittal or of receiving a suspended sentence or probation if convicted than a person who is being detailed (Foote, 1965; Nietzel & Dade, 1973; Rankin, 1964). These consequences have fallen most frequently to the indigent defendants who do not have the means to purchase their release.

The past decade has witnessed many bail reform (Nietzel & Dade, 1973) and supervised release (Oxberger, 1973) projects intended to mitigate the effects of pre-trial incarceration by developing nonfinancial methods of assuring that the accused will appear in court when required. The release of accused persons on their own recognizance (ROR) has proved to be as reliable a method as financial bail in certifying the return of criminal defendants. ROR has also reduced the amount of criminalizing incarceration to which indigents would be exposed.

The establishment of criminal restitution programs has been associated with decriminalization outcomes. Laster (1970) has described several examples of restitution at the pre-administrative (before arrest), administrative (police or prosecution), adjudicatory, and probationary levels. The goals of restitution are twofold: the crime victim's condition (either physical or financial) should be restored to the level enjoyed prior to the offense, and participation in this restoration effort should be therapeutic for the criminal. The "enforcement of responsibility" on the offender (Schafer, 1968) requires his continued presence in the community in lieu of institutional confinement. In essence, restitution offers a set of quasi-civil remedies for illegal activity. Its distinct advantage is that it can furnish the socially desirable goal of offender reform while reducing the individually ruinous result of offender stigmatization.

The decriminalization venture which has gained the widest support is the pre-trial intervention or diversion project. Diversion refers to the early suspension of the arrest-arraignment-prosecution sequence and the referral of the accused to a community-based, short-term (often 90 days) treatment program that provides resources such as individual counseling, career development, and job finding. Pre-trial diversion is innovative only in that what was formerly known as "prosecutorial discretion" has been made public and exploited for rehabilitation purposes (DeGrazia, 1974). Peterson (1973) describes a prototypical program involving a five-step process by which (1) eligible participants (usually first offender misdemeanants) are identified and interviewed by the staff shortly following arrest; (2) a rehabilitation plan is formulated by the project staff; (3) consent to the program is requested from the accused, prosecutor, arresting officer, and crime victim (if any); (4) assuming consent, the filing of criminal charges is withheld during participation in the project; and (5) at the conclusion of participation, one of four recommendations is made to the court concerning disposition of the case (dismissal of charges, filing of charges, extension of program participation, or filing of charges accompanied by a report of successful program involvement).

Despite several practical and legal imbroglios, pre-trial diversion projects have proven to be a valuable intervention strategy. More than 20 municipalities report the operation of some form of formalized diversion (Chatfield, 1974). Recidivism rates are characteristically lower for diverted individuals than for those receiving either probation or prison sentences (Peterson, 1973). Diversion is also considerably more cost-effective than probation/incarceration alternatives (Peterson, 1973). Finally, pre-trial interventions respond equally well to the often incompatible ambitions of swift, efficient case processing and judicious decriminalization.

A frequently articulated advantage of behavior modification procedures is their adaptability to *in vivo* assessments and applications (O'Leary & Wilson, 1975). In comparison with other therapeutic approaches, behavior modification is considered to be more suitable to diverse target populations (Ullmann & Krasner, 1975), more understandable to important socializing agents (Tharp & Wetzel, 1969), and more easily implemented by third-party "mediators" such as teachers, parents, or volunteers (Tharp & Wetzel, 1969). Despite these claims, behavior modification has remained disturbingly restricted to institutional settings in the adult correctional system. With the exception of the previously mentioned work on probation, correctional behavior modification has been minimally influenced by the press for community corrections.

The "ecological conventionality" of behavior modification elicits a number of appropriate concerns. First, it should give pause to the apologists who indignantly discredit criticisms that behavior modification often functions as a source of coercive control over behavior that may be compatible with administrative preferences but has little relevance to extra-institutional adjustment. It is precisely in the "total institution" context (Goffman, 1961) in which equity and competing sources of influence in adversary confrontations are minimized that the potential for coactive and irrelevant behavioral requirements is maximized. There is a monotonous regularity to prison token economies rewarding such inmate "adjustment" behaviors as cell maintenance, politeness, and promptness, a set of requirements that has been described as "convenience behaviors" (DeRisi, quoted in Geller, 1974). In this respect it is also revealing that the most systematic behavioral programs have been applied to inmate populations described by program developers in terms such as "men whose activities while not aggressive, were continually disrupting the administration of other programs and threatening 'the good order of the institution' " (Oliver, 1974, p. 2).

Anecdotal evidence suggests that the ease with which a control technology is learned is related to the ease with which it can be corrupted. Commenting on the CMP with which he was associated, Geller has been quoted as saying, "Perhaps the lawyers' most appropriate criticism of our program was that we would introduce into the penal system a new technique for manipulating behavior, a technique that would be eventually misused or abused by unsupervised prison staff" (Trotter, 1975, p. 10). In a certain sense, behavior modification has become institutionalized. In exchange for administrative acceptance, behavioral scientists often have legitimized and even routinized management techniques by the introduction of a therapeutic lexicon (Page, Caron, & Yates, 1975).

A second general concern with the orientation of correctional behaviorism is that while behaviorists and community psychologists frequently establish consensus on conceptual and theoretical alternatives to the "medical model," they remain poles apart when identifying a preferred style of service delivery (Rappaport, Davidson, Wilson, & Mitchell, 1975). Behavior modifiers have not evidenced the strong commitment to active, prevention-oriented, system-level change that characterizes the usual role models of community psychologists (Rappaport & Chinsky, 1974). Too often they have appeared to be content with making bad prisoners into good ones.

The benefits of applying behavior modification procedures to probation services (Ray & Kilburn, 1970) could be duplicated with a merger of behavioral techniques and deinstitutionalization, diversion, and decriminalization efforts. Diversion often is maligned for being unobservable, nonsystematic, and too informal (Brakel, 1971). The use of explicit contingency contracting, for example, could be effectual in specifying behaviors to be both developed and resisted. The contingencies that would support these changes would be made public and hopefully involve "naturally occurring" reinforcers such as movement privileges, employment benefits, record expungement, reductions in sentence length, and the like. Finally, contingency contracts could prescribe increased participation of significant social mediators (e.g., spouse, peers, nonprofessionals) in the offender's reparation, diversion, or restitution program.

At a minimum, behavioral programs should increase the use of functional analyses of the environmental or interpersonal situations in which an individual's unlawful conduct is most likely. This type of systematic, individualized assessment is represented infrequently in community correctional efforts. When individual assessments are utilized, they focus on the specification of behavioral "excesses" that need to be reduced. Assessment efforts might be redistributed more profitably to the identification of behavioral deficits as correctional targets (Shah, 1970).

At the societal level, corrections have yet to pursue the integration of behavioral and systems analyses which has typified recent mental health programming in other areas (Harshberger & Maly, 1974). A systems approach to crime has found expression in the suggestion that crime control would be best achieved by making unlawful behavior more difficult to accomplish. In this approach both the locus of control and the timing of interventions are altered. The "correction" of individuals is redirected to the "anticipatory prevention" (Sykes, 1972) of the criminal act itself. A collection of technological advances, environmental redesign (Jeffrey, 1971), architectural changes, improved means of surveillance, and legislative action exemplifies a type of social engineering that has been termed "hardening the target" (Sykes, 1972). (The impact of environmental redesign on educational interventions also has been investigated— see Chapters 2 and 7.) Examples of such target hardening include gun-control legislation, monetary incentives for the voluntary surrender of privately owned firearms, and payment of incentive wages to police officers contingent on decreases in the incidence of crimes in their jurisdiction (*Time*, 1974). Jacobs (1961) has suggested developing multiple social uses of unsupervised space in high-crime areas thereby diminishing the opportunities for illegal activity with low risk of detection. Schwitzgebel has developed an "electronic rehabilitiation system" (Schwitzgebel, 1968, 1972) that allows the continual monitoring of the location of parolees (or probationers, diverted offenders, or defendants released on recognizance). The system requires the subject to wear two small electronic transmitters that activate a network of repeater stations which in turn retransmit the signals to a base station. In this manner the precise tracking of individuals across large areas is possible. Supplementation of contingency contracts with the monitoring system could greatly increase the control of crucial *in vivo* behaviors. For example, a contract clause which proscribes certain high-risk areas as off-limits for the offender could be easily and reliably enforced. The common element of all these strategies is community elimination, disruption, or constraint of criminal resources. Such system-level responses to crime problems offer much promise as efficient, well-integrated control procedures. As such, they also prepresent procedures that will require persistent legal and public scrutiny of their application (see A. Miller, 1971, for a discussion of the objections to governmental surveillance of its citizens).

To date, behaviorists have demonstrated little affinity for the broad-spectrum, prevention-directed programs that would involve them in new ecological settings. Until that affinity becomes apparent, the very relevance of behavior modification to offender rehabilitation should be questioned. One hopes for the liberation of behavior modifiers from their institutions to the environments in which crime actually occurs. It is in these settings that crime can also be controlled.

Conceptual Adequacy

Procedurally, behavior modification in corrections bears little resemblance to the methods employed in other settings. This is due somewhat to marked differences in the recipient populations and the parameters of their disturbing behavior. A larger proportion of this procedural variance is due, however, to the conceptual poverty that pervades the field. Institutional settings have proven notably resistant to the conceptual advances that have been reflected occasionally in outpatient and probation services.

Often the terminology of behavior modification is used as an *ad hoc* justification for correctional procedures that are not primarily rehabilitative in intent. As Bottrell (1974) has indicated, "Any human (or animal) interaction with the environment can be conceptualized according to operant or respondent principles of learning as seen in behavior modification. This does not mean, however, that all such techniques represent behavior modification as a therapeutic technique" (p. 1). The conceptual sterility of behavior modification will continue as long as behavior principles are employed as semantic gloss for the correctional status quo. Attention to the following four issues would contribute to behavioral conceptualizations that are concerned primarily with planned principles of effective intervention.

1. *Cognitive control.* Recent conceptualizations of behavior therapy have

emphasized the importance of mediational events in the acquisition of new behavior. Procedures emphasizing attentional shifts, self-monitoring, and imaginal processes have been elaborated into such treatment packages as covert sensitization (Polakow, 1975) and methods of self-control (Thoresen & Mahoney, 1974). Systematic attempts to assist offenders enhance cognitive or self-control abilities have not been reported. Applications of covert sensitization to sex offenders (see Abel, Blanchard, Barlow, & Flanagan, 1975; Sage, 1974) and drug addicts (Polakow, 1975) are very occasional exceptions. Despite the recent social-learning emphasis on the informational value of reinforcement, the prevailing paradigm of correctional behavior modification remains a conditioning model in which contingencies are manipulated for the regulation of overt performance only.

2. *Programming of generalization.* For some time, behavior therapists have stressed that generalization and maintenance of therapy-instigated changes require the deliberate programming of generalization procedures. This issue would seem crucial for corrections whose lengthy incarcerations and intrusive treatments are justified on the basis of their supposed potency for bringing about long-term change. Review of the correctional literature revealed few programs that included deliberate generalization programming. In its last two phases, the CMP did fade the use of credits concomitant with greater reliance on social supports; however, few subjects ever progressed to those levels. Other generalization procedures such as group contingencies (see Hindelang, 1970), cognitive restructuring, delayed reinforcement, booster sessions, *in vivo* treatments, role playing, and distributed (or massed) practice have not been pursued.

3. *Individualized treatment.* The concept of individualized treatment procedures has not been adequately represented in this area. Even if one accepts the elimination of inmate aggression as a uniform target, it is not at all clear why graduated token economies would be the preferred strategy for all prisoners. Laws (1974) has attributed the failure of a token economy at the Atascadero State Hospital in part to the fact that it was applied to a heterogeneous group of patients that were not all deficient in the targeted behaviors. Uniformity of treatments reflects in most cases an earlier inattention to the assessment of conditions that are maintaining unlawful conduct. A related issue is the degree to which inmates could be paired with treatment techniques that are uniquely optimal for them. Client-techniques matching would require pre-testing to determine the nature of an appropriate pairing. Unfortunately, present conceptual understandings of patient-therapist or patient-technique interactions are minimal and provide few guidelines for the pre-intervention parameters that should be evaluated (Berzins, in press).

4. *Constructional approaches.* Goldiamond (1974) has contrasted the *pathological* and *constructional* orientations toward treatment. The former emphasizes the alleviation of distress by elimination of certain repertoires while the latter seeks solutions via "the construction of repertoires (or their

reinstatement or transfer to new situations)" (Goldiamond, 1974, p. 14). The institutional treatment of adult offenders has relied extensively on the pathological orientation. Increased attention should be directed at cultivating programs that seek to construct new lawful repertoires for those offenders requiring institutional care because of severe behavioral or self-control deficits.

Research Methodology

The research methodology in this area is at an embryonic stage of development. For the most part, the rationales of the research designs appear to be an indiscriminate amalgamation of single-subject and group methodology. In the literature reviewed, there was not a single instance in which an adequate no-treatment control group was included. Only two research programs (Milan et al., 1974; Polakow, 1975) contain enough of the rudiments of an experimental design to allow statistical comparisons. In one of these cases, the appropriateness of the comparisons that were performed was questionable. Milan et al. (1974) applied analyses of variance to data gathered in a sequential, reversal design despite the fact that the necessary assumptions of homogeneity of variance, independence of observations, and normal distribution of error are probably violated in such designs.

The minimal requirements of single-subject research are also infrequently represented. Reversal data were reported only by the Draper group and Bassett et al. (1973). In fact, very few studies even reported baseline data. Selection of multiple baselines or highly specific behaviors that could permit some functional statements did not occur (again the Draper research offers an exception).

The majority of correctional behavior modification reports have virtually no scientific value. According to Paul's (1969a) schema, they would be classified as nonfactorial single-group designs without comparative measurements. As such, the existing literature provides no compelling support for a belief in the specific efficacy of behavior modification techniques. At an anecdotal level, there is widespread agreement that offender behavior change is associated with the presence of some behavioral procedures. Isolation of the mechanisms responsible for such change, however, is not now possible. Investigations that wish to confirm a functional relationship between behavior change and some behavioral intervention will have to attend to the following *minimum* design requirements: (1) randomized or matched subject assignment to experimental and control groups (alternatively in single-subject designs reversal or multiple baseline procedures should be introduced); (2) collection of pre-intervention or baseline assessments against which later effects can be compared; (3) use of observers/assessors who are blind to the experimental status of subjects; (4) factorial representation of the domains likely to be influential in subject change (treatment techniques, "therapist" characteristics, time and physical-social environment); and (5) empirical monitoring of intentionally manipulated and unintentionally occurring independent variables.

The evaluation of social institutions is a troublesome enterprise. Outcome research in correctional environments has proven to be an especially formidable task. Political, economic, and professional limitations consistently reduce the level of product associated with program evaluation research (Wortman, 1975). One important response to this set of obstacles has been to advocate the use of quasi-experimental designs (Campbell & Stanley, 1966) that allow tentative conclusions about program effects after ruling out as many alternative explanations ("threats") for the results as possible.

One can sympathize with the plight of prison program evaluators and at the same time recognize that quasi-experimental methods have been underutilized. An illustration of this approach is Schnelle and Lee's (1974) use of an interrupted time-series design to evaluate the effects of a disciplinary intervention on the behavior of 2,000 adult inmates. The design involved an extension of a single-group "before" and "after" design. Data were collected for 7 months prior to the policy implementation (transfer of disruptive prisoners to a new institution) and for 23 months subsequent to the change. Statistical analyses were similar to those described by Glass, Wilson, and Gottman (1973) who used an "integrated moving average" model which allows probability estimates of the changes in slope and level between different treatment phases in a sequential research design.

Quasi-experimental logic is not advocated as a replacement for controlled investigations. It can provide applied behavior analysts with pilot data upon which later social experimentation can build. Unfortunately, correctional research has yet to illustrate this kind of continuity. The infrequent use of techniques such as time-series analyses may be due to their relative newness to behavioral scientists. If that is the case, efforts to become better acquainted with these methods would be a first step in upgrading the level of product obtainable from correctional behavior modification research.

Legal Challenges

Historically, the courts have been disinclined to pass judgment on what constitutes adequate or acceptable treatment. This reluctance recently has given way to a willingness to evaluate the legality of both psychiatric and correctional care. It is apparent that the courts are no longer willing to permit violations of inmate (or patient) rights despite the difficulties inherent in nonexpert review of treatment methods. Litigation designed to challenge the application of behavior therapy within prisons has been very successful (Saunders, 1974). Decisions in lawsuits (most often initiated by the National Prison Project of the American Civil Liberties Union) have resulted in the termination of several institutional behavior modification programs, including the Federal Bureau of Prison's START program, Virginia's Contingency Management Program, and the Control Unit Treatment Program in the state of Illinois.

A comprehensive review of the legal status of correctional therapy would exceed the present chapter's intentions. The reader interested in a complete exploration of the legal issues of correctional behavior modification is referred to excellent reviews by Damich (1974), Opton (1974), Schwitzgebel (1972, 1974b), Gobert (1975), Shapiro (1974), Wexler (1973, 1974a), and Spece (1972).[3] This section addresses itself to five of the most frequently cited legal principles upon which challenges to correctional behavior modification are based. Selective annotations to recent case law accompany a brief description of each of the legal precedents.

Right to treatment. First suggested by Birnbaum (1960), the right to treatment for patients committed to psychiatric hospitals found legal support in the landmark *Rouse v. Cameron* (1966) decision. Subsequent cases have strengthened this doctrine through successful due process arguments (*Wyatt v. Stickney*, 1971; later *Wyatt v. Aderholt*, 1972; *Donaldson v. O'Connor*, 1974). *Donaldson* has been upheld by the Supreme Court, which concluded that a state cannot constitutionally confine without treatment nondangerous individuals who are capable of surviving by themselves or with the help of others outside the institution (*Donaldson v. O'Connor*, 1975). Since *Rouse*, one federal court has expanded the right to treatment for the mentally ill to a right to rehabilitation applicable to imprisoned offenders (*Holt v. Sarver*, 1970). Specifically the *Holt* court held that the absence of affirmative rehabilitation programs where there are also conditions that militate against reform and rehabilitation may violate constitutional requirements.

Important aspects of the *Wyatt* decision included the court's ban on involuntary patient labor unless compensated by the minimum wage and specification of the physical and psychological resources to which patients are entitled as constitutional rights. The thrust of *Wyatt* is found in the directive that a patient is entitled to the "least restrictive conditions necessary to achieve the purposes of commitment."

While the *Wyatt* case does not involve a direct attack on a behavior modification program, it obviously has far-reaching implications for the legally acceptable reinforcers that can be used in hospital and (by implication) prison token economies (see *Clonce v. Richardson*, 1974). While based on the principle of reward, reinforcement programs require in fact an initial state of deprivation to insure their motivational potency. *Wyatt* would require, however, the noncontingent availability of the following constitutionally protected rights:
1) payment of the minimum wage for therapeutic or nontherapeutic institutional work;
2) a right to privacy including a bed, closet, chair, and bedside table;

---

[3]Extensive discussions of these issues are also presented in recent symposiums appearing in the 1975 *Arizona Law Review* (Vol. 17) and the 1975 *American Criminal Law Review* (Vol. 13).

3) meals meeting minimum daily dietary requirements;
4) the right to visitors, religious services, and clean personal clothing;
5) recreational privileges (e.g., television in the day room); and
6) an open ward and ground privileges when clinically acceptable.

Understandably, psychologists have viewed the *Wyatt* precedents with some concern. Berwick and Morris' (1974, p. 436) view is a typical one: "The field of law is beginning to step in and demand that mental patients get fair treatment; however, they may inadvertently be undermining attempts to establish adequate treatments." There is no doubt that *Wyatt* jeopardizes traditional token economies. At the same time, the decision is not irreconcilable with all possible behavior modification programs.

Wexler (1973) has suggested the contingent use of "idiosyncratic reinforcers," nonbasic items which patients differentially prefer (e.g., eating hard-boiled rather than soft-boiled eggs, viewing *Kojack* rather than *Columbo*).

Token economies utilizing idiosyncratic reinforcers would probably be legally permissible because by definition idosyncratic reinforcers are not equivalent to general rights. Another alternative (Wexler, 1974a) would be to continue to use the *"Wyatt* basics" as reinforcers but require fully informed consent of all participants in the program. A problem with this solution is that courts have held that informed consent to "drastic therapies" can be revoked at any time. This requirement would permit residents by their own choosing to convert contingent privileges into noncontingent rights, thereby usurping the program of its motivational impact.

Informed consent. The claim that institutional residents have a right to treatment is complicated by the suggestion that they also may have a right to refuse it (Damich 1974). Operationally, the individual's control over his/her treatment often takes form via the notion of informed consent. Full informed consent involves several elements including full specifications of the nature of treatment; a description of its purpose, risks, and likely outcomes; advisement that consent may be terminated at any time without prejudice to the individual; and demonstration of a capacity to consent. Obtaining written informed consent is usually required for experimental, intrusive (e.g., psychosurgery; *Kaimowitz and Doe v. Department of Mental Health*, 1973), and aversive therapies (e.g., apomorphine-based conditioning; *Knecht v. Gillman*, 1973).

At least one court (*Kaimowitz*) has found that the process of institutionalization affects an inmate's decision-making abilities to the extent that truly voluntary informed consent cannot be obtained from involuntarily confined individuals. The court claimed that neither knowledge of the process nor voluntary consent could be ensured with institutionalized persons. The court held in principle that participation in programs without necessary subject knowledge and voluntariness was in part coercive and therefore illegal.

As of yet there is no legal doctrine that an inmate could refuse all rehabilitation or even refuse all but his most preferred mode of treatment (Wexler, 1974a). There is clear precedent that inmates can refuse methods which violate their privacy (Spece, 1972), which are unduly drastic (Damich, 1974), or which are no more than cruel and unusual punishment (*Knecht v. Gillman*). However, any extension of the reasoning of the *Kaimowitz* court could result in the doctrine that institutionalization robs the inmate of volitional decision making with respect to participation in less drastic therapies—for example, group therapy or token economies. Wexler (1974b) has commented on the irony of such a development: "If involuntary confinement itself creates coercion, administering any therapy to the patient violates his right *not* to be treated without consent—which obviously vitiates entirely the right *to* treatment" (p. 679).

The very existence of the informed consent requirement in this area bespeaks the often coercive nature of rehabilitation and psychiatric treatment. However, from the legal point of view, coercion is acceptable when it is "reasonable" or "constructive" and limited (Wexler, 1974b)—for example, the legality of plea bargaining has been upheld. If it is the courts' desire to prohibit only unreasonable coercion in offender rehabilitation, they will need to exceed the level of precision evidenced in the *Kaimowitz* decision. From the standpoint of the mental health professional, the problem might be mitigated by attempts to replace the consensual model of treatment with the more ethically appealing contract model (Schwitzgebel, 1974a), or with a hierarchy of protections requiring differential levels of consent (Davison & Stuart, 1975).

Due process of special program assignment. The successful litigation brought by the ACLU National Prison Project against the START program has been based in part on a due process attack. Problem prisoners in other institutions of the Federal Bureau of Prisons were transferred for treatment to START. Given the very restrictive nature of the first level of the START program (e.g., limitations on visitation, exercise, etc.), petitioners argued that placement in START was tantamount to placement in a segregation unit and actually constituted a form of punishment. The procedural issue involved "Whether, in the absence of notice, charges and hearing, the selection and forceable transfer of a prisoner into START violates the Constitutional rights of the prisoner by denying him due process and equal protection of the law" (Saunders, 1974, p. 9).

In *Clonce v. Richardson* (1974, summarized by Saunders, 1974) the court found that because of the changes in the condition of confinement, the "START prisoners were entitled, prior to administrative transfer, to a due process hearing guaranteed by the 5th amendment" (p. 24). In this case the court rejected respondent's claim that because START was a treatment program due process criteria were obviated.

Violation of substantive constitutional rights. Petitioners in the START case also claimed that the following constitutional rights were violated by the imposition of the START program upon them (Saunders, 1974; see also *Sanchez v. Ciccone*, 1973):

1) freedom of speech and association;
2) freedom of religion;
3) freedom from search and seizure; and
4) freedom from invasion of privacy.

For its part, the government argued that the contingent availability of such "rights" was the most essential component of the treatment because that constituted the most powerful reinforcers.

While the court held that these points were moot because of the termination of START, its analyses of petitioners' claim portends the success of future litigation based on such attacks. Of future importance was the court's rejection of the government's claim that assignment to START was an internal matter of the Bureau of Prisons not reviewable by the court.

Treatment as punishment. A developing legal-medical controversy is the contention that the distinction between punishment and some forms of "treatment" (e.g., aversive conditioning, timeout, token economies, and the indeterminate sentence) is spurious (Opton, 1974). Preservation of a treatment-punishment distinction is not without important consequences. While courts are reluctant to intervene in practices classified as treatment, punishment is regulated constitutionally, statutorily, and administratively. Elimination of the distinction could result in First, Fourth, Fifth, Eighth, and Ninth Amendment attacks on coercive or violent therapies (Opton, 1974).

Case law reveals absence of treatment to be legally unacceptable (e.g., *Wyatt*). Yet Opton (1974) contends that there has not been "a single case in which a treatment has been ruled an unconstitutionally cruel and unusual punishment" (p. 609). The issue has been raised to some degree in several cases (*Adams v. Carlson*, 1973; *Clonce v. Richardson*, 1974; *Knecht v. Gillman*, 1973; *Mackay v. Precunier*, 1973; *Sanchez v. Ciccone*, 1973; *Wyatt v. Aderholt*, 1972). The *Knecht* court did find injection of apomorphine for behavior such as swearing or not getting up when ordered to be cruel and unusual punishment but did not object to the procedure when used for rule violators (Opton, 1974).

The goal of treatment-as-punishment arguments would seem to be that aversive treatments be subject to the same judicial scrutiny and legal control as acknowledged punishment. Realization of this objective might be attained best by adhering to Opton's (1974) suggestion that "opponents of involuntary, punitive therapy oppose it not on the grounds that it is 'really' punishment rather than therapy, but on the grounds that it is both punishment and therapy, hence meriting the constitutional and other legal safeguards of both" (p. 644).

Ethical Considerations

Behavior modification is acknowledged by a public that is becoming increasingly apprehensive about the ethics of its use. Historically, in the area of adult corrections, tolerance for intrusive techniques has been high because of the promise of controlling behavior which has high threat properties and is negatively sanctioned by most of us. Yet recent discussion of the morality of behavior modification in both the professional (e.g., Schwitzgebel, 1974a; Wexler, 1973, 1974a) and lay media (Hilts, 1974; Mitford, 1973) has aroused new skepticism and concern from a public whose ethical sensibilities have been tenderized in this post-Watergate era. Clearly this ferment has removed ethical considerations from a "merely academic" context to a position where vested and public interests have been mobilized into legislative or executive action. At this time, at least two federally funded prison token economies have been disbanded by their originating agencies or local officials, and several more face impending discontinuation. In addition, the Law Enforcement Assistance Administration has announced that it no longer will support any program involving behavior modification, psychosurgery, or chemotherapy research.

Ethical objections to behavior modification techniques are in fact only part of a larger concern with a host of behavior control or behavior influence (Krasner & Ullmann, 1973) technologies. Most potent sources of control (e.g., economic, political, surgical, pharmacological, and genetic) have evoked heated debates. The association of behavior modification with these influences has been a two-edged sword. On the one hand, behavior modification is attributed a degree of influence which has not been empirically demonstrated. At the same time, some of the more objectionable aspects of organic interventions (irreversibility, intrusiveness, etc.) have been inaccurately associated with behavioral methods. Bandura (1974) has argued that behavioral technology is not the puissant, irresistible source of control often portrayed by both its advocates and detractors. Neither is it irreversible, subliminal, or especially intrusive. The professionals' disclaimers aside, ethical challenges to behavior modification do continue to be vigorously expressed. For purposes of this discussion, these ethical objections are addressed under the following five topics: behavior control, ethical misconceptions, behaviorist's "image" of man, aversive techniques, and ethical "prompting."

The control of behavior. A frequently articulated objection is that behavior control procedures can and may be used for totalitarian, freedom-limiting ends. Kazdin (1975a) in a more general discussion of behavior modification morality has identified three issues related to this generalized fear: "the *purpose* for which behavior is to be controlled, *who* will decide the ultimate purpose and exert control, and whether behavioral control entails an abridgement of individual *freedom*" (p. 230). While this set of concerns is more intense for intentions such as the redesign of society (Skinner, 1971) or educational reprogramming (Winett & Winkler, 1972), questions about rehabilitation goals are increasingly encountered by correctional officials.

A continuing problem is the feeling that professionals are used to legitimize control, retribution, and induced passivity by making them appear to be instruments of treatment (Opton, 1974). Conrad (1965) has referred to the constant accommodation of therapeutic programs to the overriding requirements of public protection and safety as the "irrational equilibrum." The disturbing fact is that virtually anything within a prison can be made to look like treatment. Often the equilibrium is maintained by a strategic substitution of informal means of control for a more formalized, centralized set of disciplinary rules. Informal control may take the form of interpersonal or material rewards and deprivations from staff to inmate (Cressey, 1969).

The facility with which line staff can acquire the principles of contingency management portends the possibility of informal means becoming much more systematic in application. The fate of the Contingency Management Program provides an example of this outcome. Following legal challenges from the ACLU, the supervisory psychological staff has been removed from the Virginia program; "(t)he CMP has now been converted into a static program without graduated steps, whose intent is to modify the behavior of inmates who disrupt institutional routine by venting aggression, cowering or simply refusing to obey rules and regulations according to the latest description by prison officials" (Trotter, 1975, p. 10). Certainly it would be unfair to characterize all guards as "villains" or all psychologists as "saints" to use Skinner's (1971) terminology. Nonetheless, the use of behavior control techniques by prison guards has been shown repeatedly to further self-serving aims of managerial control and inmate docility.

Behavior control is often equated with a loss of freedom or a diminishing of personal autonomy. From a forensic perspective, this sentiment has found expression in the "right-to-be-different" ideology (Shapiro, 1974) and its "right-against-treatment" corollary (Damich, 1974). The ethical considerations involved in "treat" versus "no-treat" decisions are more complex than the rhetoric of mandatory-treatment proponents and opponents has allowed. Philosophical discussions of whether there "really is" freedom or not have yielded agreement only on the position that the *perception* of freedom is crucial to human adjustment (Lefcourt, 1973). The extent to which correctional behavior modification has enhanced or weakened the perception of individual freedom has yet to be empirically determined. Hopefully it is a question that will persist.

Control via behavior modification is not without its defenders. The hackneyed claims that behavior modification is value free or morally neutral are not as frequently heard today as in the past. There is, of course, no value-free intervention (Kazdin, 1975a). The very decision to work in a correctional institution reflects a number of moral decisions regarding what constitutes changeworthy behavior and what are the best procedures for changing it. Frankly it would be best to put to rest the pretense of ethical neutrality. It does not appease critics. Neither does it potentiate thoughtful considerations of the ethical dilemmas necessarily encountered by practitioners.

Behavior modifiers no doubt are accurate in asserting that their procedures are consonant with public norms and preferences. Indeed behavior modification possesses the unique capacity to simultaneously satisfy advocates of both correctional "permissiveness" and "harshness." At a conceptual level, thera-peutic principles are emphasized; however, the ensuing procedures are not so nurturant as to offend law-and-order sympathizers. There is at least tacit societal endorsement for current correctional practice. However, professional interest and discussion of the ethics of intervention should not be restricted to instances in which an often apathetic public's tolerance is exceeded.

One advantage over other sources of control which behavior modification may possess is its explicitness and overtness. Manipulation of environmental/ interpersonal consequences typically results in an individual's cognizance of the operative contingencies. In fact, there is a growing literature which suggests that behavior is not changed much by contingencies of which subjects are unaware (e.g., Dulany, 1968). Therefore, regulation of behavior through reinforcement procedures can be of informational value to clients (Bandura, 1974). This type of cognitive influence may be of special import to lawbreakers whose behavior is troublesome often because of its situational inappropriateness.

A distinguishing feature between several technologies of control is the degree to which they allow reciprocal control to be exercised. For example, the methods of medical or genetic influence are largely inaccessible to the public and thus restricted to a small number of users. On the other hand, we are taught that our society extends a degree of political influence to each adult. In principle, behavior modification provides methods of countercontrol against controllers. Certainly people can learn to be systematic in their attempts to modify the systems in which they live. However, countercontrol will be effective only to the extent that there is some equity in the distribution and possession of reinforcers among system members. In this regard the prospects for inmate efforts at (nonviolent) countercontrol in correctional institutions remain illusory. Reciprocity of control is more tenable for offenders whose intended rehabilitation occurs in a more open community setting.

Perhaps the greatest restriction on personal freedom is a limited behavioral repertoire and the attendant reduction in attainable outcomes (Bandura, 1974; Kazdin, 1975a). An overarching goal of most behavior modifiers is to increase the number of functional, adaptive skills from which an individual may choose. Such "repertoire expansion" can free the person from his own behavioral deficits and allow for the development of greater competence in living. The notion of limited repertoires is obviously salient to offender populations who are largely uneducated, unemployed, and unsocialized. Behaviorists can argue persuasively that their emphasis on enhancement of performance actually amplifies rather than stultifies individual freedoms.

Misconceptions. Ethical objections to correctional behavior modification are frequently generated by descriptions in the media that are best outdated and at worst distorted. It would be tempting to diminish the import of such misconceptions by representing them as merely differences in the semantic preferences of behaviorists and their adversaries. The temptation should be resisted because it obscures the basis upon which many of the most fundamental protests are founded.

Professionals have victimized, in part, their present formulations of behavior modification by their earlier nonjudicious choices of terminology. One of the most unfortunate and misleading of designations has been that of "conditioning." The term suggests a procedure of behavior change which is insidious, reflexive, and mechanical. In fact, as Bandura (1974) has indicated, behavior theory has outgrown the conditioning model and now emphasizes such processes as mediation (Bandura, 1969), self-regulation (Thoresen & Mahoney, 1974), and attentional control (Maher, 1975).

These advances aside, "conditioning" has been the appellation of choice for many publicists of behavior corrections. Descriptions of behavior modification programs have been linked inappropriately with the ethics and outcomes of psychosurgery (Gorbert, 1975) and pharmacological treatments (Shapiro, 1974). Heldman (1973) was moved to describe behaviorists as "come-lately technocrats, who see all the world as their laboratory and individual man as little more than a rat in a maze" (p. 13). Following some attempts to associate Skinner with Hitler and Mao, Heldman concludes, "In one naive stroke, he [Skinner]would destroy the edifice of protection we have built up against totalitarianism" (p. 18). Thankfully, positions as gratuitous and poorly reasoned as Heldman's are infrequent. Other less strident attributions persist however.

One connotative implication of the conditioning paradigm has been that behaviorists are reluctant to consider (if not deliberately inattentive to) internal events. In fact, systematic desensitization, modeling, and covert sensitization are techniques which conceptually and procedurally require the self-regulation of imagination, cognition, and attention. Careful philosophical scrutiny of even the extreme operant orientation of Skinner reveals a reliance on distinctly intentional, teleological, and purposive constructs (Rychlak, 1973).

Behaviorists increasingly are acknowledging man's ultimate intentional nature and at the same time maintaining that intentions are explainable and modifiable (Nietzel, 1974). This position requires the generating of empirical laws of behavior which do not violate a belief in individual responsibility for particular actions (Caplan & Nelson, 1973). As psychologists have progressed in efforts to understand and modify subjective experiences (Thoresen & Mahoney, 1974), the goals of some behavioral interventions have come to emphasize the development or facilitation of an individual's repertoire of self-regulation skills. The best example of this emphasis in corrections would be Shah's work with nonincarcerated offenders. It is also unfortunately true that almost all institutional programs have continued relatively unencumbered by such self-control developments.

Even successful attempts to correct some of the misattributions directed at behavior modifiers will not eliminate the ethical dilemmas posed by their treatments. Indeed, revised attributions will stimulate new and potentially more intense concerns. For example, effective modification of mediational behavior appears to be much more intrusive than the alternation of discrete responses. Shapiro (1974) has argued that a constitutional protection exists for the protection of cognition and the right to mental privacy. If the expectation that behaviorists will increasingly identify self-control processes as treatment targets is veridical, then one could also anticipate a replacement of charges of "simple-mindedness" with ones of "invasion of privacy."

Image of man. The foregoing set of ethical objections may converge upon the realization that many people find behaviorism's implied image of man to be objectionable. One very good indication of a profession's view of human nature is the degree of concern evidenced for the process of change as well as the final outcomes. Despite this fact, behavior modifiers have been selectively inattentive to the *process* of change which their correctional efforts have illustrated. Shapiro (1974) has distinguished between procedures intended to do something *for* or *with* an individual and those intended to do something *to* him. Commenting on the treatment of Alex, the "hero" in *Clockwork Orange*, Shapiro suggests, "Something was done *to* Alex, not *for* him, and his conforming conduct is not something for which he is likely to be praised. The way in which the conformity was achieved was an assault on personal autonomy rather than an enhancement of it" (p. 299).

In this respect correctional psychologists have not explored sufficiently the opportunities to exploit such ethical requirements as informed consent or treatment contracts for the goal of maximizing client inputs into change processes. Behavior therapists in other areas have recognized the importance of a collaborative relationship between professional and client. This collaboration is often operationalized by a therapeutic treatment contract (Karoly, 1975) that specifies desired changes, procedures to be employed, potential risks and the accompanying responsibilities of client and therapist. The client then becomes an active agent, a planner of his/her own change. If "consent" were obtained within the context of a negotiated contract that would allow the offender to reach informed decision about his own rehabilitation, it could function as a strong therapeutic tool.

The issue is not simply that for rehabilitation to be ethical it should be voluntary. What is required are interventions that take seriously the notion that offenders assume "roles as active, informed and informative participants rather than as passive recipients of programs"(Brodsky, 1973b, p. 18).

Active collaboration in rehabilitation programming could be promoted by any one of a number of procedures. For example, Brodsky (1973b) advocates the use of a prison voucher system similar to those demonstrated in public schools (Weiler, 1974). The voucher system would allow inmates to purchase the form of rehabilitation they prefer among several competing alternatives. Distribution of vouchers to inmates would increase their freedom of treatment choice and at the same time offer incentives to correctional professionals for treatment innovations. Other recommendations designed to increase inmate participation in the treatment process are participatory management (Brodsky, 1973b), employment of ex-offenders as correctional staff (Nietzel & Moss, 1972), and peer-group decision making (Schoen, 1972).

A more deliberate concern with the process by which unlawful behavior is changed is justified on both ethical and therapeutic grounds. Such a concern is also likely to foster a view of man that is more appreciative of both his abilities and desire for self-modification.

Aversive control. Despite the fact that most of our existing social systems (e.g., educational, legal, military) have institutionalized the use of aversive control, the application of aversive procedures in correctional settings typically arouses the most energetic of ethical protests (see Opton, 1974; Saunders, 1974). Aversive control is manifest in diverse ways. *Punishment* can take one of two procedural forms: the application of an aversive stimulus contingent on the occurrence of unwanted behavior or the withdrawal of a positive reinforcer following proscribed behavior. Modal prison punishment is of the latter type, although "direct" punishment is not unknown (see Opton, 1974). *Aversive counterconditioning* is a third variety of aversive control involving the application of a negative reinforcer simultaneous to either the perception of the stimuli that elicits the problem behavior or the actual performance of that behavior. It is typified by components of some penal programs and the outpatient treatment of sexual, drug, and alcohol-related problems.

Behaviorists are fond of indicating that the majority of their interventions eschew aversive control and rely instead on the use of positive influences. While this may be true in many clinical settings, it is not the case with adult corrections. Most institutional programs, behaviorally oriented or not, abound with punishable behaviors running the gamut from cursing (Opton, 1974) to a noncooperative attitude (Saunders, 1974). This misuse of aversive techniques is compounded by the fact that the stimuli used on prisoners are among the most potent available. At a time when most clinicians have sought to use minimal levels of aversive stimulus intensity or replace actual stimulus presentations with imaginal versions of the noxious event—e.g., covert sensitization, (Polakow, 1975)—prisoners are being subjected to injections of succinylcholine and apomorphine.

A continued conceptual criticism of punishment procedures is that they merely suppress behavior and do not promote the new learning of more acceptable responses. Based on the work of Estes (1944), this view has been tempered somewhat by the recognition of Solomon's work (1964) on punishment that suggests that new instrumental behaviors are learned in response to the classically conditioned fear that may accompany punishment (See Rimm & Masters, 1974, for a clinically oriented discussion of two-factor learning theory). Nonetheless it has become accepted clinical lore that the maintenance of punishment-generated behavior change is related to the extent that alternative responses are required which can replace those that were suppressed. Unfortunately, few prison programs have combined efforts of building desirable repertoires with their efforts toward eliminating undesirable ones.

Another common objection to aversive procedures is that their consistent administration results in negative side effects for the recipient population. Side effects frequently attributed to punishment include fear, anger, and helplessness. There is no reason to assume inmates to be any more resistant to punishment side effects than other target groups. Neither is there any reason to believe inmates are any more tolerant of punishment as a method of control. Indeed, the special history of prisoners probably presages their ability to execute very effective counteraggression against their punishers (see Sage, 1974).

It is paradoxical that the parameters of aversive treatments are used both to justify and condemn their use. Many aversive stimuli are quite painful; not a few introduce the risk of injury. For those reasons, aversive techniques introduce the greatest potential for human harm of all the techniques in psychology's armamentarium. At the same time, the intensity of many aversive procedures accounts for one of their main advantages. They are capable of bringing behavior under rapid, complete, and resolute control. In some instances (e.g., inmate violence), decisive control is required. It is probably the case, however, that the "successful" use of necessary aversion procedure makes future application in nonessential situations more likely. The question of how to limit the escalation of punishment is a critical one for those professionals who advocate even its very circumscribed use.

A reliance on professional ethics for the control of punishment procedures would appear to be an insufficient restraint. Numerous objectionable aversive methods have been sustained in prisons with professional succor (Sage, 1974). It would be just as futile to argue for an across-the-board prohibition of aversive techniques. In lieu of these two extremes, adherence to a set of formal guidelines for the use of aversive methods with offenders might be the most reasonable alternative. Imposition of those guidelines could be the responsibility of citizen review boards, judicial panels, local bar associations, or specially created advisory boards composed of inmates, lawyers, and correctional agents. A basis for these guidelines is suggested by Kazdin's (1975a) discussion of minimal ethical requirements surrounding the clinical use of aversive techniques. He identifies four issues that should be confronted seriously in advance of any decision to proceed with an aversive technique: careful determination of the stimulus intensity level to be used (ideally this might be between detection and pain thresholds), specification of the temporal limits of an aversive program, prior examination of the availability of nonaversive procedures for change of the targeted behavior, and empirical demonstration of the correctional utility of the proposed method. In light of a prison system that has yet to document the efficacy of 200 years of punishment, this last requirement is likely to prove particularly onerous.

Ethical prompting. The ethical questions posed by correctional behavioral modification should not remain restricted to adversarial debates between special interest groups be they prisoners or operant psychologists. Correctional policy has yet to elicit the concern and involvement that the public has demonstrated on other issues related to criminal justice. Similarly, many behavioral scientists have not evidenced an enthusiasm for contingencies that increase the likelihood of broader public participation in the development and review of correctional programming.

A much needed "ethical" contribution from professionals would be a behavioral analysis of the means by which the public can increase its inputs into discussion of ethics, values, and policy as they relate to offender rehabilitation. With respect to the implementation of community corrections, a solicitation of the local milieu's involvement in program definition is essential (Atthowe, 1973a). This prescription is based on the assumption that programs which commence with maximal citizen input are likely to yield the most meaningful outcomes. A number of related procedures could contribute to the realization of this goal. They include: early prompting of citizen participation in program development, the establishment of citizen-professional review boards for local correctional programs, entreatment of positive community resources in an attempt to develop creative, alternative social systems (Rappaport et al., 1975), and local publication of the process and outcomes of local programs.

Legitimate behavior modification programs should have no qualms about exposure to public, legislative, or judicial inquiry. If concerns or criticisms are the result of misunderstandings, misinterpretations, or inaccurate information, educative efforts are indicated. If, on the other hand, the program is revealed to be misapplied, ineffective, inadequate, or destructive, there would be a need for corrective action perhaps to include negative sanctions against program administrators and advisors. Another suggestion would be that behavior modification funding decisions should be consequated on the basis of demonstrated adherence to a codified set of ethical standards for correctional treatment (see Braun, 1975, for guidelines for such a code).

Finally, the recommendation that behavioral scientists should be about the business of shaping specific ethical decisions that increase governmental and public acceptance of behavior modification procedures seems ill-conceived. For example, Bornstein, Bugge, and Davol (1975) contend that the task for behaviorists is "formulating an intervention program to increase governmental and public acceptability regarding the practice of and research in behavior modification" (p. 65). It might behoove behaviorists to consider ethical debate as desirable independent of the ultimate opinions reached by the participants. One's doubts about the ethics of systematic behavioral control are unlikely to be mitigated by professionals who attempt to reinforce the "right values."

Chapter 5
DRUG ABUSE

The magnitude of societal concern about opiate drug addiction and abuse in this country is disproportionate to the absolute number of addicts and abusers. The National Institute of Mental Health estimated that there were 250,000 addicts in 1971, while Brecher (1972) identified the most likely range to be 250,000-315,000. Recent evidence suggests that the early 1970s has seen a reversal of the heroin "epidemic" that was feared during the 1960s (Ullmann & Krasner, 1975), and there are indications that there may now be a decrease in the rate of heroin addiction.

The incidence or prevalence of nonopiate drug abuse is much more difficult to determine. It is certain that abuse of and experimentation with "soft drugs" is much more prevalent than opiate abuse. For example, a survey by the 1971 National Commission of Marijuana and Drug Abuse revealed that 15% of the general population had used marijuana (Abelson, Cohen, Schrayer, & Rappeport, 1973).

The nonmedical use of psychostimulants and sedatives is a problem that exceeds opiate dependency in terms of frequency and complicating sequelae. Nathan and Harris (1975) cite claims that barbiturate addiction is second only to alcoholism in terms of associated medical, social, and financial problems. Barbiturates lead to physical dependence and increased tolerance; the withdrawal symptoms of barbiturate addicts can be very severe and potentially fatal.

Amphetamine and methamphetamine abuse appear to have declined since their peak in the late 1960s. While the amphetamines are not physically addictive, abusers rapidly increase their dosage levels in an attempt to achieve maximum subjective effects. As a result, amphetamine abuse often precipitates a number of medical and quasi-medical complications including exhaustion, decreased sexual responsiveness, depression, and amphetamine psychoses. There is some disagreement about the present level of hallucinogen abuse (LSD, mescaline, and psilocybin). McGlothlin (1975) indicates that unobtrusive measures (e.g., hospitalizations for "bad trips") show a decline, while surveys (Blackford, 1974) indicate a stable rate over the past 6 years.

Little is known about the use/abuse of cocaine in this country, although it is considered in the popular literature and news media to be a high status drug. Its use, though sporadic due perhaps to its high cost (Cohen, 1970) and the fact that it is not physiologically addictive (Ullmann & Krasner, 1975), has been estimated to be double that of heroin (McGlothlin, 1975). Cocaine is thought to produce strong psychological dependence.

From a numerical perspective, society's concern may seem excessive given the number of hard-core addicts (probably less than .2% of our population). The concern however, is not disproportionate to the numerous and serious social consequences associated with drug abuse. Fifty percent of urban crime is thought to be narcotic related (Wald & Hutt, 1972). It is suspected that addicts steal as much as two billion dollars in merchandise each year (Wald & Hutt, 1972). Historically, most addiction-related crime has been directed at property; however, recent trends suggest the appearance of more violent forms of addict offenses.

Many health problems surround the addict lifestyle. Malnutrition is common. DeLong (1972a) estimates the death rate of the addict population to be somewhere between 1.5% and 2% per year as a result of hepatitis, tetanus, infections, and other diseases. Other sources of addict deaths are attributed to overdoses, which may cause suppression of respiration or an idiosyncratic allergic reaction.

Finally, there is a recognition that in many ways addiction is ultimately a "social disease" (Cohen, 1970). Elevated rates of heroin use are reliably associated with high poverty areas, where rates of unemployment are high, levels of education are below national norms, and familial and peer incidence of substance abuse is high. Aversive social consequences of opiate dependency for the individual include unemployment, likely incarceration, and the social ostracism that attends criminal conduct.

Strategies of Drug Control

The history of drug control programs in this country has been one of sustained ineffectiveness. This legacy of failure belies both the broad range of control policies and the fervor with which these policies have been pursued. Anti-drug strategies have been promoted energetically by moral, legal, medical, and mental health advocates, often in competition but occasionally in conjunction with each other.

Legal Controls

For the larger part of this century, the dominant American response to unwanted use of drugs has been legal prohibition. Legal controls have taken one of two basic directions. One approach has involved international control of poppy cultivation and opium production. Early anti-drug legislation in this country was intimately tied to foreign policy (McNamara, 1973). For example, the Secretary of State was the initiator of the Opium Exclusion Act of 1909, which forbade the importation of opium for other than medical purposes. As early as 1833, the United States signed a treaty with Siam that made it illegal for Americans to traffic in opium with the Siamese. Simmons and Gold (1973) identify 30 countries with whom the United States has bilateral drug control agreements and another six with whom multilateral drug control treaties have been signed. Recent strategies have emphasized the manipulation of economic and political incentives for the eradication of the poppy crop in Mexico, Turkey, and Southeast Asia (Raskin, 1974).

There is general consensus that this international control tactic has been a failure. The problems of enforcement are legion. For example, it is estimated that enough opium to supply the American market for one year (about 175 pounds of opium) could be produced from as little as four to five square miles of land. At this time, the world's illicit production of opium is probably in the vicinity of 1400 metric tons (Simmons & Gold, 1973). As a consequence, even massive increases in surveillance and crop eradication would fall short of the level needed for complete control.

The second direction of legal controls has been to criminally sanction individuals who sell, possess, or use elicit drugs. Criminalization of drug use began in this country in the early 1900s with the passage of the Harrison Act in 1914. Since that time, the United States has relied on the criminal law to suppress drug use. In 1960 there were 31,752 arrests for drug offenses; 10 years later there were over 230,000 such arrests (Wald & Hutt, 1972). In 1972 over one-fourth of the federal monies spent on drug abuse programs were spent for the enforcement of drug laws by four federal agencies (Bureau of Narcotics and Dangerous Drugs, the Law Enforcement Assistance Administration, the Department of Justice, and the Internal Revenue Service).

Anti-drug laws continue to be enacted despite the fact that most observers of the American drug scene regard legal controls to be ineffectual. No intellectually satisfying evidence exists for the deterrent efficacy of any single piece of punitive legislation. Drug use has not been made less likely; it has been made criminal. Unfortunately, in addition to being ineffective, drug laws have had many deleterious effects. Lindesmith (1965) has evaluated the impact of our criminalization policy: "Before 1915 there was no significant elicit traffic, criminality and addiction were not linked as they are now, the number of addicts in jail and prisons was negligible, and there was no problem of juvenile addiction" (p. 128).

In addition to the criminal status of drug possession, distribution, and delivery, drug use is unequivocally related to other criminal behavior. Most addicts must turn to criminal means of acquiring the money necessary to support $100 to $200 a day habits. Further criminalization occurs as the addict-abuser is brought into contact with the skills and support of the criminals he encounters in prison. Cataloging drugs as an illegal substance fosters a black market where the cost of drugs is greatly elevated. Perhaps the most devastating effect of drug laws is their destructive impact on the legal system itself (Zinberg

& Robertson, 1972). Police corruption flourishes in the context of enforcing narcotics laws. Law enforcement resources are continuously diverted from the protection of persons and property to activities such as entrapment, surveillance, and petty seizures.

Moral Controls

The initial application of the criminal law against drug users was energized by moralistic concerns. For example, the political pressures that culminated in the Opium Exclusion Act and the Harrison Act were brought to bear through the intensive efforts of missionary and clergy lobbyists (McNamara, 1973). Both alcohol and drug use were regarded as immoral actions having sinister relations to insanity, minority groups, foreigners, strange powers, and fiendish behavior.

Moral objections to nonprescribed drug use continue to sustain our anti-drug legislation. As McNamara (1973) concludes, "Yet even today, the way in which we regard drug use and addicts bears the unmistakable trace of the temperance concepts of morality." Occasionally, moral concerns center around an endorsement of individual reliance and self-sufficiency which are viewed as incompatible with pharmacological aids or supports. More often, however, moral dissatisfaction with drug use is directed at the accompanying philosophies and lifestyles of users.

Therapeutic Controls

Therapy for the drug addict has benefited from the numerous conceptual contributions of both medical and mental health professionals as well as sociologists. This diversity of approaches has been accompanied by a long-standing disagreement concerning the appropriate goals of addict rehabilitation. Most approaches have endorsed abstinence as the only acceptable treatment goal. Alternatively, the goal of controlled, supervised, or limited drug use has been advocated mainly by those associated with "maintenance" treatments. Among all treatment strategies, there is general endorsement of two allied goals: a reduction of the criminal behavior that usually accompanies the illicit use of drugs and the development of a set of skills or attitudes described as "pro-social" or "socially productive."

Reviews of drug abuse treatments (e.g., DeLong, 1972b) typically identify six types of programs in current use or with future potential. Of the six programs briefly described in this section, the first four account for more than 90% of the addicts currently receiving treatment.

Detoxification. Detoxification involves two tasks: the supervised reduction of drug (usually opiate) intake until the individual is drug free, and necessary attention to subsequent withdrawl symptoms. Heroin addicts are usually detoxified in one of three ways: methadone substitution, tranquilizer aided reduction, and unaided or "cold turkey" cessation of drug use. Detoxification has several advantages. It can be accomplished in a multitude of settings including hospitals, clinics, therapeutic communities, and public programs. It successfully interrupts the pattern of drug dependence and the attending criminal lifestyle, albeit often for only a few days. Detoxification is a relatively inexpensive and time-limited intervention; while some ancillary symptoms of withdrawal may linger for many weeks, severe or primary withdrawal reactions seldom exceed two weeks.

These advantages are contrasted with the prevailing opinion that detoxification alone seldom results in long-term modification of drug use. Attrition among detoxification patients characteristically exceeds 50% (Gay, Matzger, Bathurst, & Smith, 1971; Smith, Gay, & Ramer, 1971). Of those patients who complete detoxification procedures, the great majority resume drug use within a short interval (Gay et al., 1971). The primary benefit of detoxification probably is achieved by its selective use as a precursor to the more complete, long-term interventions described below.

Civil commitment. Civil commitment involves the principle of therapeutic incarceration for the purpose of rehabilitation rather than punishment. Incarceration is usually for a minimum of 6 months during which the addict can be the recipient of varied treatments including detoxification, individual counseling, encounter groups, group therapy, recreation, education, job training, and therapeutic communities. More recent programs have attempted to include after-care services.

The civil commitment of addicts was a procedure first developed in the 1930s at the federal level at narcotics hospitals in Lexington, Kentucky, and Fort Worth, Texas. At the state level, both California and New York employed civil commitment procedures beginning in the 1960s. The Narcotic Addict Rehabilitation Act in 1966 legislated the use of civil commitment for federal offenders in lieu of imprisonment.

After surveying outcome data from the Lexington, Fort Worth, California, and New York programs, DeLong (1972b) concludes that the "chief function of civil commitment seems to be nothing more than to keep the addict out of circulation for intermittent short periods" (p. 190). Programs which provide after-care as an essential service tend to generate more promising results. However, civil commitment of any kind is probably too expensive—estimates range from $10,000 to $12,000 per year per addict (DeLong, 1972b)—either to justify or to allow widespread implementation.

The therapeutic community. A popular form of treatment among addicts is the therapeutic community, a residentially based program that uses a variety of therapeutic techniques to restructure the personalities or lifestyles of addicts. Estimates place the number of volunteers for therapeutic communities at 10,000 to 15,000 (McGlothlin, 1975). The origins of Synanon, one of the earliest therapeutic communities, can be found in the philosophy of Alcoholics Anonymous with its emphasis on confession and restitution and the virtues of peer support and confrontation (Yablonsky, 1965). There are now probably more than 50 therapeutic communities for addicts, the most publicized including Phoenix Houses (Biase, 1970), Synanon (Yablonsky, 1965), and Day Top Village (Casriel & Amen, 1971).

Despite a great amount of interprogram variability, there are some commonalities among therapeutic communities. The majority take an absolute stand against any form of drug use, formulating abstinence as the only acceptable therapeutic goal. Admission to therapeutic communities often takes on a ritualistic quality whereby the addict's motivation for treatment is tested in an encounter session, work assignment, or abstinence. Most therapeutic communities evidence a mistrust of professionals, preferring to employ ex-addicts as the principal change agents.

During membership in the program proper, the addict encounters a well-structured, even rigid set of rules, reinforcements, and punishments that require the renunciation of the addict culture and an acceptance of responsibility for present and future behavior. In sum, the addict is faced with a system of social control that attempts to regulate every aspect of his or her life by almost compelling adherence to new normative beliefs and a revised social role (Waldorf, 1971). Continued group pressure (most often exerted in group therapy or synanons) is directed at changing addicts' self-concepts and discouraging the rationalizations with which drug abuse is often legitimized (Brook & Whitehead, 1973). Most programs do not include a "re-entry phase" where the addict is prepared for a return to the natural community. It is often felt that such a procedure would interfere with the influence of the therapeutic community.

Synanon's methods have been given a social-learning conceptualization. Karen and Bower (1968) have identified the following similarities between "behavior therapies" and Synanon: (a) a concern with problematic behaviors rather than internal events, (b) specification of desired and undesired behaviors, (c) the use of response-contingent reinforcers (e.g., clothing) for appropriate behaviors, (d) response-contingent withdrawal of negative reinforcers (e.g., verbal abuse) for appropriate behaviors, and (e) promotion through a phase system with subsequent phases providing residents with better living conditions.

Impartial assessments of therapeutic communities are rare. Most are ambivalent if not openly hostile toward external evaluation, although there have been some recent exceptions (e.g., Aron & Daily, 1974; Collier & Hijazi, 1974; LaRosa, Lipsius, & LaRosa, 1974). The available data does not generate unbridled optimism. Attrition rates are notoriously high. There appears to be only a select group of addicts who volunteer for this type of treatment or for whom the treatment is appropriate. Brecher (1972) cites Synanon's founder, Charles Dederich, as estimating that only 5% of those who come into contact with therapeutic communities remain drug free and socially productive.

Methadone. Methadone hydrochloride is a synthetic opiate which has several properties that make it a useful agent in the treatment of heroin addicts. The use of methadone as a substitute for heroin was discovered by Dole and Nyswander (1965) who found that a daily oral dose of methadone inhibited heroin withdrawal symptoms in addicts and suppressed the physiological craving or drug urges of addicts. Another advantage is that therapeutic, oral doses of methadone are not associated with the production of either euphoria or severe side effects, although some unpleasant methadone side effects such as impaired sexual functioning and physiological complaints have been reported (Sutker, Allain, & Moan, 1974). Although higher dosage levels (usually 80 mg or more) of methadone are thought to "block" the pharmacological action of heroin and associated euophria, this effect has been disputed by some addicts (McCabe, Kurland, & Sullivan, 1974). Methadone, which itself is addicting, is used as a primary treatment for heroin addiction in one of two ways: *methadone detoxification-withdrawal*, where heroin is replaced by methadone which is then generally withdrawn resulting in fewer physical symptoms than with direct heroin withdrawal; and *methadone maintenance*, where the patient is stabilized over a long period of time on methadone as a substitute for heroin.

Despite continuing controversy (Lennard & Allen, 1973; McGlothlin, 1975; O'Malley, Anderson, & Lazare, 1972), there can be little doubt that methadone maintenance has proven to be an effective treatment strategy for decreasing heroin abuse (Brill, 1971; Dale & Dale, 1973; Dole, 1971; Dole, Nyswander, & Warner, 1968; Gearing, 1970). It currently is the major vehicle of treatment for heroin addicts with a reported 80,000 patients on methadone maintenance in 1974 (Dupont, 1974). The data concerning the efficacy of methadone detoxification-withdrawal are more complex. Some programs indicate that "narcotic hunger" returns almost immediately upon cessation of methadone, making abstinence quite difficult but not impossible, (Dole, 1970). Others (Jaffee, 1970) feel that withdrawal can be accomplished especially when supplemented by after-care services.

The alleged therapeutic effects of methadone maintenance are numerous: it allows the addict to remain in the community on a productive, usually self-supporting basis; it is associated with a reduction in urban crime for which hard-core addicts are often responsible (Dupont & Katon, 1971); it is relatively inexpensive and available to addicts who desire it—DeLong(1972b) estimates the yearly cost of methadone programs to range between $500 to $2,500 per patient; it provides a constant level of psychological and medical support and careful monitoring of drug-use behavior, all of which may be helpful in deterring abuse (DeLong, 1972a).

These numerous advantages aside, the use of methadone as a primary treatment modality for opiate addiction remains the subject of numerous questions, few of which have received suitable empirical attention. First, there is concern about the efficacy and long-term consequences of substituting one addicting substance for another (Soden, 1973). This issue is especially disquieting in light of the original introduction of heroin as a preferred substitute for morphine in the 19th century. In addition, there is some data that suggest that methadone is becoming a black market commodity in high demand by individuals other than methadone maintenance patients (Arehart, 1972).

Second, there are clear indications that methadone is not particularly successful with some types of addicts. For example, methadone programs have been unsuccessful in attracting and retaining young addicts (Bass & Brown, 1973; DeLong, 1972b). There are also indications that poly-drug abusers, particularly abusers of alcohol, fare poorly in methadone treatment. As less select populations of addicts have participated in these programs, there have been marked reductions in retention rates (Mandell, Goldschmidt, & Grover, 1973).

A third problem has been the determination of optimal dosage levels. The general maxim seems to be to administer the minimum amount of methadone consistent with treatment success. This preference was influenced initially both by moral choice and economic consideration. At the same time, there was the claim that success was more likely with higher, "blocking" doses. There is now an accumulation of independent evidence which indicates that addicts maintained "blindly" on low, moderate, and high doses do equally well in terms of program retention, drug use, employment, and arrest rates (A. Goldstein, 1971; Williams, 1970).

Finally, there is the suggestion that reductions in crime rates and increases in self-supporting addicts associated with methadone have been overestimated (Vorenberg & Lukoff, 1973). In a similar fashion, the data on economic productivity may be inflated by the fact that much addict employment involves methadone programs' hiring of "maintained addicts."

Opiate antagonists. A recently researched treatment modality has been the use of opiate antagonists which, when administered prior to opiate injection, block the opiates from having any effect. The antagonists precipitate withdrawal symptoms if taken after opiate use. Cyclazocine, naloxone, and naltrexone are the major antagonists. All can be taken orally and are effective in small to moderate doses.

Although opiate antagonists are still in the experimental stage of development, there is evidence that these compounds have potential utility in the management of narcotic addiction (e.g., Altman, 1974; Jaffe & Brill, 1966; Kurland, Hanlon, & McCabe, 1974; Martin, Jasinski, & Mansky, 1973). A number of disadvantages of current antagonist regimes make it unlikely that they will be used extensively in the near future. First, the antagonists do not reduce drug hunger; therefore, the addict is tempted continually to skip his deterrent dose and use heroin. Currently, they are expensive—$3,000-$5,000 per addict per year (DeLong, 1972b). Some produce numerous aversive side effects. The antagonists have a relatively short duration of action making it necessary to take some of them more than once a day. Finally, because the antagonists are not addictive and often have side effects, it is more difficult to maintain addict motivation and continuation in antagonist programs. The development of a depot antagonist represents an attempt to minimize this latter problem; however, the medical, legal, and social impediments to this solution have yet to be overcome.

Heroin maintenance. A final approach to heroin addiction involves maintenance of addicts on heroin or morphine. This approach, while used in the United States on a very limited and experimental basis as early as 1921 (Cohen, 1970), is the basis for the British system of treatment. England claims to have stabilized its addict population by a plan in which addicts receive free drugs from government-supported clinics (May, 1972). Proponents claim that heroin maintenance in the United States would both reduce addict-related crime and reach a number of addicts who have failed in other programs. Critics (e.g., Chinlund, 1973) have pointed to the expense, the difficult administrative problems (e.g., heroin would have to be injected several times daily), the many differences between the American and British populations, and the moral objections to providing a substance which is addictive.

Treatments for nonopiate dependencies. The treatment of other drug dependencies are both more varied and less systematically evaluated than the treatment of narcotic addiction. With the exception of barbiturate addiction (in which withdrawal symptoms can be severe), the treatments of nonopiate drug dependence for the most part do not require long-term medically supervised treatments. This, in turn, has resulted in a greater freedom of intensity, duration, location, staffing, and philosophy of these treatment programs. A rich array of preventive and ameliorative efforts have appeared.

A major attempt at prevention has taken the form of drug education programs. While an occasional program has been educational in its intent, the majority of them have sought to inculcate anti-drug attitudes and insist on the dangers of all drug use often at the expense of factual accuracy. It has been difficult to evaluate the impact of drug education programs. There is widespread doubt that the programs are effective in reducing drug use in the young (Stuart, 1974).

Among young drug abusers, crisis intervention is a popular form of treatment which provides emergency assistance for the adverse medical or psychological reaction that users sometimes experience. Crisis services are provided in a variety of settings: community health centers, "hot lines," free clinics, and campus counseling centers. Abstinence is seldom a treatment goal; most often the intervention is intended to reduce the risk of self-destructive behavior and assist the client in recovering from a problematic drug reaction. An additional purpose of some crisis interventions is the development of new problem-solving resources for the drug user.

Users of both narcotic and "soft" drugs often receive individual psychotherapy, psychoanalysis, or group therapy. In most cases, these treatments are directed at the reconstruction of the addict's personality, the cultivation of new forms of behavior, and a self-understanding that will make drug relapse unlikely. No objective evaluations of these services with this type of client have been provided.

Social Learning Factors in the Development of Drug Abuse

There are numerous theoretical formulations of drug dependence; most with a plenitude of intuitive appeal but few with the necessary empirical support (Mensh, 1970; Nathan & Harris, 1975). Three etiological perspectives are most often emphasized. The first is sociological, in which official abuse patterns are associated with cultural, racial, economic, and socioeconomic backgrounds (e.g., Chein, Gerard, Lee, & Rosenfeld, 1964). While it is evident that such factors do allow discriminations between drug users and nonusers, it would be a mistake to represent the link between demography and drugs as a causal one. A second approach has been the psychodynamic notion that abusers are frustrated by strong oral needs (Fenichel, 1945) which likewise characterize other incorporative syndromes such as obesity and alcoholism. A third theoretical position is that drug dependence has a biophysical basis whereby a predisposition to drug use is linked with metabolic irregularity, neurological vulnerability, or the actions of chemical neurotransmitters.

The contribution of learning mechanisms to the development of drug abuse has been emphasized by behaviorally oriented theorists (e.g., Cahoon & Crosby, 1972). In many ways social-learning formulations of drug abuse and alcoholism are similar (see also Chapter 6). Both emphasize the role of positive reinforcement associated with ingestion of a substance. The use of drugs is instrumentally reinforced by pharmacologically produced effects such as euphoria, relaxation, "expansion" of reality, pain reduction, and the easing of depression. Drug dependence also is secondarily maintained by the social reinforcement which peer groups provide for drug use. Related to this social influence is the rather extensive socialization process by which the person becomes a part of a drug culture. As allegiance to this culture increases, attitudes, values, and rationalizations favorable to increased drug use are strengthened (Ullmann & Krasner, 1975).

The role of modeling is emphasized in most behavioral accounts of pharmacological dependencies (Cahoon & Crosby, 1972). In its simplest form,

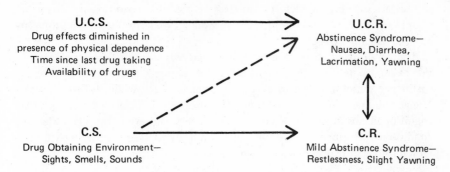

Fig. 5-1. Example of Classically Conditioned Withdrawal Syndrome (From O'Brien, C. P. The role of conditioning in narcotic addiction. In E. Chirines (Ed.) *International Symposium on Behavior Modification*, in press. Reprinted by permission.)

the notion of observational learning stresses the fact that adolescents imitate use of drugs which they observe in their parents, important socializing agents, revered heroes, or symbolic figures (Bandura, 1969). There are data which support this view for some drugs (Smart & Fejer, 1972), although the relationship of these data to the development of narcotic habits, for example, is less clear.

Independent of the original impetus to their abuse, certain drugs (e.g., the opiates and barbiturates), when repeatedly used, result in the person's becoming physically dependent on them and requiring greater quantities of the drug to avoid withdrawal symptoms such as perspiration, nausea, vomiting, diarrhea, and tachycardia. Continued and intensified drug use is thereby negatively reinforced because it results in the removal and/or avoidance of the quite aversive withdrawal syndrome.

It is well known that (1) abstinence symptoms are experienced long after successful and complete detoxification and withdrawal (O'Brien, in press) and (2) drug relapses occur frequently and rapidly after release from institutions in which the addict was drug-free for an extended period (O'Brien, in press). Wikler (1961, 1965, 1973) has introduced the concept of *conditioned abstinence syndrome* to account for the high rate of relapse among formerly abstinent addicts. Wikler's model emphasizes the classical conditioning of abstinence symptoms (see Fig. 5-1) and the incomplete extinction of previously reinforcing drug-seeking behaviors. Over time, addicts will repeatedly experience initial signs of withdrawal sickness. During these times, their symptoms are associated with numerous environmental stimuli: drug peers, the smells and sights of drug-use locations, areas where they "hustled" for drugs, the sight and feel of drug paraphernalia, encounter of a successful pusher, etc. These pairings result in associative learning whereby abstinence symptoms become conditioned to such stimuli. Following reexposure to these cues (usually after a period of enforced incarceration), the addict experiences classically conditioned abstinence symptoms. It is hypothesized that the addict relieves these symptoms by abruptly resuming drug use.

The conditioned abstinence model has received substantial empirical support. For example, it has been demonstrated that it is possible to condition opiate abstinence symptoms to neutral stimuli in animals (e.g., Wikler & Pescor, 1967). Using volunteer subjects, O'Brien (in press) has been able to generate conditioned abstinence in a laboratory setting. However, the role which the conditioned abstinence syndrome plays in precipitating relapse and thereby reestablishing drug dependence remains unclear.

Social Learning Treatments of Drug Abuse

Behavior therapy techniques are being applied increasingly to a wide range of drug abuse problems. Specific treatments are described under three general therapeutic paradigms: classical conditioning, contingency management, and a mixed or combined approach.

Classical conditioning treatments represent the most frequently used behavioral approach to drug abuse, and have taken one of two forms. The first is aversive conditioning in which either the eliciting stimuli for the problem behavior or drug ingestion behavior itself is paired with a noxious stimulus. Theoretically, this association results in a decrement of the positive value of the supportive stimuli to the point where consumptive behaviors are reduced if not eliminated.

The second form of counterconditioning treatment is the repeated association of the stimuli eliciting the maladaptive behavior with some incompatible response. The pairing of anxiety-eliciting cues (theorized to be related to incidents of drug abuse) with responses incompatible with anxiety has been used quite extensively with drug abusers. Systematic desensitization with relaxation as the conditioned incompatible response has been the procedure of choice.

A second behavioral strategy for drug abuse involves the programming of positive reinforcers contingent on the occurrence of specified behavior change. Social skills are among the most frequently targeted behaviors reflecting the pervasive view that drug-dependent individuals possess limited social-skill repertoires. Negative reinforcers are often utilized, in conjunction with positive contingencies, to suppress drug-procurement activities (e.g., drug use, association with other abusers, and criminal activities).

When applied on an individual level, contingency management is typically operationalized through contingency contracts in which an agreement is made between client and treatment personnel concerning therapy goals. These agreements usually specify critical behaviors to be developed or avoided as well as the consequences for each. Many contracts list the responsibilities of both client and staff and place time limits on contract duration. Token economies are a prevalent means of implementing contingency programs with groups of institutionalized abusers who have similar drug problems and drug-competing abilities.

The third general treatment strategy has been to combine an assortment of behavioral techniques into an integrated treatment plan for the drug abuser. A common pattern involves applying an aversive procedure to reduce drug use in association with some form of social skill-training program intended to strengthen pro-social alternatives to drug dependence. Also included in this category are those programs that employ behavior modification as an adjunct to a methadone maintenance regime. While methadone maintenance would not characteristically be regarded as a behavior modification procedure, its use can prevent the negative reinforcement (associated with withdrawal symptoms) that functions to maintain drug use.

Aversive Procedures

The most frequently applied behavioral treatments to drug abuse are ones in which the major therapeutic component is some form of aversion therapy. Of the 10 aversive treatments reviewed in Table 5-1, four have used electrical stimuli, three have used chemical stimuli, and three have employed verbal or covert stimuli.

Wolpe (1965) reported the use of electrical aversion with a 31-year-old physician who reported an addiction to demerol of 3-years' duration. He was instructed to self-administer shock with a portable apparatus contingent on the occurrence of drug "urges." In addition to counterconditioning, assertion training was provided to strengthen interpersonal skills that were thought to be incompatible with drug use. The client was abstinent for 3 months but following treatment termination resumed drug use apparently in response to repeated stress.

At least three other studies have used electrical aversion as a component in a varied therapeutic package. Lesser (1967) treated a 21-year-old male college student who was a frequent morphine user with electrical aversion in combination with assertion training and relaxation. Shock was administered contingent on the client's visualizing one of five typical steps in preparing a fix and terminated contingent on the client saying "stop," indicating that he had stopped visualizing that step. After 16 sessions, shock was applied on an intermittent schedule in an attempt to improve the durability of treatment effects. While there were two drug relapses during the treatment, the client reported no drug use at a 10-month reassessment. Other therapy goals, such as obtaining employment and reduction of anxiety, were also successfully maintained.

Lubetkin and Fishman (1974) identified three stages in the drug-taking sequence of a 23-year-old heroin user. Painful electric shock was delivered during

Table 5-1
Aversive Procedures: A Review of Target, Treatment, and Methodological Criteria

Treatment	Subjects					Treatment					Methodology			
	Study	N	Age	Sex	Drug Use	Setting	Duration	Adjunctive Procedures	Generalization and Maintenance	Staff	Design	Dependent Measures	Targets	Follow-up
Electrical aversion	Wolpe, 1965	1	31	M	Demerol 3 yr. addiction	Out-patient	8 sessions 4 months	Psychoanalysis	In vivo, self-administered shocks	Prof.	CS	SR	Drug Use	None
Electrical aversion	Lesser, 1967	1	21	M	Morphine (2-3 times/week)	Out-patient	33 sessions 4½ months	Relaxation and assertion training	Aversion faded to partial reinforcement schedule	Prof.	CS	SR	Drug Use anxiety/social skills	10 months
Electrical aversion	Lubetkin & Fishman, 1974	1	23	M	Heroin (3 yr. user)	Out-patient	20 sessions 2½ months	Group therapy and marital counseling	Partial reinforcement during last session	Prof.	CS	SR and report by wife	Drug Use	8 months
Electrical aversion	Spevak, Pihl, & Rowan, 1973	3	Adolescents	M	Amphetamines	Hospital (2) out-patient (1)	3½-5 months	Psychotherapy, group and milieu therapy for hospitalized patients	Fading of reinforcement schedule	Prof.	CS	SR and subjective ratings of drug-related stimuli, frequency of drug-related cognitions	Drug Use and drug thoughts	7 months
Chemical aversion	Raymond, 1964	1	30	F	Physeptone (6 yrs.)	Hospital	17 days	ECT, outpatient therapy (6 mo.)	—	Prof.	CS	SR and clinical observation	Drug use, later depression	30 months

Chemical aversion	Liberman, 1968	2	24, 38	M, F	Heroin (8 yrs., 5 yrs.)	Hospital	38 sessions (male patient)	Psychotherapy and milieu therapy	Booster treatments and outpatient therapy (female patient)	Prof.	CS	SR	Drug Use	12 months
Chemical aversion	Thompson & Rathod, 1968	15, 2	16-38 x̄ = 19.5	M, F	Heroin	Hospital	5 sessions; 5 days	Methadone, individual and group therapy, occupational and parental therapy	—	Prof.	Group design with untreated controls	Urine analyses clinical observation, SR	Drug Use	Unsystematic (longest 30 weeks)
Covert sensitization	Anant, 1968b	1	32	F	"Addicted to tranquilizers"	Outpatient	—	Systematic desensitization	—	Prof.	CS	SR	Drug and alcohol use, anxiety	3 months
Covert sensitization	Steinfeld, 1970	8	S_1 (mid-20s) S_2 (36) 5 subjects (unspecified)	M	Heroin (6) Cocaine (2)	Federal correctional Institute	8 sessions	Encounter groups, seminars, group therapy	Relaxation training	Prof.	CS	SR and reports from aftercare services	Drug Use	none
"Assisted" covert sensitization	Maletsky, 1974	13, 7	x̄= 27.4 (M) x̄=33.9 (F)	M, F	Paint (1), heroin (2), alcohol (10), marijuana (2), hallucinogens (1)	Army outpatients	12 sessions; 8 weeks	Group and individual counseling	Booster sessions; in vivo conditioning trials	Prof.	Group design with alternative treatment controls	SR, chemical analyses, and reports of authorities	Drug use and urges	6 months

CS = Case study   SR = Self-report   Prof. = Professional the client's visualization and verbal description of the *intention* phase (initial thoughts about heroin), *precipitation* phase (preparation of a fix), and *action* phase (injection and the feeling of the rush). Fifteen conditioning trials were presented per session. Drug abstinence and improved marital relationships were reported by the client and his wife at an 8-month follow-up.

Spevack, Pihl, and Rowan (1973) report the successful use of electrical aversion with three adolescent, male amphetamine abusers, two of whom also had received inpatient psychotherapy, group therapy, and milieu therapy prior to aversive conditioning.

Within the context of examining conditioned abstinence, some investigators have reported the existence of "pseudo-addicts" who, while not physically dependent on drugs, report periodic drug hunger and sickness when given low doses of narcotic antagonists (Blachly, 1973; O'Brien, in press). Because of the adulterated quality of street heroin, it is hypothesized that a number of "addicts" actually are using insufficient amounts of heroin to be physically dependent. In these cases it is suggested that the self-injection ritual has become a conditioned reinforcer which supports drug habits. Blachly (1971) has proposed an electrical aversion procedure to directly treat the "needle addiction." An addict is instructed to prepare a fix (in this case a saline solution) in front of other addicts. At the time of injection, the "executive" addict receives a shock from the electric needle. At times, the entire group of addicts is attached to the apparatus and a shock is received as the "executive" addict injects. Blachly's report did not include any outcome or case study data so the efficacy of the electric needle treatment has yet to be investigated.

Chemical aversion is not presently advocated as a preferred treatment modality. The last reports of chemical aversion for drug addicts appeared in 1968. Raymond (1964) produced aversion to physeptone in a 30-year-old hospitalized female who had been abusing the drug for 6 years. Apomorphine was injected 7 minutes prior to self-injection of physeptone. This timing resulted in the pairing of drug abuse with apomorphine-produced nausea, dizziness, and vomiting. Aversion was supplemented with outpatient therapy and later the use of ECT for depression. At a 30-month follow-up, the patient had not resumed drug use. Liberman (1968) also used apomorphine in a hospital setting to produce aversion to heroin with two patients. Thirty-eight conditioning sessions were used. Periodically, the patients were asked to choose between a fix and consumables such as coffee, cigarettes, and candy. If the former were chosen, conditioning trials ensued. If something other than the drug was chosen, the patient was reinforced by the therapist with praise and extended conversation. While one patient relapsed, the other remained abstinent at a 1-year follow up. The maintenance of the second subject's improvement may have been related to the provision of numerous "booster sessions" in the treatment-reassessment interval. "Boosters" were not used with the first patient.

Thompson and Rathod (1968) report the aversive conditioning of 17 hospitalized heroin addicts with scoline-produced apneic paralysis paired with heroin injection. Admonishments about the negative effects of heroin were repeated to the patient during the paralysis. Five conditioning sessions were supplemented with individual, group, and occupational therapy. Of the 10 patients who completed treatment, eight remained drug-free at follow-ups that were as long as 30 weeks and included urinalysis as well as patient reports. Six "control" patients who left the hospital and did not receive aversion therapy had resumed their drug abuse at follow-up.

Covert sensitization offers several advantages over the use of shock or chemically induced aversion (Cautela & Rosenstiel, 1975; see also Chapter 6, this volume). Few side effects have been noted although some investigators have reported a tendency for aversive responses to generalize to nontargeted stimuli (Ashem & Donner, 1968). Special equipment or medical personnel is not required, and the procedure can be applied repeatedly in multiple environments. An additional asset is that "because the subject's own visualized experiences are used, a wide variety of conditioned and unconditioned stimuli are available and the conditioned stimuli presented in imagery may better approximate his behavior in the natural environment" (Droppa, 1973, p. 147). These advantages are balanced by the facts that some patients report difficulty in maintaining vivid imagery thereby necessitating imagery training and that precise therapist monitoring of imagery is problematic.

Anant (1968b) reported the first use of covert sensitization with a drug abuser, a 32-year-old female "addicted to tranquilizers," and with a history of alcohol abuse. Visualization of nausea was repeatedly paired with imagination of drug use and the desire for drugs. Another stage of treatment involved "aversion relief" in which imagery of drug-control behaviors was paired with termination of visualized illness. The client reported no drug use at a 3-month post-treatment assessment.

Steinfeld (1970) and his colleagues (Steinfeld, Rautio, Rice, & Egan, 1973) have used group covert sensitization with correctional inmates (primarily heroin users). Evaluation of this approach is difficult because some patients were receiving multiple treatments (e.g., encounter and traditional group therapy) (Steinfeld et al., 1973) and no follow-up was collected. Self-reports revealed no drug use at the end of treatment in seven of eight patients.

Maletzky (1974) reported an innovative supplement to covert sensitization in the treatment of 20 army outpatients, 10 of whom were abusers of alcohol with the remainder evidencing a varied history of drug dependence including paint, heroin, valium, cigarettes, marijuana, and hallucinogens. Patients were assigned to either a control group (individual counseling) or a covert sensitization procedure (in addition to counseling) in which the imagined noxious stimuli were paired with the presence of valeric acid, a chemical that produces an extremely foul odor described as having "almost human fetid properties." Comparisons at treatment termination revealed the "assisted" covert sensitization group to be significantly superior to the counseling group on self-report, authority-report, and chemical measures of drug use. Group differences were maintained at a 6-month follow-up, although the difference favoring the sensitization group on the chemical analyses was no longer significant. Unfortunately, it appears that assessments were conducted by individuals who were not "blind" to the treatment status of the participants.

Systematic Desensitization

An alternative counterconditioning approach involves the attempt to condition drug-incompatible responses to stimuli that elicit drug use. Kraft (1968) has proposed that drug use is a response intended to mitigate the social anxiety that many addicts experience. From this perspective, treatment which reduces the patient's anxiety to social stimuli also will be successful in reducing drug use (see Table 5-2).

Systematic desensitization in which the client learns to maintain a state of deep relaxation while visualizing a hierarchy of stress-eliciting scenes has been employed with some success. Kraft (1968, 1969c, 1970a,b) has reported the treatment of two hospital patients who had been addicted to drinamyl for 4 and 5 years, respectively. The basic treatment modality was systematic desensitization, although several procedures designed to facilitate generalization and maintenance of treatment effects were included. For example, *in vivo* desensitization for hierarchy items was programmed by the therapist who also gradually lengthened the intervals between treatment sessions, thus preventing clients from becoming overly dependent on the therapy contacts. A "Post-Behavior-Therapy Club" provided an opportunity for supportive interventions from both the therapist and peers. Self-report and psychometric measures converged on a judgment of substantial alleviation of social distress and elimination of drug use. Follow-up data supported the durability of these improvements. Kraft (1969b) has successfully applied a similar treatment package to a 50-year-old female with a long-standing barbiturate addiction.

Desensitization also has been applied to a young boy who was experiencing sleep disturbance and severe anxiety associated with a stressful LSD experience (Spevack et al., 1973). Multiple hierarchies were constructed and desensitization was used to reduce anxiety associated with attendance at dances, rock music, and sleep. Anxiety reduction and sleep improvement as measured by self-report, two rating scales, and a physiological measure were maintained at a follow-up 1 year after treatment.

Contingency Management

Contingency contracts. Contingency contracting has become a recently popular treatment modality with addicts. In addition to its responsiveness to the legal mandate of informed consent, contingency contracting is especially

Table 5-2

Systematic Desensitization: A Review of Target, Treatment, and Methodological Criteria

| Treatment | Study | Subjects | | | | | Treatment | | | | | | Methodology | | | |
		N	Age	Sex	Drug Use	Setting	Duration	Adjunctive Procedures	Generalization and Maintenance	Staff	Design	Dependent Measures	Targets	Follow-up
Systematic desensitization	Kraft 1968, 1969 c & 1970a, b	2	18, 20	M	Drinamyl (5, 4 yrs.)	Hospital	3 months 26 sessions and 5 months 52 sessions	—	*In vivo* practice, fading of treatment sessions, post behavior therapy club	Prof.	CS	SR and personality inventories	Drug use and social anxiety	9 months
Systematic desensitization	Kraft, 1969b	1	50	F	Phenobarbitol (12 yrs.)	Hospital	8 months 72 sessions	ECT, group psychotherapy, chemotherapy	—	Prof.	CS	SR	Drug use and social anxiety	—
Systematic desensitization	Spevack et al., 1973	1	17	M	LSD	Outpatient	2 months 10 sessions	—	—	Prof.	CS	SR, physiological measures, self-rating scales	Anxiety reduction and sleep improvement	12 months

CS = Case study   SR = Self-report   Prof. = Professional

163

well-suited to control of relevant client behavior in the natural environment. (See Table 5-3.)

Boudin (1972) employed contingency contracting to control amphetamine and barbiturate use by a black, female graduate student. Behavior of both the client and therapist for the 3-month duration of treatment was specified in a detailed treatment contract. The client was required to (a) prepare a weekly schedule of her activities, (b) contact the therapist three times each day to allow his monitoring of her activities, (c) solicit the therapist's advice regarding her handling of any "potentially dangerous situations" (ones in which the probability of using drugs was increased), (d) formally and publicly commit herself to total drug abstinence, (e) self-administer shock from a portable dispenser contingent upon drug-procurement behaviors, (f) establish a joint bank account with the therapist in which all of her money was deposited, (g) forfeit $50.00 for each instance of actual or suspected drug use (forfeiture checks were to be made payable to the Ku Klux Klan). For his part, the therapist agreed to arrange his schedule so that he was accessible to the client at all times and to countersign checks necessary to meet her living expenses.

The success of contractual arrangements depends, in part, on the therapist's willingness to enforce the agreements with the specified contingencies. In this case, the therapist exercised decisive control at three points: refused to permit the client to discontinue therapy upon her request on the fourth day of treatment; promptly paid the Ku Klux Klan $50.00 when the client reported the use of amphetamines; and established firm contingencies and stimulus control that allowed the client to complete an important research report. Follow-up 2 years later revealed the client to be drug-free.

Boudin, Valentine, Inghram, Brantley, Ruiz, Smith, Catlin, and Regan (1974) report an impressive community-based extension of the contracting approach with a large group of drug-dependent individuals the majority of whom were opiate addicts. Four types of contracts were employed as clients progressed through the treatment program. The first was a *pre-contract agreement* in which the clients were asked to make a material commitment to the project (e.g., deposit of money or some highly valued personal item) as a demonstration of their motivation. At this time, the client was asked to assume several responsibilities including frequently contacting the project by phone and in person, writing daily diaries, supplying several urine samples per week, and seeking or continuing employment.

Following this phase, which also functioned as a baseline period, a *managerial contract* was written that established an "individualized behavior program" in five areas: responsibilities, consequences, privileges, bonuses, and special considerations. Client responsibilities included behavioral requirements such as job procurement or job maintenance, drug abstinence, attendance at all meetings with treatment staff, self-monitoring of several dependent measures, making frequently scheduled phone contacts with staff, daily preparation of a diary, and adherence to a urine collection schedule. Clients were also required to establish a joint bank account with their contract manager. Contract breaches resulted in specific penalties (usually a fine) while privileges and bonuses were earned by contract compliance. Special considerations involved necessary changes in client status (e.g., treatment furlough). Krasnegor and Boudin (1973) reported the adjunctive provision of aversive conditioning, behavioral rehearsal, and marital counseling as individually needed throughout the project.

Transitional contracts were introduced as a means of reducing project structure and increasing individual responsibility for those clients who demonstrated successful performance with the managerial contract. In the final stage of treatment, clients were asked to construct *personal contracts* that established long-term objectives and the behavioral means for their attainment.

Four criteria were used to determine case outcome: (1) work and school performance, (2) personal and social adjustment, (3) drug use, and (4) arrest and conviction history. Multiple sources of criteria evaluation were employed, including self-report, clinical observation, urinalyses, agency records, peer report, and client diaries. For a client to be judged a positive case outcome, satisfactory performance must have been evident in at least three of the four criterion areas. Any incidence of extremely maladaptive adjustment (e.g., felony arrest) precluded a judgment of positive case outcome.

Data were reported for 33 clients who had participated in the project for at least 15 days. Of these, 14 were current clients while 19 had terminated treatment. Of the terminators, six were program graduates. All were evidencing positive case outcomes. Eleven clients terminated treatment against staff advice. Of these, seven were meeting positive case criteria, two were classified as negative outcomes, and the status of the other two was unknown. Two clients terminated treatment for "other reasons"; both were classified as negative outcomes. The successful adjustment of the self-terminators was especially interesting in light of the fact that some "occasional discreet use" of drugs was reported by this group while drug use was very rare among program graduates. This difference may have been an artifact of the drug preferences of the two groups; graduates were all primarily opiate users, while self-terminators tended to prefer barbiturates which are both more easily obtained and less subject to severe social surveillance and sanction than opiates, particularly heroin. Whatever the explanation, the results do suggest that abstinence and controlled use might be indicative of equally positive treatment outcomes with different types of addicts. Follow-up of program graduates (with a range of 12 to 453 days) indicated maintenance of positive effects.

Two aspects of the Florida project are particularly important. First, the program demonstrated that a comprehensive, well-integrated treatment package could be applied to a large group of quite diverse drug abusers in a natural, noninstitutional setting. Second, this is the only behaviorally oriented program that has systematically prepared paraprofessional volunteers to implement the

Table 5-3

Contingency Management: A Review of Target, Treatment, and Methodological Criteria

Treatment	Study	Subjects				Treatment					Methodology			
		N	Age	Sex	Drug Use	Setting	Duration	Adjunctive Procedures	Generalization and Maintenance	Staff	Design	Dependent Measures	Targets	Follow-up
Contingency contracting	Boudin, 1972	1	Graduate student	F	Amphetamines and barbiturates	Outpatient	3 months	—	Crisis management and phone contacts	Prof.	CS	SR	Drug use	24 months
Contingency contracting	Boudin et al., 1974	33	16-33	F	Heroin and other opiates and multiple drugs	Outpatient	Minimum of 15 days	Psychotherapy, aversive conditioning behavior rehearsal	Crisis management, in vivo monitoring of drug behaviors	Prof. & paraprofessionals	Group design	Work/school performance, urine analysis, arrest records, client observations, SR client diaries	Work/school performance, drug use, arrests, personal and social adjustment	12-453 days $\bar{x}$ = 278 days
Contingency contracting	Polakow & Doctor, 1973	2	21, 23	M F	Barbiturates	Probation	36 sessions 9 months	—	Couple-negotiated contracts	Probation official	CS	SR	Drug use new social behaviors	12 months
Token economy	O'Brien, Raynes, & Patch, 1971	150		M (135) F (15)	"Proven narcotic addition"	Hospital	30 days/group	Detoxification	—	Nonprof. (some addicts)	Group design	Behavior ratings	Self-care, social interactions, compliance and motivation, attendance	—

	N	Age	Sex	Drug	Setting	Duration	Concurrent treatment		Unit staff	Design	Outcome measures	Dependent variables	Follow-up
Token economy, contingency management Melin & Gotestam, 1973	16	$\frac{16\text{-}44}{\bar{x}=25}$	F	Amphetamine (6 mos.-13 yrs.)	Hospital	8 months	Detoxification	—		Group design with no treatment controls	Behavior observations	Ward behaviors	—
Token economy Eriksson, Gotestam, Melin, & Ost, 1975	52	$\frac{16\text{-}41}{\bar{x}=22}$	M (37) F (15)	Opiates, stimulants, and hallucinogens	Hospital	2-204 days $\bar{x}=17$ days	"Therapeutic community system"	—	Prof. and paraprofessionals	Reversal	Staff observations, urine analyses	Ward behaviors	—
Token economy Glicksman, Ottomanelli, & Cutler, 1971	32	$\frac{16\text{-}35}{\bar{x}=20.5}$	M	Heroin	Hospital	Average: 4 months	Group therapy and educational classes	—	Prof. and paraprofessionals	Group design	MMPI, staff ratings	Therapy participation, ward behaviors, educational achievement	—
Token economy Coghlan, Dohrenwend, Gold, & Zimmerman, 1973	70	12-17		Heroin (80%)	Institution	4 months	Group, milieu, and individual therapy, recreation and education services	Fading to symbolic/self-monitored reinforcement	Prof. and paraprofessionals	CS	Self-esteem survey, IE scale, staff evaluations	Self-esteem, internal control, drug use	—
Covert extinction Gotestam & Melin, 1974	4	16, 25 30, 47	F	Amphetamines	Hospital	—	—	—	Prof.	CS	SR	Drug use	9 months

CS = Case study   SR = Self-report   Prof. = Professional bulk of the intervention. The conjunctive use of paraprofessionals and an ecologically representative treatment setting is likely to increase the range of the addict population that perceives the program to be a viable one. In fact, Boudin et al. (1974) reported data that the percentage of younger and nonwhite participants subsequently has increased over the levels reflected in their initial report.

An innovative contractual agreement was introduced by Polakow and Doctor (1973) in an attempt to decelerate a young married couple's use of barbiturates and marijuana. A contingency contract was drawn between the therapist and the couple which specified that the couple must engage in one nondrug-related social activity per week, the verifiable completion of which would be reinforced by shortening total probation time by a matching week. The wife further agreed to reinforce her husband's efforts to reduce drug use and gain employment; he in turn contracted to attempt to procure a job. This was accomplished successfully 2 weeks later. Over the 36 sessions of treatment, the number of required nondrug activities was increased gradually to seven per week. The couple also received group-based training in social skills and instructions on how to negotiate their own marital contracts. At a 1-year follow-up, neither individual reported any drug use; the husband had retained his employment and marital adjustment was satisfactory.

Token economies. The institutional management of groups of addicts has been accomplished by token economies which provide for the systematization and stabilization of a contingency management system. Of the five token economies reviewed in this section, three have dealt primarily with the control of ward-adjustment behaviors (Eriksson et al., 1975; Melin & Götestam, 1973; O'Brien et al., 1971). Two token programs (Coghlan et al., 1973; Glicksman et al., 1971) have attempted to reinforce a set of behaviors that might be regarded as directly rehabilitative in nature.

O'Brien et al. (1971) employed a staff, approximately 50% of whom were ex-addicts, to apply a reinforcement program to 150 addicts. Their study included a 2-week baseline followed by a 34-week contingency phase in which patients were given access to high-frequency behaviors (passes, entertainment privileges) contingent on the performance of low-frequency behaviors such as self-care, meeting attendance, and social interactions. The contingencies in effect required that the patient perform nearly all of the specified low-frequency behaviors to receive the available reinforcers. During the treatment phase, the days on which a patient performed all targeted behaviors increased fourfold over the baseline level.

A similar program (Melin & Götestam, 1973) was developed for 16 female amphetamine addicts. During the first 4 months of its operation, the project proceeded in essentially an all-or-none fashion where the patient had to perform nearly 100% of the low-frequency behaviors to gain access to reinforcers. For the second 4-month period of the program, a procedural modification was introduced whereby the patients received a predetermined number of points for each targeted behavior performed. Twenty-five points per week were necessary to receive the privileges. This quantification of activities increased flexibility for both the patients and the staff.

Treated patients evidenced significant increases in certain ward behaviors and decreases in the doses of prescribed psychotropic drugs over their own baseline levels. At a 1-year follow-up, a higher percentage of the treatment group had remained drug abstinent than a comparison control group. However, this comparison is confounded by two factors: (1) treatment and control status of the patients were not randomly determined and therefore the two groups may have differed systematically from each other; (2) while the control group consisted of all ward members during the period immediately previous to the project, only 25% of the available and eligible patients participated in the experimental program, introducing the possibility that factors relevant to self-selection also may have influenced outcome criteria.

A second study by the Swedish group (Eriksson et al., 1975) employed an A-B-A-B-C design (A_1 and A_2 = baseline, B_1 and B_2 = token economy, and C = noncontingent reinforcement) to evaluate a refined version of their former program. Fifty-two detoxified hospitalized patients participated, although no patients were in all phases of the study and 60% participated in only one phase.

Predictably, prescribed ward behaviors such as exercise, bed-making, and total activities increased from baseline to the treatment phase, decreased upon reversal, increased with introduction of the second treatment phase, and decreased during the noncontingent reinforcement phase. During treatment phases, the proportions of drug intoxication as measured by urinalyses was lower than during the nontreatment phase. A follow-up was not conducted.

Glicksman et al. (1971) reported a program in which involuntarily committed addicts could purchase their release from the facility by accumulating a large number of points. Points were earned by the achievement of "satisfactory" performance in three areas: group therapy, educational achievement, and quality of ward behavior. The necessary points were earned in an average of 4 months by program participants; this contrasts with 7.5 months average duration of stay for residents on other wards of the institution at the same time.

Despite the author's categorization of the program as a token economy, it appeared not to include several of the expected components of a token economy. First, there were no immediate consequences or back-up reinforcers for acceptable behaviors, only the promise of release upon the attainment of the final point total. Neither were there well-specified criteria for what constituted acceptable behaviors. This deficit was illustrated by the apparent widespread disagreement among the staff concerning the quality of residents' performances. Finally, the report did not indicate that either baseline or control data were collected that could have allowed an evaluation of the program's relative impact.

Coghlan et al. (1973) combined a psychodynamic treatment model with a token economy structure to treat adolescent (age range: 12-17) drug abusers in New York City. Residents moved through four levels of the program with progress determined by staff evaluation meetings. Initial emphasis was placed on the development of behavior patterns consistent with the requirements of group, institutional living. The later stages faded out the use of a point system because of the expectation that the resident had internalized the program values of working on problems in therapy, helping peers, and participating in occupational and educational training.

Assessment of change was based on psychometric instruments (e.g., Rotter's I-E scale) and weekly or biweekly staff evaluations. The only evaluation datum reported however was the case history of one 16-year-old resident. Despite the frequent feedback which residents allegedly received, the phase-level system appeared to lack the quantification that is essential to most token economies. Behavioral targets appeared to be vaguely defined. For example, the case-study resident's behavior was defined variously as "unreasonable and irrational" (p. 775) and reflecting "negative transfer" (p. 775). Progression and demotion through the phases were determined apparently not by specific performance levels but by staff consensus that "progress" was occurring. At the time of the published report, there were no program graduates, therefore data concerning post-treatment drug use were not available.

Extinction. As previously mentioned, one principle often proposed to account for the reported success of opiate-blocking or antagonist agents is extinction of drug-produced positive reinforcement. Götestam and Melin (1974) discussed the treatment of four hospitalized amphetamine addicts using a "covert extinction" procedure in which the patients repeatedly visualized their injection ritual but were instructed to imagine that they received no "flash" or positive effect whatsoever, After 1 week of treatment, with approximately 100 extinction trials, patients reported experiencing no autonomic reactions to addiction situations. All four patients experienced some drug use during this time. At a follow-up 9 months later, three of the four patients reported no drug use; relapse of drug abuse occurred for the fourth patient 2½ months after treatment.

Multimodal Treatments

Multifaceted treatments of addicts no doubt reflect an increased appreciation of the fact that drug dependence is multiply determined, and that addicts usually are characterized by a diversity of problem complaints including physiological dependence, interpersonal deficits, social anxiety, and impoverished self-concept. Treatment strategies that respond effectively to each of these areas are likely to be associated with the greatest rehabilitative success. (See Table 5-4.) The most common multimodal behavioral approach involves the use of some form of aversion therapy to reduce drug use in combination with other procedures designed to develop or enhance the addict's functioning in other critical areas (similar programs for alcoholics are discussed in Chapter 6). O'Brien, Raynes, and Patch (1972) successfully used a multimodal behavioral approach to treat a poly-drug user and a heroin addict. Following detoxification, the patients were trained to relax themselves to reduce the tension that often preceded drug use. Electrical aversion also was used to decelerate drug use. Extensive verbal descriptions of the patients' usual drug craving, procurement, and use sequence were associated with painful shock. At a later point, electrical aversion therapy was replaced by a form of covert sensitization. Finally, systematic desensitization was administered to reduce the arousal properties of stimuli that were elicitors of anxiety and craving.

Treatment was effective in eliminating drug use in both clients at follow-up (14 months for one person and 6 months for the other). The follow-up status of the first person was noteworthy. While on a hospital pass, she was forcibly injected with Numorphan and later self-administered an injection of heroin. Despite this setback, the subsequent use of three booster sessions following treatment facilitated drug abstinence in this patient as assessed at follow-up.

O'Brien and Raynes (1972) used a similar combination of therapy components in the treatment of three heroin addicts. Two of the patients were drug-abstinent at 6- and 9-month follow-ups, respectively. The third patient resumed drug use shortly after treatment termination.

A variety of covert techniques was used by Wisocki (1973) for the outpatient treatment of a heroin addict with a history of multiple drug abuse. Three behavioral goals were identified: elimination of heroin use, improvement of self-concept, and development of "pro-social behaviors." Across 12 treatment sessions, the therapist applied covert reinforcement, covert sensitization, and thought stopping to the appropriate targets. Follow-up at 18 months revealed substantial improvements in all three areas. Drug use had not occurred.

Polakow (1975) treated a probated barbiturate addict with the simultaneous use of covert sensitization, behavioral rehearsal, and contingency contracting. This contract was similar to that of the Polakow and Doctor (1973) report in which successful completion of therapy assignments resulted in 1-week reductions in total probation time. Self-report and agency records indicated that the client was drug free and had maintained employment 18 months after treatment.

A few studies have combined methadone maintenance with behaviorally based procedures for the treatment of heroin addicts. Failure in methadone maintenance programs often is attributed to multiple drug use, especially alcohol (Perkins & Bloch, 1971). In addition, it is suspected that methadone treatment may result in increased use of alcohol. In an attempt to reduce the possibility of an alcohol-related failure in a methadone maintenance program, Liebson and Bigelow (1972) supplied methadone contingent on continued disulfiram therapy

Table 5-4

Multimodal Treatments: A Review of Target, Treatment, and Methodological Criteria

Treatment	Study	Subjects					Treatment				Methodology			
		N	Age	Sex	Drug Use	Setting	Duration	Adjunctive Procedures	Generalization and Maintenance	Staff	Design	Dependent Measures	Targets	Follow-up
Relaxation training electrical aversion, SDS covert sensitization	O'Brien, Raynes, & Patch, 1972	2	24, 30	M, F	Heroin, multidrug use	Hospital	19, 27 sessions	--	Booster sessions for one patient	Prof.	CS	SR, self-ratings of drug craving	Drug use and anxiety	6, 14 months
Aversion therapy, SDS, relaxation training	O'Brien & Raynes, 1972	3	--	--	Heroin, at least 10 yrs.	Hospital	17-46 sessions	--	Booster sessions, partial reinforcement schedule	Prof.	CS	SR	Drug use	6, 9 months
Covert reinforcement, thought stopping, covert sensitization	Wisocki, 1973	1	26	M	Heroin and other drugs	Out-patient	12 sessions; 9 months	--	Homework assignments	Prof.	CS	SR, clinical observations	Drug use, self-concept, social functioning	18 months
Covert sensitization, behavior rehearsal, contingency contracting	Polakow, 1975	1	24	F	Barbiturate	Probation	15 months 60 sessions	--	Home practice, promotion of nondrug activities	Probation official	CS	SR	Drug use	18 months

Technique	Author	N	Age	Sex	Problem	Setting	Duration	Comparison	Procedure	Staff	Design	Measures	Dependent variables	Follow-up
Methadone; contingency management	Liebson & Bigelow, 1972	1	36	M	Alcohol, barbiturates, amphetamines	Outpatient	3 years	--	Daily administration of drug regime and contingency program	Prof.	CS	Urine analysis, informal observations	Drug use and drinking	3 years
Methadone maintenance, and contingency management	Bigelow, Lawrence, Harris, & D'Lugoff, 1974	80	20-25	M (80%)	Drug abuse "over 5 yrs. duration"	Outpatient	1-39 weeks	"Supportive counseling"	--	6 counselors	2 X 2 group design	Urine analysis, arrests, employment	Drug use, arrests, social productivity	--
Methadone maintenance SDS, self-image training, behavior rehearsal, assertion training	Cheek, Tomarchio Standen, & Albahary, 1973	21 / 12	x̄=26 / x̄=26	M / F	Heroin	Inpatient methadone program	8 sessions; 4 weeks	Psychological, vocational, and legal supports	In vivo practice, "take-home" workbooks	Prof.	group design	Test scores, Program Evaluation questionnaire	Anxiety control, self-image, assertion, internal control	3, 6 months

CS = Case study   SR = Self-report   Prof. = Professional

173

by a client with an 18-year history of alcohol abuse and a 12-year history of opiate addiction. The reinforcing properties of methadone rendered it an ideal consequence for the contingency management of disulfiram-taking. Despite previous failures with AA, hospitalization, and disulfiram therapy, the client had not resumed opiate or alcohol use after 3 years on the contingency schedule.

Bigelow et al. (1974) have evaluated the contributions of contingency management (the major reinforcer being medication take-home privileges) and "behavior therapy" (anxiety reduction techniques) to a methadone maintenance and supportive counseling program. A factorial study of these approaches yielded the following four treatment cells: behavior therapy, contingency management, combined behavior therapy and contingency management, and supportive counseling only.

At the time of the report, 80 volunteers had participated in the program; however, the majority of clients from whom preliminary data had been gathered had been in their assigned treatment for less than 20 weeks. Therefore, small group size and truncated treatment precluded meaningful between-group comparisons. Some suggestive evidence of relative treatment effects were discussed. First, the percentage of clients engaged in such activities as work or school increased as time in treatment increased. For those persons participating in their assigned treatment for at least a duration of 20 weeks, the two modalities which utilized contingency management were associated with the largest percentage of full-time employment. Urinalysis results indicated that the rate of poly-drug use remained quite high in the population and was not reliably differentiated between treatment modalities. However, the great majority of positive tests were sedative-tranquilizer positives rather than narcotic-quinine positives. Parametric evaluations and subsequent reassessments of these outcomes must await the enlargement of sample sizes and the passage of sufficient post-treatment time for adequate follow-up.

Cheek, Tomarchio, Standen, and Albahary (1973) have used a rich variety of behavioral techniques to facilitate self-control in a group of inpatient methadone-maintained addicts. Male and female residents took part in similar but separate group sessions in which the procedures of relaxation training, desensitization, behavioral rehearsal, self-image training, and assertion training were presented. Group discussion and practice of the techniques were emphasized, and daily practice sessions were also provided.

Measures of anxiety, locus of control, self-image, and assertiveness were employed to determine the immediate effects of the program. Thirty-three residents were assessed. Pre-post comparisons of "treatment subjects" revealed a significant decrease in anxiety level, a significant increase in level of self-esteem, and significant enhancement of internal control. There were no control or comparison groups.

Outcome status at 6 months for those residents who participated in the behavior modification program was compared to a group of addicts who graduated from the facility prior to implementation of the behavioral project. Fifty-eight percent of the behavior modification group was rated by social workers as achieving a successful adjustment while 40% of the comparison group was so rated. This difference was not statistically significant.

Evaluation

The history of behavioral treatments of drug dependency is relatively limited. Only 13 years have passed since Raymond's report of aversion therapy with an opiate addict, an account representing the first published, well-circulated documentation of behavior therapy as the principal intervention for drug abuse. All but one (Thompson & Rathod, 1968) of the studies employing either a group or within-subject design have appeared since 1971. Given this abbreviated ancestry, it should not be surprising that behavioral drug treatments have yet to achieve the clinical or methodological maturity that should typify future programs. The remainder of this chapter presents five recommendations for bolstering both the empirical status and clinical sophistication of behavior modification with drug abuse.

Patient Characteristics

The modal recipient of behavioral treatments can be distinguished on multiple dimensions from the general population of drug abusers or specific subsamples of that population. In his assessment of the generalizability of behavioral drug treatment research, Callner (1975) concluded that, for the most part, the research "did not select subjects that represented good examples of 'street addicts' or addicts entering treatment programs under duress from the courts" (pp. 153-154). Estimates of racial characteristics, for example, suggest that more than 50% of hard-core addicts come from nonwhite populations (Cohen, 1970). Only 21% of the reviewed behavioral treatments reported the racial composition of the subjects. Based on this somewhat inadequate sample, the percentage of nonwhite treatment recipients was only 34.1%.

In general, patients in behavioral programs are characterized by a set of features that is not only discrepant from the historical background of most addicts but is also associated with a clinically favorable prognosis. This has been especially true of single-subject case studies. The participants in two programs were a college graduate (Wisocki, 1973) and a college senior (Lesser, 1967). Wolpe's (1965) patient was a young physician, while Boudin's (1972) and Lubetkin and Fishman's (1974) were graduate students. Over 50% of the 33 participants in the Boudin et al. (1974) program had obtained at least a high school education. Approximately 25% of these persons had attended college. Few reports include sufficient descriptions of participants' educational background, occupational status, criminal record, financial resources, and marital status to allow any assessment of the generalizability of treatment effects. Increased attention to such variables is necessary for an appraisal of the extent to which demographics place boundary limitations on the efficacy of behavioral treatments.

Descriptive information relevant to the pattern and intensity of drug abuse among patients is seldom included in the behavioral literature. While behavioral treatments have been applied to a wide array of abused drugs, the literature has failed to discuss how these treatments interact with a number of drug-use parameters. Length of abuse, daily dosage level, pharmacological effects of the abused drug, expense of habit, quality and duration of withdrawal symptoms (if any), and extent of poly-drug use are variables that are likely to affect drug abusers' motivation and ability for changes as well as clinicians' strategies for generating and maintaining them.

Setting of Treatment

In Chapter 4 the concept of "ecological conventionality" was introduced as a description of the tendency for behaviorally oriented corrections to be restricted to institutional settings. In the drug abuse area there has also been an extended inattention to the effects of the treatment environment as it relates to the outcome and durability of behavioral treatment programs. Over 50% of behavioral treatments have been applied to inpatients in either a hospital, correctional institution, or special residential facility. The great majority of these appear to involve voluntary admissions to general or psychiatric hospitals; only occasionally are these programs administered to involuntarily committed patients (Glicksman et al., 1971) or correctional institution inmates (Steinfeld et al., 1973). Approximately 41% (12 studies) of the programs delivered services to outpatients or were conducted in a natural setting. In most of these cases, outpatient status refers to the one-to-one delivery of psychological services to a client by a psychotherapist.

While there is virtual unanimity of preference for the community-based treatment of other types of offenders, there is a lack of consensus on the recommended setting for the rehabilitation of drug abusers. Many claim that hospitalization and/or civil commitment is a desirable, if not necessary, condition for addict treatment. The argument for involuntary or coerced treatment is predicated on the observation that few addicts voluntarily become abstinent (Vaillant, 1970). From this perspective, hospitalization allows complete detoxification, medical supervision of the withdrawal syndrome, interruption of a pro-drug lifestyle, diminution of anti-social behavior if even for a short period, and the introduction of a usually multifaceted rehabilitation program. On the other hand, the development of programs such as methadone maintenance has increased substantially the prospects for successful treatment of heroin addicts in the natural environment. Outpatient programs allow the abuser to obtain or maintain employment as well as avoid the stigma which commitment produces. A methadone- or narcotic antagonist-aided community placement is also likely to increase the likelihood of directly extinguishing the conditioned abstinence syndrome which is thought to potentiate resumption of drug use in many cases. Forced treatment procedures may have some face validity for addictive substances, however they appear unnecessary or undesirable for abusers of nonaddictive substances where the risks of adverse physical sequelae are not as great.

Together with the aforementioned demographic descriptions, the typically utilized treatment settings suggest that participants in most behavioral programs are a somewhat "sanitized" subsample of the abuser population. This is particularly ironic in light of the frequent championing of behavioral treatments' suitability for non-YAVIS (Young-Attractive-Verbal-Intelligent-Successful; Schofield, 1964) patients. if there is a unifying feature of these patients, it is that most of them possess a level of motivation for treatment which is not found in the totally or partially coercive contexts of many drug programs.

Behavioral programs should begin to examine empirically the intuitively suspected interactions between treatment techniques and the environments in which they are delivered. As with factorial investigations of psychotherapy (e.g., Paul, 1969a) the goal of this research would be a determination of maximally effective treatment-ecological setting combinations for specific classes of abusers. For example, procedures designed to promote social skills or reduce social anxiety in individuals who are dependent on nonaddicting drugs and who lack a history of criminal activity might be implemented successfully in community settings. On the other hand, individuals whose treatment includes an initial period of detoxification or who are unable to resist continued drug use might benefit most from a period of sojourn in an inpatient facility.

Ideally, the residential component of any drug rehabilitation program could be kept to a minimum. The sequential programming of residential treatment followed by nonresidential after-care services would have several therapeutic advantages and could be easily achieved within a behavioral framework. Rate of progress through the inpatient portion of the program could be individualized and made contingent on the attainment of specific behavioral objectives (e.g., Glicksman et al., 1971) while after-care could be structured along the lines of the contractual model of probation (e.g., Polakow, 1975).

Maintenance and Generalizability of Treatment Effects

The effectiveness of behavior therapies in bringing about short-term, relatively circumscribed improvements in the behavioral functioning of drug abusers has not been established conclusively, although the existing pattern of results is consistent with the prediction that properly designed research will allow such a conclusion. A remaining problem in the field is the failure to develop and systematically assess procedures deliberately designed to promote transfer of recently developed repertoires to natural settings and maintain these repertoires over time.

A consistent omission of most behavioral treatments of drug dependency has been the failure to train clients to deal effectively with the environmental and interpersonal pressures for resumption of drug abuse. This deficit is critical because the consequences which follow a client's post-therapy performance of newly developed and uncertain skills (e.g., assertion, refusal of drugs) certainly will affect both maintenance and generalization of reduction of drug use. Of these 29 studies, 18 (62%) included treatment procedures intended to institute or enhance the maintenance and/or generalization of treatment effects. The most frequently employed generalization procedure has been to instruct the client in the *in vivo* use of such techniques as relaxation (Steinfeld et al., 1973), aversive counterconditioning (Wolpe, 1965), and covert sensitization (Wisocki, 1973). "Booster sessions" involving the reintroduction of conditioning trials (e.g., Liberman, 1968) following treatment termination have been used to fortify prior treatments and make post-therapy change more permanent. Kraft (1969c) attempted to insure the permanence of drug abstinence by combining several generalization/maintenance procedures including *in vivo* desensitzation, the gradual fading of treatment sessions, and the provision of a "Post-Behavior-Therapy Club" where ex-clients could meet to discuss mutual problems. It is possible that durability of behaviors incompatible with drug abuse could be enhanced by procedures which attempt to develop complex, sequential repertoires that allow clients to maintain a desired position in spite of social pressures to the contrary. For example, Nietzel, Martorano, and Melnick (1976) demonstrated that unassertive subjects who received a covert modeling treatment supplemented by "reply training" (learning effective responses for noncompliance to initial assertive behaviors) improved significantly more on post-test and generalization measures than untreated subjects or those who received covert modeling without the reply training. Addicts frequently find themselves in situations where refusal of offered drugs requires sustained assertion across verbal exchanges. The addition of a reply training component to larger drug-treatment packages might enhance the addicts' ability to confront peers with whom the risk of relapse is greatest. The establishment of complex sequential social skills also is discussed extensively in Chapter 8.

At this point, there have been no evaluations of the impact generated by the preplanned application of generalization/maintenance procedures derived from social learning principles. The need for such evaluation is obvious. In addition to directing researchers' attention to the methodological issues involved in follow-up assessments, such evaluations hopefully can assist clinicians develop treatment packages that are effective, not only in reducing drug abuse and related problems, but insuring the transfer and preservation of these outcomes.

Methodology

The empirical evaluations of behavioral drug-abuse programs display little methodological excellence. The only scientifically defensible conclusion to be drawn from the current literature is that a series of consistently confounded studies yield consistently optimistic results about the efficacy of behavioral treatments. At this time, there is not a single study in the area with the research design sufficient to eliminate numerous threats to the internal validity of the results.

The state of research affairs has changed little from that observed in previous reviews (Callner, 1975; Droppa, 1973; P. Miller, 1973a). Of the 29 studies summarized in Tables 5-1 to 5-4, 20 (69%) were case studies, eight (28%) were group designs, and one study (Eriksson et al., 1975) was a reversal design. Callner's (1975) review of 22 studies classified 75% as case studies and 26% as single-subject or group designs. While the additional studies included in the present review increase slightly the percentage of group designs, this increase does not reflect an increment in the level of research product. Of the eight group designs, four were nonfactorial single-group designs in which all subjects were assigned to the experimental condition. Two studies compared treated subjects with a group of untreated controls; however, in neither of these were subjects randomly assigned to their group status or drawn from the same population. One study (Maletsky, 1974) compared subjects who were assigned randomly to either a covert sensitization treatment or individual counseling. Only one factorial study has been reported (Bigelow, Lawrence, et al., 1974), but the small number of subjects who had completed the program disallowed any parametric comparisons. While one study (Eriksson et al., 1975) was described as a within-subjects reversal design, none of the subjects was exposed to all of the sequential manipulations, thereby disqualifying its justification as a true within-subject design.

The use of case studies to generate and evaluate low-level treatment hypotheses has been pursued sufficiently. The area is in need of well-controlled single-subject designs employing either reversal or multiple baseline procedures. Tactically, these studies would precede the use of factorial designs which would allow an unconfounded evaluation of numerous independent domains.

Assessment of the permanence of treatment-instigated alteration in drug use is an absolute necessity of research seeking to evaluate the efficacy of any therapeutic technique. Sixty-nine percent of the reviewed studies included a follow-up assessment of drug use and related changes. The median follow-up interval was 10 months. While 80% of the case studies reported systematic follow-up data, only 50% of the group-design studies did so. This difference may be due to the fact that follow-ups of several individuals multiply the administrative-logistical impediments to these types of assessments.

The advantages of long-term assessment must be weighed against practical disadvantages, increased subject attrition, and consequent unrepresentativeness of the remaining sample. However most criteria would require a more extensive follow-up than the year or less interval evidenced by the typical behavioral investigation. Vaillant (1970) has suggested that final remission of drug dependency occurs only after the passage of lengthy intervals of time, perhaps 5 years or more. The necessity for the abuser to establish and refine a drug-free pattern of life may render short-term follow-ups inadequate for a determination of the ultimate success of behavioral treatments. Perhaps the best solution to the follow-up problem is a longitudinal-type compromise suggested by Collier and Hijazi (1974) in which follow-up data are collected and reported periodically at regular intervals over an extended period of time.

For the most part, behavioral drug-abuse treatments have not been evaluated by diverse sources of outcome measurement. The development and use of multisource measures are essential for evaluation of various interventions (Berzins, Bednar, & Severy, 1975) and are particularly needed in instances in which the problem to be modified manifests itself in diverse manners (criminal record, unemployment, social functioning, physical health, and psycho-pathology). Thirty-four percent of the 29 studies reviewed employed only self-report measures of such criteria as drug use and social adjustment. While the reliability of self-reports of drug use tend to be quite high (Cox & Longwell, 1974), and while the reports from the direct consumer of services may be the single most important source of outcome evaluation, the multifaceted nature of therapeutic change (Cartwright, Kirtner, & Fiske, 1963) would seem to require that researchers concern themselves with multimethod assessments. Only 52% of these studies supplemented self-reports with peer ratings, third-party observations, or psychometric assessments. Despite the recent proliferation of chemical analyses (DeAngelis, 1973), only 21% of these reports utilized any form of this type of assessment.

In addition to the use of preplanned, sequential follow-ups and the expanded use of chemical analyses, Callner (1975) has offered three other recommendations for the enrichment of dependent measures related to drug dependency. First, researchers could increase the number of dependent measures by partitioning the concept of drug dependency into smaller behavioral, cognitive, and emotional components. For example, Boudin et al. (1974) monitored drug urges, ratings of social discomfort, etc. by having patients record drug-relevant behaviors in a personal diary.

Second, quality of outcome assessments would be bolstered by the development of either *in vivo* and/or unobtrusive measures of patients' responses to naturalistic problem situations. For example, refusals of drug offers, assertive solutions to peer pressure, and avoidance of high-risk situations or associates are discrete behaviors likely to make sustained reductions of drug use more probable.

Callner's final recommendation is that researchers increase their use of "ongoing program performance measures." These would include either naturalistic or contrived assessments of "observable and verifiable performance of tasks while the patient is in treatment, designed to assess his ability to deal with the difficult problems likely to occur after treatment termination" (p. 158).

Patient-Treatment and Patient-Therapist Matching

While the rhetoric of behaviorally oriented clinicians bespeaks at least their token appreciation of the need to tailor treatments to clients' individual differences, behavior modifiers of drug abuse seem to have relegated "personality variables to the domain of error or nuisance variance in making psychotherapy more effective" (Berzins, in press). Kiesler (1966) has referred to this failure to distinguish between the personological lineaments of psychotherapy recipients as the "patient uniformity myth."

The existing literature indicates that drug abusers are best characterized by their heterogeneity. Marked variability has been demonstrated empirically for such psychological factors as field dependence (Arnon, Kleinman, & Kissin, 1974), time perspective (Stein & Rozynko, 1974), and value preferences (J. Miller, Sensenig, Stocker, & Campbell, 1973). Similarly, the stereotype of the drug abuser as a psychopath has been disputed by research that reflects drug dependence to be associated with neurotic, characterological, and psychotic symptomatology (Monroe, Ross, & Berzins, 1971; Stein & Rozynko, 1974). Finally, numerous demographic characteristics distinguish abusers of different drugs (Lewis & Trickett, 1974).

It is not possible to discuss all the practical implications which abuser heterogeneity raises for the design of drug rehabilitation programs. However, an example will illustrate the variance-reducing potential that might be developed from more deliberate attention to patient-technique or patient-therapist matching.

One clear trend in most nonbehaviorally oriented drug treatment programs is the use of volunteers and nonprofessionals in the delivery of program services (Dwarshuis, Kolton, & Gorodezsky, 1973). Despite the widespread use of nonprofessionals, there are few empirically established principles to indicate when their use would be most appropriate.

One study has addressed the issue by producing data relevant to the purposeful and selective use of nonprofessionals in drug rehabilitation. Berzins and Ross (1972) required 60 female addicts to make a forced choice between two very similar stimulus items (e.g., state a preference for a tan versus a maroon car). Subjects were tested twice within a 3-day interval. During the retest period, subjects were given information that allegedly portrayed the choices made by either the professional staff or an addict peer. The influence agents' choice was represented as being consonant or dissonant (an equal number of times) from the addicts' initial choice. Addicts were trichotomized into low, moderate, and high subgroups on each of four psychological measures (the Ego Strength scale,

Acceptability for Psychotherapy scale, and Identification with Addicts scale, and a Maladjustment Index based on elevated MMPI clinical scales).

The major findings indicated that low ego strength or, conversely, high scores on the Maladjustment Index predicted greater reactivity to the alleged choices of addict peers than of a professional. The patients who were better adjusted responded significantly more frequently to professional than to peer influence. The fact that addict subgroups responded differentially to professional and peer influences in an analogue situation led the authors to suggest "the potential desirability of adding rehabilitative addicts to the treatment when the patient population includes seriously maladjusted addicts" (Berzins & Ross, 1972, p. 147).

Only a handful of behavioral treatment programs have utilized para- or nonprofessionals on any systematic basis. In none of these cases was there a concern for the deliberate, optimal matching of patients with professional versus nonprofessional. The Boudin et al. (1974) project did develop an extensive training program which enabled nonprofessionals to ultimately assume the majority of treatment responsibilities. An interesting question would be whether such training might also have attenuated some of the advantages which nonprofessionals may have with particularly deviant patients.

This last issue is illustrative of many of the problems in the drug abuse area. The provision of data upon which treatment decisions can be based must await the formulation of the necessary research questions. At this time, there is little indication of a strong commitment to the asking of such questions. Both researchers and clinicians seem to be content with case-level demonstrations of short term treatment success. In the absence of more ambitious empirical goals, behavioral approaches to drug abuse will likely fail to emerge as anything more than a set of techniques whose suitability is limited to a narrow range of patients, treatment settings, and therapeutic personnel.

Chapter 6
ALCOHOLISM

Alcoholism is one of our most demanding social-health problems. Estimates of the number of alcoholics range from 5,000,000 (Chafetz, 1967; Ullmann & Krasner, 1975) to 10,000,000 (O'Leary & Wilson, 1975; Wilkinson, 1970). Disagreements over the defining criteria of "alcoholic," "problem drinker," and "social drinker" probably account for this widely discrepant range (Franks, 1970). Even the largest estimates substantially underestimate the impact of alcohol abuse. It has been suggested that for every alcoholic five to six additional persons are exposed to the disruptive, destructive consequences of alcoholism (O'Leary & Wilson, 1975). Further, the number of alcoholics is rapidly growing; approximately 200,000 additional cases are added per year (Ullmann & Krasner, 1975).

Alcohol abuse has been associated with diverse indicators of social malaise and disruption. Up to 50% of the first admissions to psychiatric hospitals are alcoholics (Ullmann & Krasner, 1975). More than half of fatal and/or injurious traffic accidents involve at least one drunken driver (Wilkinson, 1970). A number of chronic and severe illnesses have been associated with alcoholism—for example, heart disease, cirrhosis of the liver, and alcoholic psychosis (Sanders, 1970; Wallgren & Barry, 1970). Criminal behavior and life-threatening activities also are related to drunkenness (Haberman & Baden, 1974). For example, one of every three arrests in this country is for public drunkenness (Morris & Hawkins, 1970). It is estimated that one-third to one-half of all felons were to some degree under the influence of alcohol when they committed their crimes (Kittrie, 1971). Homicide and suicide are more frequent among alcoholics than nonalcoholics (Blum & Braunstein, 1967; Goodwin, 1973). Annually, thousands of cases of irreversible birth defects are linked to fetal alcohol syndrome occurring in about 50% of the births to alcoholic mothers.

The economic reverberations of alcoholism are staggering. The cost of alcoholism to our economy is somewhere between $10-15 billion per year. These costs include losses due to absenteeism, illness, industrial accidents, lessened productivity, and the expense of social control practices such as arrest, treatment, and hospitalization.

The widespread abuse of alcohol is due in part to the fact that use of alcohol is socially approved. Approximately 70-80 million Americans use alcohol on a recreational, ceremonial, or routine basis, spending over $25 billion to consume more than 400 million gallons of alcohol annually (Licensed Beverage Industries, 1973). Historically, society's responses to alcohol have been ambivalent. While the overuser generally is condemned, principled abstainers are mistrusted or ridiculed. In this regard, Ullman (1958) has concluded that there is a relationship between inconsistent, poorly integrated cultural attitudes toward drinking and high rates of alcoholism.

As one illustration, alcohol has been vigorously disapproved and selectively prescribed in religious writings. The Old Testament warns, "Wine is a mocker, strong drink a brawler; and whoever is led astray by it is not wise," and later instructs, "Drink no wine nor strong drink, you nor your sons with you, when you go into the tent of meeting, lest you die." However, the New Testament writer, Timothy, advised, "No longer drink only water, but use a little wine for the sake of your stomach and your frequent ailments."

While our culture continues to provide conflicting conditions that simultaneously proscribe and prescribe alcohol use, society's approach to alcoholism appears to have become progressively more objective (Nathan, 1976). Temperance and prohibition movements have gradually given way to conceptualizations which emphasize medical, physiological, and social-psychological factors and treatments which have become progressively more comprehensive and elaborate. Many of these developments are illustrated well by the social learning programs which are the primary focus of this chapter.

Classification of Alcoholics

Two major systems exist for the classification of alcohol abusers. The more official schema is provided by the Diagnostic and Statistical Manual of the American Psychiatric Association (DSM-II; 1968) where differential diagnosis of alcohol-related problems is made on the basis of presenting physical and social-psychological complaints. Heavy drinking resulting in tissue impairment (either acute or chronic) is categorized under "psychoses associated with organic brain syndromes" as "alcoholic psychoses." This category is subdivided further into "delirium tremens," "Korsakov's psychosis," "other alcoholic hallucinosis," "alcohol paranoid state," "acute alcohol intoxication," "alcoholic deterioration," "pathological intoxication," and "other (and unspecified) alcoholic psychosis."

When alcohol use is great enough to interfere with health, personal or social functioning, or has become a prerequisite to normal functioning, the syndrome is classified as "alcoholism" under the general category of "personality disorders and certain other nonpsychotic mental disorders." DSM-II describes the following four subcategories of alcoholism: "episodic excessive drinking" (intoxicated as often as four times per year), "habitual excessive drinking" (intoxicated more than 12 times per year or "under the influence of alcohol" weekly), "alcohol addiction" (direct or presumptive evidence that the person is dependent on alcohol; dependence can be of either a psychological nature in which alcohol use is the typical response to a diversity of situations or of a physiological nature in which withdrawal symptoms and habituation are present), and "other (and unspecified) alcoholism."

Jellinek's (1960) classification schema is a widely cited one and is based on a description of the patterns which excessive drinking may take in different individuals or cultures. Four major varieties of alcoholism are described. The *Alpha* alcoholic uses alcohol frequently to reduce bodily or emotional stress but has not lost control over his drinking. The *Beta* alcoholic suffers physical complications such as malnutrition and cirrhosis of the liver. Loss of control may not have occurred. *Gamma* alcoholism is characterized by loss of control over drinking, increased tissue tolerance to alcohol, and withdrawal symptoms. American and Canadian inebriates are predominantly *Gamma* alcoholics. *Delta* alcoholism is also represented by loss of control despite the fact that intake can be regulated at any given point. Wine drinking countries (e.g., France) frequently contain many *Delta* alcoholics.

Theories of Alcoholism

Reviews of alcoholism (Nathan, 1976; Nathan & Briddell, in press; Nathan & Harris, 1975) have identified four major theoretical approaches to the etiology of alcoholism. Nonetheless, confusion and disagreement concerning the causative factors of alcoholism are likely to plague us for some time; Nathan's concise evaluation, "no definitive etiology of alcoholism has been established" (1976, p. 5) does not appear to face impending refutation.

Physiological Theories

Chafetz and Demone (1962) have discussed a food addiction theory which proposes that certain people are particularly sensitive to specific food grains capable of producing temporary tension reduction. Some of these grains happen to be ones from which alcoholic beverages are derived.

Alcoholics have been hypothesized to differ from nonalcoholics in their ability to metabolize alcohol. One theory identified the adrenal cortex as the site responsible for metabolic disturbance (J. J. Smith, 1949). While such theories are logically defensible, recent empirical evidence (e.g., Mendelson, 1968) has failed to document different rates of alcohol metabolism between alcoholics and nonalcoholics.

Alcohol abuse also has been linked to the notion of nutritional deficiencies (R. J. Williams, 1959). Early animal research on the topic indicated that vitamin-deficient rats' intake of alcohol in a choice situation was reduced by provision of a nutritional diet. However, other data (e.g., Lester & Greenberg,

1952) have suggested that choice of alcohol may be an artifact of taste preferences.

Nathan (1976) reports an active interest in possible genetic predispositions to alcoholism. Support for such a view stems from the convergence of twin studies, adoption research, and animal experimentation upon the conclusion that genetic factors are implicated in the development of alcoholism.

Sociocultural Theories

Several reliable differences in rates of alcoholism have been found among persons with different geographic, demographic, and cultural-religious backgrounds. Individuals from countries such as China or Italy in which alcohol use is endorsed only in well-defined, circumscribed, or ceremonial settings evidence low rates of alcoholism. On the other hand, the rates of alcoholism are high in some Western European countries (e.g., Ireland) where alcohol is used in a diversity of social settings and is viewed as instrumental in producing individual gratification. The importance of cultural influences is supported further by data indicating that rates of alcoholism become more similar among second- and third-generation, immigrant Americans; alcoholism rates increase in groups formerly displaying low rates, while the reverse is true for groups whose initial incidence was low.

Numerous types of demographic variables have been related to the prevalence of alcoholism. For example, males are classified as alcoholic much more often than females, although females may develop chronic alcoholism more quickly than men (Rosen, Fox, & Gregory, 1972). Members of certain occupations, notably bartenders, housepainters, cooks, restaurant workers, and seamen have elevated rates of alcoholism (Hitz, 1973).

While sociocultural influences may predispose individuals to excessive drinking, more specific social learning variables probably are involved in the determination of actual alcohol addiction (Nathan & Harris, 1975). Bandura has concluded in this regard that, "Normative injunctions alone do not explain either the relatively low incidence of *addictive drinking* in social groups that positively sanction the use of alcoholic beverages, or the occurrence of chronic alcoholism in cultures prohibiting intoxicants" (Bandura, 1969, p. 534).

Psychological Theories

The attempt to identify an "alcoholic personality" appears to be a futile pursuit (Lemere, 1953; Syme, 1957; Zax & Cowen, 1972). While some reviewers remain sympathetic to the validity of the concept (e.g., Franks, 1970), the major problem appears to be a continuing failure of pre-morbid personality descriptions to be cross-validated against new samples of alcoholics.

A wide array of psychodynamically oriented theories have speculated on possible relationships between problem drinking and a number of psychological determinants. The alcoholic's basic conflict has been viewed variously as the outgrowth of a too nurturant mother-child relationship (Knight, 1937), a too deprived mother-child relationship (Abraham, 1926), the revenge of an adult toward a malicious mother (Bergler, 1946), and a repressed mother fixation (Fromm & Maccoby, 1970). Other theorists have viewed alcoholic behavior as a form of suicide motivated by deep-seated guilt or hostility (Menninger, 1938). Several interpretations of drinking have emphasized its defensive functions with respect to such conflicts as repressed homosexuality (Freud, 1930), feelings of inferiority (Adler, 1941), and interpersonal insecurities and inhibitions (Schilder, 1941).

Behavioral Theories

Behaviorally oriented approaches to alcoholism etiology have sought to respond effectively to some of the deficits associated with sociocultural and psychodynamic theories. For this reason, emphasis has been placed on the formulation of concepts which (1) allow empirical verification, (2) identify specific antecedents and consequences likely to influence drinking parameters, and (3) can be linked to the development of treatment techniques capable of some demonstrable regulation of aberrant drinking   Learning-based formulations initially explained excessive drinking in terms of the reinforcing properties of alcohol. The rewarding qualities of alcohol have been divided into three general categories, each of which illustrates what has become perhaps the most basic tenet of behavioral theories of alcoholism: "Alcohol consumption is a widely generalized dominant response to aversive stimulation" (Bandura, 1969, p. 536).

1.   The most widely endorsed view of alcohol's reinforcing effects is the tension-reduction hypothesis, which holds that alcoholics drink to help mitigate tension states (e.g., fear, approach-avoidance conflict) or to avoid situations which they perceive as particularly aversive. Evidence for the tension-reduction hypothesis has been derived from animal experimentation on conditioned avoidance behaviors (Conger, 1956; Masserman & Yum, 1946; Smart, 1965), human research on the disinhibiting effects of alcohol (Bruun, 1959), the relationship between drinking and interpersonal stress (P. M. Miller, Hersen, Eisler, & Hilsman, 1974), self-reports by problem drinkers on the precipitating effects of stress (Hershenson, 1965), and the widely recognized ability of central nervous system depressants to reduce emotional arousal.

2.   Intoxication also is seen as reinforcing by virtue of the fact that otherwise inappropriate or disapproved behaviors are legitimized by the supposedly disinhibiting effects of alcohol. From this perspective, intoxication functions as a discriminative stimulus for the performance of behaviors which if displayed under sober conditions (S^Δ) would be either socially condemned or considered incompatible with pre-existing self-concepts. The pattern and existence of alcohol-disinhibited behaviors may be culturally determined (MacAndrew & Edgerton, 1969); in the United States alcoholics are most likely

to selectively display examples of seductive, aggressive, dependent, or unexpected sexual behaviors.

3. Sustained heavy use of alcohol will be maintained secondarily by the
person's attempt to avoid the unpleasant physical reactions associated with
lower blood-alcohol concentration levels. Following the development of physical
dependence, use of alcohol will be negatively reinforced because of its ability to
alleviate and/or prevent the severe symptoms of the withdrawal syndrome.

While the emphasis on the reinforcing properties of alcohol is blessed by a
certain logical appeal and intuitive charm, more recent behavioral approaches
have attempted to enrich what is a rather conceptually sterile position as well as
reconcile behavioral accounts of alcoholism with data that have failed to support
some of the early tenets. For example, a large amount of research has
accumulated which challenges the validity and generality of the tension-
reduction hypothesis. The animal data has been reinterpreted as being artifactual
(Freed, 1971) or equivocal (Cappell & Herman, 1971). Research with human
alcoholics has indicated consistently that alcohol consumed in other than small
doses tends to actually *increase* levels of anxiety and depression (McNamee,
Mello, & Mendelson, 1968; Mendelson & Mello, 1966, Nathan & O'Brien, 1971;
Nathan, Titler, Lowenstein, Solomon, & Rossi, 1970). Others have found
alcohol consumption to be unaffected by stress manipulations (Higgins &
Marlatt, 1973) or related differentially to physiological and subjective tension
indices (Steffen, Nathan, & Taylor, 1974). Sobell and Sobell (1973c) have
argued that these results may be due to lower levels of anxiety among
institutionalized subjects and the fact that these "drinking experiments"
eventually end in the subjects' having to return to institutional life. However, the
existing data are far from compelling with respect to the tension-attenuating
functions of alcoholic drinking.

A second objection to reinforcement explanations of alcoholism is that they
overestimate the rewarding properties of alcohol relative to its severely negative
social, medical, and personal consequences (e.g., Chafetz & Demone, 1962). If
drinking is controlled by its consequences, one would expect that alcohol-
generated aversive effects would ultimately prove to be a deterrent to
drunkenness. Most behavior therapists invoke the gradient of reinforcement
concept as an explanation (or description) of the fact that behavior is more
influenced by immediate rather than long-term consequences. However, there
has been little attention to what allows some people to internalize delayed
consequences (thereby making them more immediately salient) while others are
unable to regulate behavior via self-produced cues.

Finally, the "alcohol-as-reinforcer" theory fails to account for the fact that
most people encounter stress without becoming alcoholic and, secondly, that of
those individuals who may have periodically reduced tension via alcohol
consumption few go on to become habitually excessive drinkers.

As learning theorists have attempted to confront these limitations, behavioral formulations of alcoholism have become more complex, increasingly emphasiz-ing social, interpersonal, or environmental contingencies in the etiology of alcohol abuse. Two of the more important developments are summarized below.

1. Heavy drinking serves a number of instrumental purposes which can be distinguished from the reinforcing properties of alcohol itself. The operant view of alcohol abuse stresses contingencies involving such drinking-produced consequences as elevated levels of verbal and nonverbal marital communication (Hersen, Miller, & Eisler, 1973), the anonymity and protection of alcoholic subcultures (Bandura, 1969, p. 550), and reinforcers involving recreational, rehabilitative, social, financial, and medical resources (Hunt & Azrin, 1973). Simultaneous with the maintaining of heavy drinking, these patterns of reinforcement also are likely to result in systematic extinction of the vocational, social, and educational competencies which are necessary for even minimally effectual modes of behavior.

2. Several social learning mechanisms have been considered influential in the production of alcoholism. The distinctive ethnic-subcultural differences in alcohol use suggest that cultural norms potentially determine parameters of drinking and the consequences for deviations from these patterns. Transmission of cultural influences is attributed to modeling experiences based on observa-tional learning involving important socializing agents—family, peer, or symbolic (Bandura, 1969). For example, the probability of excessive drinking is significantly greater among individuals who have at least one alcoholic parent (McClearn, 1973). Caudill and Marlatt (1975) demonstrated that collegiate social drinkers exposed to a "heavy drinking" (large sips, frequent refills, consumption of 700 ml of wine) model consumed significantly more alcohol during an analogue "taste test" than subjects exposed to either a "light drinking" model (small sips, consumption of 100 ml of wine) or no model. The precise means by which modeling variables may influence drinking have not been isolated. In ambiguous situations, a model's behavior may serve as a source of information which provides persons with data about prevailing drinking norms. A model's influence also may be experienced as social pressure or as a challenge to bouts of competitive drinking (Caudill & Marlatt, 1975). While Marlatt's research has demonstrated consistently the influence of models' behavior on social drinking, documentation of modeling effects in naturalistic drinking situations and with clinical-level consumption needs to be pursued. A particularly important area for future inquiry is the social learning history of individuals who (1) practice abstinence or control drinking despite exposure to multiple, alcoholic models or (2) become alcoholic despite membership in social groups which discourage any or all but very circumscribed alcohol use (Bandura, 1969, pp. 534-555; O'Leary & Wilson, 1975, p. 356).

While these conceptual advancements are crucial to the construction of a more comprehensive view of alcoholism, their greatest impact may be at the level of treatment innovation. Subsequent presentation of alcoholism treatment interventions will reveal a pattern of progress that in many ways parallels some of these theoretical emendations. As this chapter will reveal, behavioral clinicians have progressed from a preoccupation with Pavlovian nullification of alcohol's positive valence to an appreciation of the need for treatments "aimed at the modification of [the alcoholic's] whole life pattern if need be" (Franks, 1970, p. 460).

Modification of Alcoholism

The pursuit of an effective solution for alcoholism has been largely a futile exercise. Psychotherapeutic approaches including psychoanalysis (Blum, 1966), transactional analysis (Steiner, 1969), family therapy (Esser, 1971), and group therapy (Gazda, Parks, & Sisson, 1971) have been applied to alcoholics repeatedly despite numerous reviewers' agreement that evidence for significant effects of psychotherapy is equivocal (Emrick, 1975; Gerard, Saenger, & Wile, 1962; Hill & Blane, 1967; Wallgren & Barry, 1970) or indicative of "moderate successes with preselected, good pre-morbid cases" (Costello, 1975).

Clinical lore often has identified Alcoholics Anonymous as the treatment of choice for chronic alcoholics. The reported success of AA may be due to its ability to combine effectively a wide range of behavior-change techniques (group therapy, religious conversion, social control, reinforcement of new "abstinence" behaviors, modeling, and auxiliary attention to members' families, employers, and friends) in its resocialization effort. While AA claims a 75% abstinence rate (Ullmann & Krasner, 1975, p. 458), this figure may be inflated since attrition from AA is very high, screening and self-selection factors may result in the pretreatment deselection of many high-risk alcoholics, and relapses are reported to be quite common occurrences. Related to this last problem is the frequent objection that AA's inflexible insistence on abstinence as a treatment goal conflicts with *in vivo* contingencies in which moderate drinking is positively sanctioned (Sobell & Sobell, 1973c).

Several pharmacological agents have been used to reduce alcoholic drinking. The drug with the most extensive therapeutic history is Antabuse (disulfiram) which, when present in the body, will interact with alcohol to produce very strong aversive physical reactions that may continue for up to two hours. While empirical comparisons between Antabuse therapy and other treatments are rare, there appears to be decrements in the use and popularity of Antabuse. At least two factors may account for this pattern. First, Antabuse-based abstinence requires self-administration of a chemical which has numerous unpleasant side effects apart from disulfiram-alcohol interactions and which requires a continuous, rather cumbersome regime often involving a period of hospitalization. Second, abstinence rates following disulfiram treatment are approximately the same as those reported for aversive conditioning procedures which are time-limited and generally less intrusive than chemical deterrents to drinking (Bourne, Alford, & Bowcock, 1966; Epstein & Guild, 1951). In Europe, the use of disulfiram implants has been directed at some of these limitations, especially the ease with which alcoholics can discontinue oral administrations, but the implant procedure has not gained much popularity in the United States (Wilson, 1975). While chemical restraints on alcohol consumption have been identified as an important element in some successful rehabilitative programs (Costello, 1975), Motin (1974) has concluded, after a very thorough review of the literature, that drug treatments of alcoholism including antidipsotropics, aversives, ataractics, and hallucinogens have not yielded evidence of pharmacological therapeutic effectiveness.

Alternatives to traditional treatments of alcoholics have proliferated in the form of numerous learning-based techniques which typically aim at either the suppression of drinking or the establishment of behaviors incompatible with drunkenness. Suppression of the drinking response has been the goal of aversion therapies which have been the most extensively applied of currently available behavioral treatments.

Aversion Methods

Aversion procedures are not particularly new in the treatment of alcoholics (e.g., Voetglin, Lemer, & Bros, 1940). However, interest in investigating procedural variations and supplementary therapeutic components as well as the comparative efficacy of alternative aversive techniques have been recent developments. As was the case with other addictive problems (Chapter 5), aversion procedures for alcoholism can be divided into chemical aversion, electrical aversion, and covert sensitization. In the following presentation of this research, each technique has been subdivided according to the design used, in ascending order of sophistication. These subdivisions will involve case studies, single-group designs, and control group designs.

Chemical aversion. Nausea-inducing (e.g., apomorphine, emetine) and apnea-inducing (succinylcholine chloride) agents are the most frequently used drugs to produce chemical aversion. In some cases, repeated conditioning trials are utilized; in others, one-trial pairings are employed.

Case studies. Raymond (1964) reported the successful use of apomorphine-based conditioning with a 63-year-old, hospitalized, male alcoholic. Following regular production of the nausea reaction, intermittent choice trials were introduced in which selection of a nonalcoholic drink did not result in nausea. Chemical aversion was supplemented with other techniques (occupational and group therapy). Follow-up indicated continued abstinence after 3 years. Gordon (1971) also presented a case study in which an emetic was paired with alcohol use. While the subject reported experiencing conditioned nausea, a follow-up of treatment effects was not made.

Single-group designs. The most comprehensive chemical aversion program (referred to as "conditioned reflex therapy") was conducted at the Shadel Sanitarium in Seattle, Washington (Shadel, 1944). Potential clients were evaluated for genuineness in their desire to stop drinking. If it was felt that their desire was an earnest one, they were informed concerning the aversion procedures to be used, their likely effects, and that a brief period of hospitalization and booster sessions would be required for 1 year. Treatment consisted of four or five trials of pairing nausea with their favorite alcoholic drink. Subjects were encouraged to talk among themselves about alcohol-related experiences in what could be characterized as "Alcoholic Anonymous type" group support of abstinence. A goal of complete abstinence was stressed, and periodic booster treatments were included after discharge.

A series of evaluations of this treatment approach resulted. The first (Voetglin et al., 1940) was a 3-year follow-up study of 685 patients; it showed a 64% abstinence rate. The second (Voetglin, Lemere, Bros, & O'Hollaren, 1941) examined the effect of the follow-up booster treatments. Follow-up treatments were made available at 30-, 60-, and 90-day intervals. Results indicated: (a) 90% (n=130) abstinence among those subjects accepting booster treatments, (b) 100% (n=25) abstinence among those subjects accepting booster treatments who were, however, unavailable to return for it, (c) 75% abstinence among those subjects who were offered booster treatment but refused it, and (d) 70% abstinence among those subjects not offered booster treatment. Measures of abstinence were made in each instance after 1 year. The third study (Lemere & Voetglin, 1950) involved a survey of 4,468 subjects treated over a period of 13 years. Of 4,096 persons available for the survey, 44% had remained totally abstinent. This figure increased to 51% with the inclusion of subjects who had been retreated. Over 100 charity cases had been treated with poor results and the authors concluded that aversive conditioning was of value only for the "better-off" patients.

Other investigators have presented similar findings. Thiman (1949a, 1949b), in a 1- to 3-year follow-up of 245 subjects, found 51% abstinent. They had been treated with emetine, while continuing under a traditional institutional and psychotherapeutic regime.

Group aversive conditioning procedures have been suggested for more efficient handling of large numbers of patients. Beaubrun (1967) used group aversion treatment to increase subjects' suggestibility for conversion to Alcoholics Anonymous groups. Subjects were released from an institutional setting to local AA groups. While some subjects developed a genuine aversion, others did not but their drinking was reduced anyway. Of 231 subjects available at follow-up approximately one-half were abstinent or drinking only socially. Another report of the use of group aversion techniques without adjunct psychotherapy was concerned with studies of 20 male alcoholics in a hospital setting (E. C. Miller, Dvorak, & Turner, 1960). All subjects reported a conditioned aversion to alcohol. Of 10 subjects available at an 8-month follow-up, five had remained abstinent, three were drinking periodically, and two had returned to alcoholic patterns.

More recently, succinylcholine chloride has been used to induce apnea as the basis of conditioned aversion. In a laboratory examination of the effects of succinylcholine chloride, five male alcoholics received single-trial pairings with an auditory stimulus (Campbell, Sanderson, & Laverty, 1964). Physiological measures showed a presence of conditioned responses after one trial and no extinction over a large number of unreinforced trials. One investigation (Sanderson, Campbell, & Laverty, 1963) applied this technique to 15 non-voluntary alcoholics from lower socioeconomic classes. A single conditioning session constituted the treatment. According to a 1-year follow-up, half were drinking heavily and half were abstinent. Less encouraging results have been reported more recently. Holzinger, Mortimer, and Van Dusen (1967) reported that 81% of their participants had returned to heavy drinking after 4 months; and Farrar, Powell, and Martin (1968) reported that 77% of their sample were drinking again after 1 year.

Control-group designs. Application of more sophisticated designs has been made only with the succinylcholine respiratory arrest technique. In one study (Madill, Campbell, Laverty, Sanderson, & VanderWater, 1966), 45 subjects were randomly assigned to one of three groups. All were inpatient volunteers. The treatment group received a one-trial pairing of succinylcholine-induced apnea with alcohol, the pseudotreatment group received the induced apnea but not paired with alcohol, and the placebo group was presented with the alcohol in the "treatment room." Physiological recordings and a fear-rating schedule indicated that conditioning took place in both treatment groups but that some conditioning also took place in the placebo group. All three groups showed a significant pre-post reduction in alcohol intake. A similar study failed to find significant differences between subjects receiving succinylcholine injections and those receiving saline solution injections (Clancy, VanderHoff, & Campbell, 1967).

Electrical aversion.

Case studies. McGuire and Vallance (1964), in a brief description of a portable shocking device, presented a case of a 40-year-old male alcoholic. The treatment involved presenting the subject with slides of alcoholic stimuli and actual glasses of alcoholic beverages, followed by shock. Both sets of stimuli were interspersed with neutral stimuli. A follow-up at 6 months showed complete abstinence.

Attempting to use procedures which had been successful in treating sexual deviations, MacCulloch, Feldman, Orford, and MacCulloch (1966) reported failure with four cases. An avoidance training paradigm involved pairing electric shock with slide presentations of increasingly attractive alcoholic stimuli. The shock was terminated by the subject's switching off the slide presentation of alcoholic stimuli. Results indicated a wide variability in response latencies and avoidance responses. Short-term follow-up demonstrated an immediate return to heavy drinking in all cases.

Single-group designs. Blake (1965) described a multiple-component, learning-based approach to alcoholism. The treatment regime included: (1) relaxation training, (2) instructional motivation arousal about the negative effects of drinking, and (3) electrical aversion and avoidance training. The subjects were shocked half the time when they sipped alcohol. Termination of the shock was contingent upon the subjects' spitting out the alcohol. Thirty-seven subjects (10 female, 27 male) from essentially middle and upper class backgrounds received the full treatment. Follow-up interviews indicated 54% abstinence after 6 months and 52% abstinence after 1 year.

Hsu (1965) investigated a more extreme electric shock procedure. With electrodes attached to the subject's head, levels of shock just less than those that would have rendered the subject unconscious were administered when alcoholic beverages were selected and sipped (three alcoholic and three nonalcoholic beverages were available). Daily treatments took place for 5 days, with 1- and 6-month follow-up booster sessions included. Of the 40 original male volunteers, only 16 completed the full sequence. Four of five cases presented remained abstinent for 1 year.

Control-group designs. A subsequent investigation by Blake (1967) made use of relaxation training in addition to the usual electrical escape-training procedures. The experimental group (n=37) received the escape-training procedure and separate relaxation training to reduce general anxiety. The control group (n=25) received only the electrical avoidance training. The groups were comparable on demographic variables. A 6-month follow-up study of the abstinence of improvement rates showed 62% and 60% for experimentals and controls, respectively. At 1 year, the rates were 59% (experimentals) and 50% (controls); neither difference was statistically significant.

Results from a number of studies have suggested that aversive techniques per se are possibly not the essential elements in successful treatment. For example, Regester (1971) performed a well-designed experiment with 60 male Veterans Administration alcoholics. Four treatments were conducted. The first treatment paired alcohol intake with electric shock. Under a second condition, the participants were given information about the dangers of alcohol as well. Under the third, shocks were administered randomly in addition to giving the negative information. The fourth condition, a treatment-as-usual control, consisted only of general inpatient care. Only the first two groups showed signs of physiological conditioning to alcohol stimuli, but wide variations occurred. All groups showed a significant reduction in alcohol consumption in a 6-month follow-up study, and no significant differences between the four groups were found.

A further analysis of the function of conditioning in the use of certain aversive techniques was undertaken by Hallam, Rachman, and Falkowski (1972). They postulated that if conditioning in fact takes place, subjects should be expected to display certain physiological reactions and to report anxiety in relation to alcohol intake. They used a typical strategy—pairing electric shock with deviant stimuli. Three groups of subjects were studied: (1) alcoholics of middle socioeconomic status with good prognosis (n=6), (2) alcoholics of lower socioeconomic status with poor prognosis (n=5), and (3) sexual deviates (n=5). Ten days after treatment, interviews were conducted which yielded the following results: five-sixths of group 1 and two-fifths of group 2 decreased intake markedly, while three-fifths of group 3 were classified as showing improvement to a more limited extent. Assessment of subject distaste of the deviant stimuli showed that while four-sixths of group 1 reported a distaste, only one-fifth of groups 2 and 3 reported this. It was also found that the subject's optimism concerning the potency of the treatment appeared to be related to positive outcomes. A second study by the same authors, using a similar strategy, reported that continued autonomic sensitivity to alcohol was the best predictor of successful outcome.

A very well-controlled investigation of Blake's escape-conditioning paradigm was conducted by Vogler, Lunde, Johnson, and Martin (1970). Chronic alcoholics (n=73) were assigned to one of four treatment conditions: (1) *conditioning only* subjects received escape-conditioning trials but did not participate in outpatient booster sessions, (2) *booster conditioning* participants received both inpatient escape conditioning and outpatient reconditioning trials, (3) *pseudo-conditioning* alcoholics sipped alcohol but received random as opposed to drink-contingent shock, and (4) *sham-conditioning* participants received no shocks. *Ward control* subjects, receiving routine hospital treatment, were added to this study later.

Initial follow-up data revealed that the booster-conditioning group had maintained the longest period of abstinence when compared to all other groups. However, a clear interpretation of this difference is precluded by the fact that subject attrition was differentially distributed across the treatment conditions; a comparatively large number of conditioning-only and booster-conditioning participants terminated treatment prematurely and were not included in the outcome comparison. A 1-year follow-up (Vogler, Lunde, & Martin, 1971) on such criteria as days to first hospitalization, proportion of year hospitalized, and number of rehospitalizations revealed that conditioned subjects (combined booster and conditioned only groups) showed significantly greater improvements than ward controls. However, the members of the conditioned groups did not differ significantly on any criteria from pseudo-conditioned subjects.

Miller, Hersen, Eisler, and Hemphill (1973) failed to find a significant difference on alcohol consumption or attitudes toward alcohol between an electrical aversion treatment and two control groups. Chronic alcoholics were matched on demographic characteristics and then assigned to the aversive treatment group in which an escape-conditioning paradigm (Blake, 1965) was used, a control-conditioning group in which shock was set at a barely detectable level, or a group-therapy condition oriented toward confronting subjects with the inappropriateness of their behavior. Percentage reductions in alcohol consumption during a "taste test" assessment were 36% (electrical aversion), 32% (control conditioning), and 30% (group therapy). These outcomes were not significantly different from one another, lending support to the authors' conclusion that nonspecific elements associated with conditioning (e.g., instructions, demand characteristics) rather than conditioning itself may be responsible for the positive outcomes sometimes attributed to aversive conditioning.

Claeson and Malm (1973) assigned 26 chronic alcoholics to two forms of electrical aversion treatment. Group 1 participants (n=17) were conditioned to alcohol-relevant stimuli presented via directed activity, imagination, tape recorder, and slides, while alcoholics in group 2 (n=9) were conditioned to behavioral and imaginal stimuli. The authors claimed "better results" for group 2, a fact which may have been due merely to the greater number of sessions for that group. Neither condition appears to exert a clinically significant effect on drinking; after 1 year, 64% of all participants had relapsed, 12% were not located, and 24% had remained sober.

Wilson, Leaf, and Nathan (1975) examined the effects of two types of aversive control contingencies on alcohol consumption in a well-controlled laboratory setting. Subjects were *Gamma* alcoholics who had shown no substantial improvement as a result of previous therapeutic efforts. In the first two studies reported, an escape-conditioning procedure was compared to a control procedure in which shocks were administered *prior* to drinking. Neither procedure was effective in reducing alcohol consumption in either study.

In contrast to the negligible effects of the conditioning procedure, a third study reported that electric shock, administered contingently on consumption of alcohol, suppressed drinking substantially below baseline levels. As predicted, withdrawal of the punishment contingency was associated with increases in alcohol use. A fourth study was designed to provide an evaluation of contingent versus yoked, noncontingent shock as well as the efficacy of self- versus experimenter-administered punishment. Contingent shock was found to be significantly more effective than noncontingent stimulation, and self-controlled punishment was found to be as effective as experimenter-controlled shock for two of four subjects. This latter finding is consistent with data to be reviewed which indicate that *some* alcoholics are able to develop self-control over their formerly uncontrolled drinking patterns.

Covert sensitization.

Case studies. Several case studies have reported the use of covert sensitization (Cautela, 1967) or verbal aversion therapy (Anant, 1967) in which imaginal stiumli are used instead of electrical shocks or chemicals for the conditioning of aversion to alcoholic stimuli. The theoretical and practical advantages which covert sensitization are purported to have have been discussed in Chapter 5. Direct empirical support for these contentions has not been provided for treatments of alcoholics and the clinical popularity of verbally induced aversion appears to be uncertain (Nathan & Briddell, in press).

Cautela (1967) claimed success with a covert sensitization procedure involving the following elements: determination of typical drinking patterns, training in progressive muscle relaxation, and instructions to imagine drinking a favorite beverage in a customary setting followed immediately by the experience of nausea and vomiting also imagined in the most vivid of details. In a more recent form of this treatment, Cautela (1970) supplemented the imaginal aversion scene with a number of aversion-relief scenes wherein the client imagines his desire to drink attended by physical discomfort which is then relieved by a feeling of pleasure as the client decides not to drink. Clients also are taught to employ covert sensitization outside of the therapy setting through the practice of various homework assignments.

Single-group designs. Anant (1967) claimed well-maintained abstinence following verbal aversion therapy with 26 alcoholics treated in either individual or group contexts. However, the status of these results would appear to be quite equivocal since a later report (Anant, 1968a) indicated that few of the clients treated in groups had remained abstinent, and the disposition of the individually treated clients was not specified clearly.

Control-group designs. In one of the few experimental studies of covert sensitization, Ashem and Donner (1968) compared untreated controls (n=8) with alcoholics assigned to a covert sensitization treatment (n=15) in which suggestions of sickness and vomiting were presented immediately after the client's signal that the taste of alcohol had been imagined. Feelings of relief and relaxation were contingent on imagined rejection of alcohol or performance of activities incompatible with drinking. All subjects participated in the general activities of their treatment unit. The covert sensitization treatment consisted of nine 30-40 minute sessions. At a follow-up 6 months later, six of the treatment participants (40%) were abstinent while none of the untreated controls had been able to stop drinking.

At present, the clinical utility of covert sensitization has not been determined. However, ongoing research on such issues as introducing actual nonalcoholic beverages during imagination of aversion-relief scenes, physiological responses during training, and individual differences in achieving conditioned nausea (Costello, 1975) may provide the data base from which an effective covert sensitization package could evolve.

While a detailed evaluation of aversive treatments for alcoholics exceeds the present chapter's intentions, a critical consideration of some selected issues will be presented. Most research designs employed to evaluate aversive techniques have not allowed definitive conclusions about the relative contribution of specific aversion treatment components or the expected outcomes associated with application of intact treatment packages. In many instances, treatment variables are confounded with nonspecific treatment influences, subject mortality, subject selection, and instrumentation effects. While the literature has demonstrated a broadening of the means by which the conditioning treatment takes place (e.g., groups, outpatient, etc.), practically no systematic monitoring of the treatment process has taken place.

While investigators of aversive conditioning treatments apparently share a theoretical bias that the "learning" occurring in the treatment is the primary determinant of behavior change, the lack of consistency in the literature suggests that outcome variance may be controlled by other influences. Subject factors may be one such class of influence. Aversive procedures have a positive impact primarily on clients who are in good circumstances; indigent, uncooperative, psychopathic, or unintelligent patients are not viewed as good candidates for aversive techniques (Franks, 1963). No meaningful, practical information concerning significant characteristics of the therapist has been presented. If patient characteristics in various treatment approaches are found to have an important relationship with positive outcome, designation of therapist characteristics and mode of service delivery which interact in a predictive fashion with outcome are also needed.

It is difficult to justify a preference for chemical, electrical, or verbal treatments on the basis of currently existing evidence. For a time, the prevailing sentiment appeared to favor electrical methods although this preference was justified more on the basis of procedural efficiency and control than on outcome comparisons. Davidson (1974) has discussed seven such advantages usually associated with electrical methods: (1) greater temporal precision, (2) more suitable to frequent repetitions, (3) fewer medical complications, (4) fewer apparatus requirements, (5) fewer staff needed, (6) less traumatic implementations for staff, and (7) more widely applicable.

However, recent reviews (Elkins, 1975; Wilson & Davison, 1969) have suggested that the positive effects of chemical aversion (especially emetine) may have been underestimated in early investigations. For example, it appears that some unsuccessful applications of chemical aversion may have been due to the use of backward conditioning (alcohol consumed after nausea onset), a type of conditioning which is difficult to develop but easy to extinguish (Elkins, 1975; Franks, 1966). The reemphasis of chemical aversion also may be attributed to the view that certain types of aversion are differentially appropriate for behaviors involving a particular sensory-motor system. Intuitively, it would appear that associations between consumption and nausea would be biologically and psychologically easier to establish than connections between drinking and tactile pain.

At this time, it is not possible to evaluate whether covert sensitization is as effective as its advocates claim. Its practical advantages (e.g., flexibility, generalizability, and ease of administration) are numerous; however, the existing data on outcome are conflictual and have been generated from studies lacking the necessary controls.

Reviews of aversion-based treatments of alcoholics (Costello, 1975; Davidson, 1974; Franks, 1963, 1966; Laverty, 1966; Rachman & Teasdale, 1969) have converged on the conclusion that aversion techniques have at best a limited impact on uncontrolled drinking. Therapy-instigated aversions appear to extinguish rapidly, resulting in large decrements of generalization and maintenance of improvements observed or reported at treatment end. Studies with the highest success rates are typically ones in which high-risk clients were eliminated prior to treatment or dropped shortly after treatment had begun (Costello, 1975). Finally, aversion therapy does nothing to promote the acquisition of competencies commonly thought to be lacking in alcoholics. Recognition of these substantial limitations has had the encouraging effect of prompting behavioral clinicians to develop increasingly sophisticated treatment packages which have been less concerned with altering alcohol's stimulus value or merely suppressing alcohol use and more involved in increasing the probability of alternatives to drinking in high-risk situations. These developments have occurred on three dimensions, which can be considered essential for behavioral methods that attempt to remediate comprehensively a community problem such as alcoholism.

One important trend has been to select treatment goals that are likely to be supported maximally by the post-treatment environment. The treatment objective of controlled drinking reflects the decision that certain alcoholics can be taught to maintain a pattern of controlled drinking and that such a goal may be more easily maintained by *in vivo* contingencies than abstinence.

A second development has been to bolster the social contingencies which would maintain sobriety in the community. Regulation of familial, legal, social, and vocational consequences of drinking has proven that sobriety can be achieved effectively through the mobilization of resources and deterrents which would reduce the probability of uncontrolled drinking.

A group of "broad spectrum" behavior therapies have sought to reduce alcohol abuse by establishing new interpersonal behaviors (e.g., assertion), vocational skills, and general problem-solving abilities thought to lessen the probability of uncontrolled drinking. Related to these techniques are ones which seek to modify frequently suspected elicitors of alcoholic drinking such as anxiety.

In the remainder of this chapter, treatment programs which illustrate each of the above three developments will be reviewed and evaluated with respect to their potential for the community-based treatment of alcoholics.

Promotion of Controlled Drinking

The prevailing belief among experts in the field of alcoholism is that the alcoholic suffers from an irreversible disease characterized by an inability to regulate alcohol intake during a period of drinking (Jellinek, 1960; Williams, 1948). The disease model of alcoholism has identified loss of volitional control of drinking as a primary diagnostic feature of the disorder. For this reason, total abstinence has been viewed historically as the only acceptable, medically defensible treatment goal for the alcoholic. This dogma has been supported by nonmedical treatment orientations (e.g., Alcoholics Anonymous) as well.

The past 10 to 15 years have seen a challenge to the conviction that alcoholics are incapable of controlled drinking. Evidence from clinical and research perspectives has converged on the conclusion that *some* alcoholics are capable of "regulated," "controlled," "moderate," or "social" drinking. Davies (1962) reported long-term (7-11 years) follow-up data on 93 alcoholics, seven of whom were successfully controlling their drinking after abstinence-oriented treatment. Pattison (1966) reported controlled drinking among some alcoholics who had received minimal or no treatment. McNamee et al. (1968) found no evidence for irresistible craving or uncontrolled drinking in 12 volunteer alcoholics across a 7-day experimental drinking situation. Sobell, Sobell, and Christelman (1972) examined data from over 200 hospitalized alcoholics who had participated in experimental drinking sessions where they could consume between 1 to 16 ounces of 86-proof liquor (or its equivalent.) Less than 4% of the participants left the hospital to obtain more liquor or go on a drinking spree; further, no subjects, even those consuming the maximum of 16 ounces, reported experiencing withdrawal symptoms after drinking sessions. Data from other laboratories have confirmed the occurrence of controlled drinking among chronic alcoholics (M. Cohen, Liebson, Faillace, & Allen, 1971; Cutter, Schwaab, & Nathan, 1970; Marlatt, Demming, & Reid, 1973; Merry, 1966).

This pattern of results suggests that the loss-of-control phenomenon may be best understood not as a physiological mediated symptom of an addictive state but as a learned behavior whose parameters are discernibly different from social drinking (Schaeffer, Sobell, & Mills, 1971; Sobell, Schaeffer, & Mills, 1972). Numerous factors may be influential in support of uncontrolled versus controlled drinking; for example, operant contingencies (Cohen, Liebson, Faillace, & Allen, 1971) and expectancies (Marlatt et al., 1973) have been found to contribute to the development of different drinking patterns.

The implication that drinking patterns are subject to learning explanations has spawned a variety of treatment programs with controlled or social drinking as the preferred treatment goal. O'Leary and Wilson (1975) discuss the advantages associated with such an objective: (1) it provides patients with an alternative to chronic drunkenness; (2) it allows ex-alcoholics access to the social reinforcement commonly bestowed on the moderate drinker in our culture; (3) it enhances the self-esteem of patients who are able to reflect on this new accomplishment; and (4) it may increase the number of alcoholics willing to receive treatment because they perceive partial abstinence as a more obtainable and satisfying goal than total abstinence.

Nathan (1976) has classified behavioral approaches to controlled drinking into three categories: (1) blood alcohol level discrimination, (2) multimodal approaches, and (3) environmental manipulations of drinking determinants.

Blood alcohol level (BAL) discrimination. Lovibond and Caddy (1970) were the first to report a strategy in which alcoholics were trained to discriminate proprioceptive cues indicative of various blood alcohol concentration levels. The treatment, administered on an outpatient basis, was divided into two phases: *discrimination training* and *control conditioning.* The program began with a 2-hour session in which subjects were instructed through immediate feedback on the behavioral effects and perceptual cues indicative of varying blood alcohol levels. With electrodes attached to face and neck, subjects were allowed to drink their favorite alcoholic beverages in the control conditioning phase. During this drinking period, subjects were required to give repeated BAL estimates and were provided feedback on the accuracy of their estimations. Subjects were permitted to drink freely but received a varying schedule of shocks whenever their BAL exceeded .065%. A control group was employed which was procedurally identical to the experimental group, except that shocks were delivered randomly before and after the critical BAL level was reached.

A total of 44 randomly assigned alcoholics participated (31 experimentals, 13 controls). Treatment sessions lasted 2 hours and were spaced 5 to 7 days apart. At early sessions, eight to ten shocks were administered; in later sessions, the number of shocks was reduced to three or four.

The results indicated that the contingent shock group demonstrated a significantly lower rate of alcohol consumption and a significantly lower rate of BALs exceeding .065%. Follow-up data indicated that 75% of the experimental subjects completing treatment were able to control their drinking. Additional follow-up data revealed that experimental subjects tended to report an intention to stop drinking after a couple of drinks rather than a conditioned aversion to alcohol.

Silverstein, Nathan, and Taylor (1974) analyzed what they viewed as the crucial components of BAL discrimination training with four volunteer, chronic alcoholics. This study was divided into two phases (*BAL discrimination training*, 10 days; *control training*, 22 days). The BAL discrimination training phase began with a 2-day baseline during which subjects estimated BAL but were not provided feedback on estimate accuracy. On the following 6 days, discrimination training was provided to subjects who received continuous feedback on their BAL estimate accuracy (2 days), intermittent feedback (2 days), and intermittent feedback associated with social and token reinforcement contingent on accurate estimates (2 days). Training procedures were withdrawn on days 9 and 10, which constituted a second baseline period.

Phase I data revealed that estimate accuracy was much greater during the

6-day training period than during the pre-training baseline. During the post-training baseline, subjects' BAL estimates became less accurate; for three subjects, the discrepancies averaged 30 mg per 100 cc, while the fourth subject's estimates averaged 257 mg per 100 cc from his actual BAL.

The *control training* phase, intended to train subjects to use BAL estimates as discriminative stimuli for controlling their alcohol intake, began with a 3-day baseline. During this period, subjects engaged in ad lib drinking but were instructed to maintain their BAL at .08% without feedback or contingent reinforcement. Following a 2-day reinforcement sampling period in which a drink's "cost" became progressively greater as BAL increased over .08%, the core portion of the training program was implemented (days 16-28). Subjects were provided with feedback and contingent token points for maintaining their BAL within target ranges. Across the duration of the training period, control procedures were modified on the following three dimensions: (1) locus of control over drinking was gradually shifted from entirely experimenter-programmed to completely subject-controlled; (2) the range of reinforced BAL was progressively narrowed from .03-.13% to .07-.09%; and (3) feedback and reinforcers were faded out. During the last 7 days of the control training phase, feedback and contingent reinforcement were completely removed.

Data from Phase II revealed that subjects were unable to estimate BAL accurately during the initial baseline period. However, accuracy was rapidly attained during the training period for three subjects who were able to maintain their BALs within the targeted range. However, control over BALs disappeared upon removal of feedback and reinforcement contingencies during the second baseline of this phase.

An energetic follow-up of the study's effects was conducted. Subjects were asked to return a dated postcard on which they reported information about their drinking behavior. Corroborating information was sought from friends and relatives and from subjects themselves in a final interview 10 weeks after the study's termination. Two of the three subjects completing the study returned their postcards, were available for follow-up interviews, and had relatives who provided corroborative data. The third subject resided in a local Salvation Army shelter, thus allowing adequate follow-up of his drinking patterns.

The data suggested that one subject had successfully maintained controlled drinking following training, the Salvation Army resident had remained abstinent for most of the follow-up period, and the third subject had not regulated his alcohol consumption and was drinking heavily during this time. The study represents an important extension and clarification of Lovibond and Caddy's (1970) findings. It confirmed that under certain circumstances some alcoholics are capable both of making accurate BAL estimations and controlling their drinking. Contrary to Lovibond and Caddy's interpretations, however, Silberstein et al. (1974) concluded that these alcoholics were not able to accurately estimate BAL independent of external, corrective feedback.

The results of their study raised the question of whether BAL discrimination can be made reliably on the basis of internal cues alone. Nathan and Briddell (in press) report a study by Huber, Karlin, and Nathan (1975) designed to evaluate the comparative effectiveness of BAL discrimination training based on internal cues, external cues, and a combination of both types. Thirty-six social drinkers gave BAL estimates during a baseline in which no training cues were used. Subjects were matched on the basis of baseline estimation accuracy and assigned to one of three training conditions. Subjects (n=12) receiving internal cues were trained with self-report instruments that associated internal sensations with specific BALs. External cue subjects (n=12) received training based on awareness of temporal factors, drink count, and knowledge of their own metabolism rates. Subjects (n=12) in the combined internal-external group received both types of training. All subjects received feedback on their estimates.

Performance in the third and final session (no cues or feedback) revealed that subjects were able to increase the accuracy of the BAL judgments by approximately 50% following training. The three training procedures were not differentially effective in generating this improvement. Unfortunately, the design of this study did not allow a determination of possible interactions between subject differences and effective training methods. This issue is important, for the question remains as to whether alcoholics also can employ internal cues to estimate BAL or whether, as Nathan and Briddell (in press) have suggested, the phenomenon of tolerance prevents alcoholics from learning to associate specific BAL levels with certain internal, subjective cues to intoxication.

Multimodal approaches. Among the most systematic and comprehensive of behavioral interventions with alcoholics has been the work of the Sobells and Schaeffer at California's Patton State Hospital. While this research program has contributed several innovative techniques to the behavioral treatment of alcoholism, it is best recognized for its continual demonstrations that alcoholics can acquire and maintain controlled drinking patterns following exposure to a combination of behavior change techniques.

Initial studies of this group (Schaeffer et al., 1971; Sobell, Schaeffer, & Mills, 1972) compared the characteristic drinking patterns of hospitalized alcoholics and normal drinkers. Assessment of drinking pattern parameters was conducted in an experimental bar located on a hospital treatment unit for alcoholics. Subjects were studied in small groups and were allowed to engage in ad lib drinking up to a limit of 16 ounces of 86-proof liquor or its equivalent. Differences in drinking patterns of the two groups were consistent and permitted the identification of separate behavioral patterns for alcoholic and normal drinkers. The alcoholics were found to prefer straight alcohol, to take larger sips, to drink faster, to take a longer time between sips, and to drink more than normal drinkers (Sobell, Schaeffer, & Mills, 1972).

Sobell and Sobell (1973c) reported a very comprehensive study in which the separate treatment components described in previous research (e.g., aversive conditioning, videotaped confrontation, etc.) were combined into an extensive treatment plan and compared with "conventional" treatment for alcoholics. Seventy *Gamma* alcoholics were assigned to one of two treatment goals: abstinence (n-30) or control drinking (n=40). Assignment to treatment goals was a staff decision based on consideration of subject preferences, presence or absence of social supports for controlled drinking, subjects' ability to identify socially with Alcoholics Anonymous, and evidence of successfully controlled drinking in the past. Following determination of treatment goals, subjects within each goal condition were randomly assigned to either an experimental or control group. Control subjects received the hospital's usual therapeutic regime, which included AA meetings, therapy groups, somatic treatments, and industrial therapy. Experimental subjects received the conventional hospital treatment plus a 17-session, multifaceted, behavioral program aimed at developing alternatives to drinking for high-risk situations (i.e., where inappropriate drinking most often occurred). Every attempt was made to individualize subjects' treatments with respect to specific setting events for drinking and the most likely alternatives to this response. Subjects were required to generate, practice, and evaluate these alternative responses.

The design therefore involved four conditions: controlled drinking experimental (CD-E; n-20); controlled drinking control (CD-C;[n=20); nondrinking experimental (ND-E; n=15); and nondrinking control (ND-C; n=15). Treatment sessions took place in a simulated environment (cocktail lounge and/or "home" on the Patton State Hospital research ward). In all sessions except the first three and "probe sessions" (8, 12, and 16; described below) inappropriate drinking behavior (as defined by treatment goal) was punished by electric shocks on a VR2 avoidance schedule. Under the shock contingency, nondrinker subjects received a 1-second shock for ordering a drink and a continuous shock during anytime they touched the drink glass. On the other hand, controlled drinker subjects received shocks when they violated the empirically derived "rules" for social drinking—for example, ordering a straight drink, ordering more than three drinks, ordering too rapidly, or taking large sips.

The general content of the 17 treatment sessions is described below.

Sessions 1 and 2, drunk, videotaped. Subjects were allowed to drink up to 16 ounces of 86-proof liquor (or its equivalent) while staff members discussed with them several aspects of their drinking behavior—for example, in what settings it most often occurred.

Session 3, education. During this session, subjects were acquainted with their respective treatment plans, given an explanation of the shock contingencies, including instructions as to the sessions during which shock would not be given, and provided with a response repertoire for refusing drinks (nondrinker subjects) or for ordering mixed drinks (controlled drinker subjects).

Sessions 4 and 5, videotape replay. Previously recorded videotapes of drunkenness were replayed to subjects because they demonstrated subjects' behavioral ineffectiveness while drunk and because prior research had found this type of self-confrontation to maximize motivation for treatment.

Session 6, failure experience. In order to focus on the way in which subjects responded to stress and its possible influence on their drinking, subjects were asked to complete a series of tasks which were in fact impossible to complete in the allotted time.

Sessions 7 through 16, stimulus control. These sessions constituted the core of the treatment program and were devoted to "(1) elucidating stimulus control variables for heavy drinking, (2) generating a universe of possible alternative responses for those situations, (3) evaluating the probable consequences of exercising each response, and (4) practicing under simulated conditions the response decided to be most beneficial." In addition, 30 minutes of session 16 ("probe session") were videotaped (Sobell & Sobell, 1973c, p. 57).

Progress during treatment was measured by three "probe sessions" (8, 12, and 16) where no shocks were delivered for alcohol use (nondrinkers) or inappropriate alcohol consumption (controlled drinkers).

Session 17, videotape contrast and summary. Selective videotapes depicting drunkenness and sobriety were contrasted for the subject. Following a discussion of therapeutic progress, the subject was given a card on which a list of behavioral prompts ("Don't drink after fighting with your wife") specific to his treatment goal was printed. Within 2 weeks after this session, almost all subjects had been discharged from the hospital.

Evaluation of outcome was based on the following sources of data gathered in follow-up interviews:

1) drinking disposition—(a) drunk days (consumption of 10 or more ounces of liquor on any day or consumption of more than seven ounces on more than 2 consecutive days); (b) controlled drinking days (consumption of six ounces or less on any day or isolated days, no more than 2 consecutive days where seven to nine ounces were consumed; (c) abstinent days; (d) abstinent days due to incarcerations;
2) vocational status (improved, worse, or same as prior to treatment);
3) use or nonuse of community, therapeutic supports (e.g., Alcoholics Anonymous);
4) collateral report (e.g., relative or friend) on the subject's general adjustment compared to the year prior to hospitalization.

Data from treatment and probe sessions revealed that while suppression of the inappropriate drinking (controlled drinkers) or drinking per se (nondrinkers) was brought about by the conditioning procedures, the incidence of these behaviors increased almost to baseline levels during the probe sessions where contingencies were not in effect. Despite these initially discouraging results, data from 6-week, 6-month, 1-year, and 2-year follow-ups (Sobell & Sobell, 1973a, 1973b, 1973c) have indicated consistently that "alcoholics treated by the method of individualized behavior therapy were found to function significantly better after discharge than control subjects treated by conventional techniques" (1973c, p. 67).

At both the 6-week and 6-month reassessment, subjects in the experimental groups were superior to their respective control groups with regard to the number of days "functioning well" (displaying abstinence or controlled drinking). While differences between controlled-drinker experimental and control subjects were significant, the nondrinker experimental-control difference was not significant. However, by the 1-year follow-up (Sobell & Sobell, 1973a), subjects in both experimental groups were evidencing a significantly higher percentage of days functioning well than their respective controls. CD-E subjects were functioning well for 70.5% of all days during this time compared to 35.2% of all days spent functioning well by CD-C subjects. In a similar fashion ND-E subjects were functioning well for 68.4% of all days during this time compared to 38.5% of all days spent functioning well by ND-C subjects.

Table 6-1 presents a summary of follow-up data collected for follow-up months 1-6 and 7-12, and Table 6-2 summarizes this same data for follow-up intervals covering months 13-18 and 19-24. Comparison of these tables reveals that during the second follow-up year, the above differences tended to be maintained especially for CD-E subjects. Specifically, CD-E subjects functioned well during the second follow-up year for 89.6% of all days compared to 45.1% of all days for CD-C subjects ($t < .01$). For the second year of follow-up, ND-E subjects functioned well on 62.2% of all days compared to 45.1% of all days for ND-C subjects (this difference was not significant).

These data on drinking behavior were supported by the adjunctive measures which indicated that experimental subjects evidenced significant improvement in vocational status and interpersonal adjustment compared to their counterpart controls. Such differences tended to be maintained better during the second year by CD-E subjects than by ND-E subjects. Finally, data during the second year follow-up (Sobell & Sobell, 1973b) revealed that CD-E subjects when compared to ND-E subjects tended to evidence a greater percentage of abstinent or controlled drinking days and a smaller percentage of days incarcerated either in jail or hospital.

Sobell and Sobell (1973b) summarized the second year trends by concluding that "subjects treated by individualized behavior therapy with a goal of control drinking functioned significantly better over a follow-up duration of two years than did appropriate control subjects treated by the conventional state hospital treatment program oriented toward abstinence. Subjects treated by individualized behavior therapy, but with a treatment goal of abstinence, did not function significantly better than appropriate control subjects treated by the conventional hospital program. At this time, it is not totally clear whether these

Table 6-1

Mean Percentage of Days Spent in Different Drinking Dispositions by Subjects in Four Experimental Groups Displayed Separately for the First and Second 6-Month (183 Day) Follow-Up Intervals, and for the Total 1st Yr (366 Day) Follow-Up Period†

Drinking disposition	Experimental condition*			
	CD-E	CD-C	ND-E	ND-C**
Follow-up Months 1-6††				
Controlled drinking	27.81	13.83	4.05	11.83
Abstinent, not incarcerated	40.55	24.77	66.15	22.32
Drunk	18.55	48.60	15.34	39.34
Incarcerated, alcohol-related: Hospital	11.15	3.57	10.27	9.45
Jail	1.94	9.23	4.19	17.06
Total	100.00	100.00	100.00	100.00
Follow-up Months 7-12				
Controlled drinking	22.57	5.29	2.59	3.09
Abstinent, not incarcerated	50.02	26.55	64.00	39.73
Drunk	9.48	51.17	15.34	40.36
Incarcerated, alcohol-related: Hospital	11.53	7.53	10.27	3.12
Jail	6.40	9.46	4.19	13.70
Total	100.00	100.00	100.00	100.00
Follow-up Year (Months 1-12)				
Controlled drinking	25.19	9.56	3.33	6.13
Abstinent, not incarcerated	45.29	25.66	65.06	32.35
Drunk	14.02	49.88	13.99	39.85
Incarcerated, alcohol-related: Hospital	11.34	4.44	11.77	6.29
Jail	4.16	9.35	5.85	15.38
Total	100.00	100.00	100.00	100.00

*Experimental conditions were controlled drinker experimental (CD-E), $N = 20$; controlled drinker control (CD-C), $N = 19$; nondrinker experimental (ND-E), $N = 15$; and, nondrinker control (ND-C), $N = 14$.

**Does not include data for one ND-C subject who died of drug-related causes about 8 weeks after hospital discharge.

††Very minor differences between results previously reported for follow-up months 1-6 (Sobell & Sobell, 1972) and similar data appearing in this table resulted from added information not available to the authors when the earlier publication was prepared. In no case did corrected information constitute serious changes in treatment outcome conclusions.

† From Sobell, M. B. and Sobell, L. C. Alcoholics treated by individualized behavior therapy; one year treatment outcome. *Behavior Research and Therapy*, 1973a, *11*, 599-618. Reprinted by permission of Pergamon Press.

Table 6-2

Mean Percentage of Days Spent in Different Drinking Dispositions by Subjects in Four Experimental Groups Displayed Separately for the Third and Fourth 6-Month (183 Day) Follow-Up Intervals[†]

	Experimental condition			
Drinking disposition	CD-E	CD-C	ND-E	ND-C
Follow-up Months 13-18				
(N)	(20)	(17)	(14)	(14)
Abstinent, not incarcerated ($\overline{X}$ %)	61.56	38.83	59.41	41.02
Controlled drinking ($\overline{X}$ %)	21.58	4.50	2.89	1.13
Drunk ($\overline{X}$ %)	12.81	49.08	19.75	35.95
Incarcerated in hospital ($\overline{X}$ %)	2.71	2.28	6.40*	10.81*
Incarcerated in jail ($\overline{X}$ %)	1.34	5.31	11.55*	11.09*
Total	100.00	100.00	100.00	100.00
Follow-up Months 19-24				
(N)	(19)**	(17)	(13)	(14)
Abstinent, not incarcerated ($\overline{X}$ %)	66.98	38.38	62.84	46.21
Controlled drinking ($\overline{X}$ %)	24.79	8.49	3.53	1.99
Drunk ($\overline{X}$ %)	7.08	43.43	19.72	35.85
Incarcerated in hospital ($\overline{X}$ %)	0.49	2.25	6.22*	6.05*
Incarcerated in jail ($\overline{X}$ %)	0.66	7.45	7.69*	9.88*
Total	100.00	100.00	100.00	100.00

*Nondrinker incarceration data overrepresents extreme scores of a few individuals.
**The CD-E subject not located for follow-up during months 19-24 had functioned well for 1.63% of all days during months 13-18; two of the CD-C subjects not located for follow-up had functioned well for 9.29% and 19.95% of all days during the first year and one CD-C subject was never located; one ND-E subject was not located for follow-up months 19-24 and had functioned well for 77.87% of all days during months 13-18.

†From Sobell, M. B. and Sobell, L. C. Evidence of controlled drinking by former alcoholics: A second year evaluation of individualized behavior therapy. Paper presented at the 81st convention of the American Psychological Association, Montreal, Canada, 1973b.

results can be attributed more to the treatment goal of controlled drinking or to the method of individualized behavior therapy, since the subjects in the controlled drinking and nondrinking goal conditions differed in many respects" (p. 6).

The Sobells' work is distinguished by numerous factors. First, they present data which confirm the success of a multifaceted, systematic, behavioral treatment program for chronic alcoholics in generating targeted outcomes which were more substantial, durable, and extensive than those achieved by control subjects. In fact, their results can be considered as the most positive to date, regarding the impact of behavioral procedures on alcohol use. Second, their results further support the contention that controlled drinking is an attainable and maintainable goal for carefully selected participants. Finally, their attention to assessing maintenance and generalization of treatment outcomes provides an exemplary model for future researchers in this area.

While appreciative of these contributions, some reviewers (e.g., Nathan, 1976) have identified a number of as yet unanswered questions or problems that were presented by the Sobells' data. First, it is not clear what enabled subjects to function so successfully 1 and 2 years after treatment when they apparently were unable (or unwilling) to do so in the probe sessions interspersed throughout the treatment period. Second, follow-up data on drinking behavior was (1) derived mainly from self-reports, therefore subject to distortion, and (2) collected by one of the experimenters who may have introduced unintentional bias to the data. (Future follow-ups of these patients will be conducted by two groups of independent judges.) (Sobell & Sobell, 1973b). Finally, future research needs to be designed in such a way as to allow an evaluation of the contributions which specific components of the treatment package make to patient improvement. This question was not a concern in the initial study; therefore, current data do not allow a determination of which procedures were responsible for which types of subject change.

One recent investigation (Hedberg & Campbell, 1974) directly compared the effectiveness of four distinct, behavioral treatments in fostering either controlled drinking (13 subjects) or abstinence (36 subjects) in outpatient alcoholics. Two of the methods investigated (behavioral family counseling and electrical aversion) were similar to specific techniques in the Sobell and Sobell (1973c) program.

Subjects were randomly assigned to the following four treatments, each of which followed a standardized sequence over a 1-year period: systematic desensititzation (n=15), covert sensitization (n=15), behavioral family counseling (n=15), and electric shock. While 12 patients initially were assigned to this last group, all but four terminated treatment by the third session.

Data were collected at a 6-month reassessment. The percentage of subjects obtaining their specified treatment goals were as follows: behavioral family counseling (74%), systematic desensitization (67%), covert sensitization (40%), and electric shock (0%). While significance levels were not reported, it was clear that the behavioral counseling and systematic desensitization treatments were the most effective in modifying excessive alcohol use. Comparisons between this study and others are precluded because of its insufficient operationalization of outcome dispositions such as "goal attainment," "much improved," and "controlled drinking." Further, the outcome judgments were the product of interviews conducted by patients' therapists, thereby introducing numerous sources of rater bias which might have distorted such judgments.

Another ambitious, multimodal approach to effectuate controlled drinking is illustrated by the recent research of Vogler and his colleagues (Vogler, Compton, & Weissbach, 1975). Forty-two chronic alcoholics, receiving conventional hospital treatment for alcoholism at Patton State Hospital, were assigned to one of two integrated behavioral packages differing in the presence of numerous behavior modification techniques. Subjects in group 1 (n=23) received discrimination training for BAL at the 50-mg percent level, aversion training for overconsumption (drinking above the .05% level); discriminated avoidance practice (shock delivered contingent on display of alcoholic drinking patterns), videotaped self-confrontation of drunken behavior, alcohol education (intended to remove misconceptions of alcohol abuse), training in alternatives to uncontrolled drinking, and behavioral counseling (involving such techniques as contingency contracting for nonalcoholic behaviors, relaxation training, assertion training, and instruction in problem-solving methods). Group 2 subjects (n=19) received only the last three techniques: alcohol education, alternatives training, and behavioral counseling. Both groups participated in a "wrap-up" session in which therapeutic progress was summarized, and written prompts for appropriate post-therapy behavior were delivered on a small card. Both groups also received booster sessions (BAL was monitored and avoidance sessions were held) once a week for 1 month and then once a month for 11 months.

Fifteen (65.2%) group 1 subjects identified social or controlled drinking as their preferred therapy while 11 (57.9%) group 2 subjects did so. While several pre-treatment differences existed between the two groups, the most substantial difference was that median duration of treatment for group 1 was 45 days (range: 22-77 days) while for group 2 it was 22.5 days (range: 7-71 days).

At a 1-year follow-up, the two groups did not differ significantly in the percentage of subjects evidencing either abstinence or controlled drinking. Sixty-two percent of the subjects were either abstinent or drinking in a controlled fashion (less than 50 ounces of alcohol consumed per month and no more than one uncontrolled drinking episode per month). This represents a success rate that has been exceeded infrequently by either behavioral or nonbehavioral approaches to this type of alcoholic population. Pre-post differences were assessed with five other measures: alcohol intake (in ounces), preferred beverage, drinking companions, drinking environment, and absenteeism because of drinking. Both groups demonstrated positive changes on amount of alcohol intake, preferred beverage consumed, drinking companions chosen, and type of environment in which drinking took place. Between-group differences did not exist for these behaviors with the exception that group 1 subjects showed significantly ($t < .01$) greater pre-post decrements in alcohol intake (17.2-3.5 gallons per year) than group 2 subjects (11.8-6.9 gallons per year). Regression and discriminate analyses also revealed pre-treatment alcohol intake to be the single best predictor of outcome disposition.

This study's data confirmed the findings of Sobell and Sobell that some chronic alcoholics are able to maintain controlled drinking over an extended period of time. Additionally, the contribution of booster sessions to durable changes were emphasized in this study as it was by Sobell and Sobell (1973b, p. 7). While the authors speculated on which procedures were the most powerful in implementing drinking changes, such speculations were not justified by the existing results; the slightly more favorable outcome of group 1 might have been due not to component differences but to the fact that this group spent much more time in treatment than did group 2. Second, significant pre-treatment differences between the two groups on such variables as amount of alcohol intake (more by group 1), number of jobs held and lost, drinking patterns, and source of referral might have accounted for the differential pre-post change in alcohol intake. Finally, as the authors point out, the design did not allow for a separation of the relative effectiveness of specific components.

The selection of component techniques in this research was particularly well-suited to the flexible implementation of the treatment package in natural environments by a wide range of treatment personnel. Techniques were selected which could be used on an outpatient basis, could be administered by paraprofessionals, could be applied on a one-to-one basis, were economical, and were compatible with one another. Future research on these procedures could address itself to an investigation of the possibility of using controlled drinking methods to *prevent* the development of uncontrolled consumption.

Environmental manipulations. Alcoholic drinking increasingly is conceptualized as a response that is controlled by a variety of environmental and social influences. From this perspective, controlled versus uncontrolled drinking can be viewed as discriminately different operant behaviors which are developed or influenced by differential environmental, social, or interpersonal consequences.

Early research by a group of Johns Hopkins investigators indicated that (1) social interactions were more frequent during times when alcoholics had access to alcohol than when such access was restricted; (2) a brief period of social isolation contingent on alcohol consumption could reduce alcohol use by one-half of baseline levels; and (3) the suppressive effect of isolation could be partially reversed by programming minimal social interactions during the isolation period (Griffiths, Bigelow and Liebson, 1973). Other research has documented the effectiveness of contingency management of monetary (Cohen,

Liebson, Faillace, & Speers, 1971) and social reinforcers in instigating and sustaining controlled drinking by alcoholics. In an initial report, Cohen, Liebson, Faillace, and Allen (1971) investigated the impact of providing an enriched environment within the hospital contingent on controlled drinking (drinking no more than five ounces of alcohol per day). During 3 of the initial 5 weeks (weeks 1, 3, and 5) of the study, five hospitalized alcoholics were given access to a living situation which permitted remunerated employment, use of a private telephone, group therapy, visitation privileges, etc. if they engaged in controlled drinking. Drinking more than five ounces resulted in impoverishment. Weeks 2 and 4 were noncontingent weeks, during which moderate drinking was not differentially reinforced; no matter how much the subject drank, he was impoverished. All five subjects drank five ounces or less most of the time during the contingent weeks and drank more than five ounces in the noncontingent weeks.

Because the control weeks in experiment 1 consisted of continuous maintenance of the imporverished environment regardless of level of alcohol use, increased drinking during that period may have been due to either the aversiveness of the situation or the absence of the reinforcement contingencies. Therefore, a second 5-week study intended to separate the effects of the reinforcement contingencies from general aversiveness of the situation was conducted with four of the original five subjects. Study 2 consisted of the same reinforcement procedures as in study 1; however, patients were exposed to a continuously enriched environment during the control weeks. Drinking increased in all patients during control weeks as in study 1, indicating that reinforcement procedures and not general environmental factors were controlling the behavior.

Bigelow, Cohen, Liebson, and Faillace (1972) summarized the results of the enrichment-impoverishment contingencies reported in three separate studies (Cohen, Liebson, Faillace, 1971a, 1971b; Cohen, Liebson, Faillace, & Allen, 1971) as follows: (1) 19 chronic alcoholic volunteers had participated in the experiments; (2) excessive drinking (more than five ounces per day) occurred in only 9.7% of contingent subject-days; (3) during contingency periods, participants abstained on 13.7% of the days and controlled their drinking successfully 76.6% of the time; and (4) all subjects demonstrated at some time the ability to drink small quantities of alcohol and then terminate drinking.

Two research reports have investigated timeout as a possible suppressant of drinking. Bigelow, Liebson, and Griffiths (1974) found that 10 to 15 minutes of physical and social isolation contingent on taking a one-ounce drink reduced drinking to about one-half of its baseline level in 9 out of 10 alcoholic volunteers. A second study (Griffiths, Bigelow, & Liebson, 1974) investigated the environmental conditions under which timeout from social interaction only as opposed to the physical restriction used in the Bieglow, Liebson, and Griffiths (1974) study could be an effective controller of an alcoholic's drinking. A social timeout period of 40 minutes followed each drink and was replicated across three conditions during which varying levels of ward privileges were available.

During "full privileges," participants were free to engage in all available ward privileges. Under the "restricted privileges one" condition, subjects could engage in all privileges except television-watching between 12:00 noon and 11:00 p.m. The "restricted privileges two" condition did not allow subjects to watch television or use reading materials.

Results indicated that social timeout was increasingly effective as other social stimuli (i.e., privileges) were increasingly restricted. Little suppression of drinking occurred when many alternative activities (e.g., playing pool, reading) were available to persons whose social interactions were prevented. These results clarified earlier findings on operant determinants of alcoholic drinking and implied that reliable control of drinking is likely to be maintained best by manipulation of multiple contingencies involving financial, social, and environmental variables.

P. M. Miller (1972) employed behavioral contracting as a means of rearranging the social consequences of alcoholic drinking. A mutually agreeable contract was negotiated between a 44-year-old alcoholic and his wife. The contract specified the following conditions: (1) the husband was not to drink more than three drinks per day and these drinks were restricted to situations which his wife could monitor; (2) excessive or situationally inappropriate drinking was to result in a $20.00 fine payable to the wife for as frivolous a use as possible; (3) the wife was to eliminate negative responses to her husband's drinking and any occurrence of her criticism was to be punished by a $20.00 fine payable to the husband; and (4) both partners agreed to provide one another with attention and affection for desired behaviors.

Daily drink counts revealed that the husband's pre-treatment baseline consumption was seven to eight drinks per day. During the 30 days the contract was in effect, drinking stabilized (after 10 days and a few fines) within targeted limits. Follow-up at 6 months indicated the durability of the controlled drinking pattern as well as the maintenance of marital improvement.

Subsequent to this successful case history, Miller, Hersen, and Eisler (1974) attempted to analyze the relative contributions of different behavioral contracting components to the modification of alcohol abuse. Forty hospitalized alcoholics were matched on demographics and drinking patterns manifest in a laboratory assessment and assigned, following complete detoxification, to one of four conditions: (1) *verbal instructions*, which informed participants to limit their drinking to a specified level; (2) alcoholics assigned to the *written agreement* condition received the same instructions on a written form which they signed and which was countersigned by the psychologist in charge of each case; (3) the third group of participants received the *verbal instructions* plus *reinforcement* in the form of token points for adherence to instructions or token fines for failures to comply; and (4) group four received the *written agreement* which also detailed the same *reinforcement* contingencies as applied to group three.

A drinking goal (one-half of a subject's mean number of pre-test drinks with the additional requirement that the goal not be below one-half of a "shot") was established for each participant. Twenty percent of the alcoholics in the verbal instruction group attained their goal while 40% of the written agreement participants did so. This contrasts significantly with the fact that only one subject in each of the two groups receiving reinforcement failed to attain the drinking goal. As a parametric measure of treatment effectiveness, the difference between each individual's goal and his actual performance was calculated and subjected to an analysis of variance which revealed significant differences among the four groups. Participants in both groups receiving some form of reinforcement exceeded their drinking goals significantly less often then did verbal instruction participants. No other individual comparisons were significant.

The provision of consequences contingent on compliance with contractual agreements appears to be a potent ingredient in therapeutic contracts with alcoholics. Future research needs to address itself to an unconfounding of the effects of reinforcement per se versus its informational properties in the form of performance feedback. Empirical identification of the functional parameters of the contracting approach would facilitate the construction of therapy contracts with an increased potential for controlling a relatively intractible behavior such as alcoholic drinking.

Operant Modification of Drinking

A distinguishing aspect of some recent alcoholism treatment programs is their tendency to focus on important etiological factors that are not tied conceptually to the tension-reduction hypothesis (Hamburg, 1975). Similar to the previously described work by Cohen and Bigelow in establishing moderate drinking, other investigators have emphasized operant determinants of drunkenness while minimizing the attention paid to precipitating subjective conditions (e.g., tension) regardless of their plausibility as causal agents. Hunt and Azrin (1973) have described the most systematic, operant approach to the establishment of alcohol abstinence via the deliberate, careful engineering of environments in which many reinforcers were made contingent on sobriety and were temporarily withdrawn contingent on drinking.

Sixteen hospitalized alcoholics were matched on the basis of age, education, prior hospitalization, marital status, and employment, and were randomly assigned either to a community-reinforcement group (RFT) or a control group (CTL). Both groups received regular hospital services and didactic counseling aimed at inhibiting alcohol use. The RFT group involved the development of vocational, familial, and social reinforcers which were made contingent on sustained sobriety. Extensive behaviorally based training was provided in each of these areas. Patients were instructed in skills which were instrumental in obtaining a job. Special emphases were placed on preparing a resume, job interviewing, and soliciting leads for employment from friends, relatives, and employers. Upon acquisition of a satisfactory job, the patient was released from the hospital. Marital counseling was directed at three goals: (1) reinforcement of the alcoholic for performing satisfactorily in the family, (2) reinforcement of the spouse for maintaining the marital relationship, and (3) making the improved marital relationship contingent on sobriety. Marital inadequacies and conflicts were improved through the development of reciprocal marital contracts (Stuart, 1969) in which husband and wife exchanged reinforcers for specified improvements in problem areas such as the family budget, sex, and child management. All wives required complete sobriety as one condition of the contract.

Special, "synthetic" families were created for patients who had neither their own family nor a parental family with whom they could live. These families (often an employer or minister) were encouraged to have regular social contact with the alcoholic. Sobriety was made a precondition for such benefits. Because most of the alcoholics' prior social interactions were with other problem drinkers, attempts were made to reorder social relationships so that the patient would associate with friends and community groups responding to excessive drinking with strong, negative sanctions. Since many patients' drinking problems had reduced their circle of nonalcoholic friends, a former tavern was converted into a special social club where patients could engage in a wide range of social and recreational activities. The club also promoted renewed companionship with females, families, and nondrinking friends. Alcohol use was not tolerated.

Patients were provided with important communication facilities (newspaper, telephone, radio, and/or television) in an attempt to foster communication with employers, increase access to friends, and make living arrangements more attractive. Initial financial arrangements were made by the patient's counselor; however, succeeding payments became the responsibility of the patient. It was hypothesized that the continued cost of maintaining these "access activities" would act as a further deterrent to relapse.

Following discharge, a program of community maintenance was initiated. A patient was visited by his counselor who reviewed the patient's progress, reminded him of the program procedures, and assisted in solving any problems which had developed. At each visit (which became progressively less frequent), the counselor obtained information concerning the number of days unemployed, drinking days, and days spent away from home. In most cases, collateral sources such as a family member were also consulted.

Patients in the community reinforcement program evidenced significantly superior outcomes when compared to control patients. RFT patients spent less time drinking than controls, were less often unemployed, left their families less often, and were reinstitutionalized less frequently. Figure 6-1 summarizes these comparisons. In addition, the earning power of RFT participants was greater than for controls ($355 versus $190 per month per patient). Patients in the RFT Group spent a mean of 13 weekends in a structured social activity outside the home as compared to an average of four such weekends for control participants.

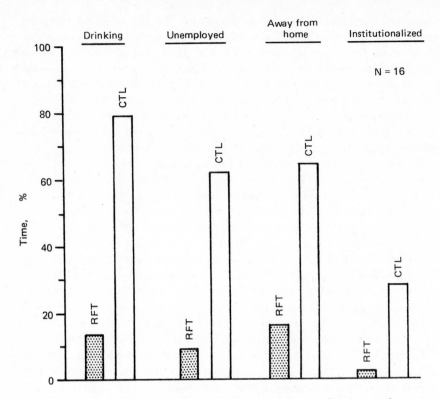

Fig. 6-1. A comparison of the key dependent measures for the reinforcement and control groups since discharge: mean percentages of time spent drinking, unemployed, away from home and institutionalized. (From Hunt, G. and Azrin, N. A community-reinforcement approach to alcoholism. *Behavior Research and Therapy*, 1973, *11*, 91-104. Reprinted by permission of Pergamon Press.)

Marital improvements were evidenced by the five married couples in the RFT group. While all of these couples initially had considered divorce, they all had remained together following treatment. In contrast, two of the four control couples had permanently separated or divorced. Figure 6-2 illustrates that treatment effects did not dissipate during a 6-month follow-up period. For every measure at each month, the RFT-CTL difference remains signficant.

This program illustrates a "movement away from the use of isolated technique such as aversion conditioning and systematic desensitization to a broader use of environmental-influence procedures which focus on training the individual and his family in ways of controlling the reinforcement contingencies in his own life" (Ullmann & Krasner, 1975, p. 456). Decisions about (1) the relative contributions of this program's components, (2) the optimal sequencing

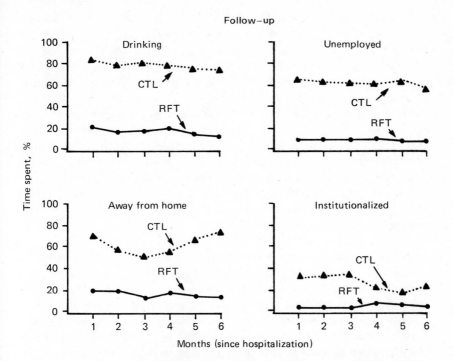

Fig. 6-2. The stable difference between groups over the 6 months after discharge of the key dependent measures: mean percentages of time spent drinking, unemployed, away from home, and institutionalized. (From Hunt, G. and Azrin, N. A community-reinforcement approach to alcoholism. *Behavior Research and Therapy*, 1973, *11*, 91-104. Reprinted by permission of Pergamon Press.)

of these components, and (3) alternative program implementation styles must await future empirical attention.

P. M. Miller (1975) developed a behavioral intervention program for chronic public drunkenness offenders (primarily Skid Row alcoholics). This project, although limited in terms of size and duration, illustrates the advantages of coordinating community agency services with systematic behavioral contingencies designed to maintain sobriety.

Contingent on sobriety as assessed by direct observation or breathalizer tests performed on a variable interval 5-day schedule, 10 chronic alcoholics were provided with required goods and services (housing, employment, clothing, medical service, meals, cigarettes, and counseling) through several community service agencies. Participants with alcohol concentrations in excess of 10 mg/100 ml of blood volume were not provided with these resources for 5 days after determination of alcohol abuse. A control group of 10 alcoholics similar to the intervention group in terms of age, education, arrests, and length of problem drinking received the same goods and services whether intoxicated or sober.

While the two groups were not different from each other on number of arrests prior to the intervention, only the contingency management group evidenced a significant pre-post decrease in arrest rates. Further, intervention participants significantly increased the number of hours employed after the introduction of the contingencies while the control group showed no employment changes.

Sulzer (1965) reported a very interesting demonstration of a limited community-reinforcement program for an alcoholic who had rejected aversive conditioning as a mode of treatment. The therapy program involved the programmed participation of two friends of the patient who were instructed to withhold social reinforcement whenever he drank alcoholic beverages. The following treatment plan was formulated:

> After working hours, they would meet in a conveniently located tavern where the three of them would drink for a time before going home. The patient could only order and drink soft beverages. If he ordered or drank hard liquor, the friends would leave immediately. However, the patient's friends might drink anything they wished. This plan was to continue on at least once a week basis for an undetermined period of time. Also, the patient agreed to invite the friends to his home on all occasions that might call for alcoholic beverages to be served to guests and the friends agreed to come and remain only as long as the patient took no alcohol. His friends would also invite the patient to their homes fairly frequently but would not serve him alcohol. (p. 196)

Initial *in vivo* occurrences of the treatment program resulted in the client experiencing a range of pre-planned and fortuitous contingencies. For example, during one accompanied visit to a tavern, not only did the client's associates provide social reinforcement for continued sobriety, but the bartender did so as well. On another occasion, the friends, having met the client who had already drunk some alcohol, improvised a contingency in which their continued presence was contingent on his use of nonalcoholic beverages in that situation. While no systematic outcome data are presented, Sulzer reported that the client experienced an improvement in his interpersonal relationships and successfully maintained his sobriety over an unspecified period of time.

Broad-Spectrum Treatments of Alcoholism

As with problems of drug abuse discussed in Chapter 5, recognition of the complex problems presented by most alcoholics has led to a growing appreciation of "broad-spectrum" or multimethod treatment approaches (Lazarus, 1965). In his well-circulated account of the behavioral treatment of a 42-year-old male alcoholic, Lazarus described the following elements of the broad-spectrum approach: (1) procedures directed at reestablishing the client's physical well being, (2) aversive and anxiety-relief conditioning to eliminate the compulsion to drink (3) evaluation of the client's social interaction with a special emphasis on determining anxiety antecedents to drinking, (4) anxiety-reduction techniques such as desensitization, assertion training, behavioral rehearsal, and hypnosis, (5) auxiliary therapy with the client's spouse, (6) socioeconomic interventions with past or potential employers, (7) establishment of new reinforcing activities including hobbies, new forms of group participation, or Alcoholics Anonymous membership, and (8) adjunctive measures including drugs or chemotherapy.

Kepner (1964) described a set of learning based procedures used at the Cleveland Center on Alcoholism. Treatments were aimed at establishing abstinence, developing a repertoire of new adjustment responses to stress, and encouraging the alcoholic to acquire new self-knowledge. The following techniques were described as components of this approach: (1) making the treatment situation a rewarding one by the creation of a nonpunitive atmosphere, (2) restoring the physical health of the alcoholic, (3) providing social reinforcement and support for sobriety, (4) using naturally occurring aversive stimuli (e.g., marital separation, hangovers, occupational setbacks) to discourage drinking, (5) teaching the alcoholic new behavioral skills incompatible with drinking, and (6) promoting the acquisition of self-control. Unfortunately, the report did not present any data upon which an assessment of treatment effectiveness could be based.

McBrearty, Dichter, Garfield, and Heath (1968) adopted a multimodal approach to problem drinking in which drinking behavior was regarded as being imbedded in a complex of maladaptive behaviors all of which should be modified in order to deal efficaciously with the target behavior. Based on previous behavioral modification data and their own anecdotal evidence, the authors suggested a program which would:

1) provide background information relevant to alcohol abuse (alcoholics were exposed in groups to principles and rationales of behavior therapy approaches in general, with specific reference to alcoholism; problem solving and counseling occurred during group meetings);

2) shape adaptive behaviors (role-playing techniques were used to increase the probability of adaptive behaviors and reduce the probability of drinking-

related responses. In addition, a token economy was suggested as a second-order technique to enhance and maintain nondrinking);

3) punish drinking (three punishment procedures involving alcohol-shock contiguity were used in addition to a covert sensitization procedure which paired "imagined" nausea with alcohol consumption); and

4) reduce anxiety to situations which were felt to trigger drinking (systematic desensitization was used if anxiety-inducing situations which provoked drinking could be isolated). It should be noted that no data were presented to support the efficacy of this program, although the authors comment that it was in operation in at least one institution. Also it was not clear whether an alcoholic received all or part of the program, and, if only a part, how that determination was made. Failure to provide any quantitative evaluation detracted from the clinical importance that this report might have had.

Miller, Stanford, and Hemphill (1974) described a broad-spectrum program in operation on a 15-bed alcoholism treatment ward at a VA hospital in Jackson, Mississippi. Following receipt of factual information on alcohol and its behavioral and physiological consequences, patients were exposed to aversion conditioning based on chemical, electrical, or verbal stimuli. The decision about which form of aversion to use was based on a determination of individual patients' requirements. A token economy was used to encourage active participation in therapeutically oriented behaviors (personal hygiene, attendance at treatment session, involvement in vocational or educational training) and to discourage irresponsible behaviors (drinking, absence from treatment sessions, violence). The program also sought to develop new adaptive behaviors in participants. Alcoholics were taught to handle responsibilities and life stresses more adaptively through a range of techniques such as group therapy, role playing, assertion training, systematic desensitization, and family therapy based on principles such as reciprocity counseling and contingency contracting.

Readjustment to community life was programmed explicitly and participants were prepared for community reentry by vocational counseling, job placement, and direct program contact with potential employers. Weekly contacts with program personnel were continued after discharge for 1 to 2 months. These contacts continued for as long as a year and were supplemented by such maintenance procedures as family therapy and provision of Antabuse. The authors claimed that the maintenance of personal contact with discharged participants was crucial to their continued community adjustment. However, since only subjective evaluations of programmed effectiveness were provided, any strong conclusions about the effects of the program or its separate components are premature.

Nathan and Briddell (in press) have summarized a recent multitechnique program by Wilson and Rosen (1975) which was intended to establish controlled drinking in a 30-year-old male alcoholic. Techniques included aversive conditioning, BAL discrimination training, assertion training, behavioral rehearsal, self-monitoring of alcohol intake, and behavioral contracting for controlled drinking and improved familial and social functioning. Controlled drinking was maintained successfully at a 6-month follow-up.

The integrated application of broad-spectrum techniques within a single treatment program is rare, although some examples in addition to those just reviewed have been described in other contexts of this chapter (Hunt & Azrin, 1973; Lovibond & Caddy, 1970; Sobell & Sobell, 1973c; Vogler et al., 1975). However, a number of investigators have reported the application of certain individual components typically associated with the multimodal or broad-spectrum approach. Investigation of these components has been concentrated in two areas: anxiety-reduction techniques and the establishment of alternatives to drinking.

Anxiety-Reduction Techniques

Related to behaviorists' long-standing conviction that alcohol use is maintained by its tension-reducing qualities is the popularity of anxiety-modification techniques for the treatment of alcoholics. Kraft (1969a) and Kraft and Al-Issa (1967) have used systematic desensitization with a number of alcoholic clients who reported alcohol use as a high probability response to social anxieties. Evidence of clinical improvement was reported in all cases although rigorous follow-ups of clients' post-treatment status were not provided.

Newton and Stein (1974) evaluated the contribution of implosive therapy when combined with a typical milieu treatment program. Male alcoholics were assigned to one of three conditions: detoxification and inpatient milieu treatment (n=26); detoxification, milieu treatment, and implosion (n=16); detoxification, milieu treatment, and brief psychotherapy (n=16). Results revealed no significant treatment differences on either observational or self-report measures of outcome. Even those measures most likely to be affected by implosion (e.g., distress, anxiety) were not differentially related to subjects' treatment condition.

Steffen (1975) compared the effects of EMG feedback-assisted relaxation training to an attention-placebo condition on the drinking behavior and subjective mood of four chronic alcoholics. A pair of participants was assigned initially to 14 one-hour sessions of either relaxation training assisted by EMG feedback or attention placebo ("contemplation" condition). Following training, a 4-day period permitting free drinking in a laboratory-treatment setting was introduced. During a second treatment phase, subjects were assigned to the alternative treatment condition, which was followed by a second free-drinking phase. Analysis of variance revealed that EMG-aided relaxation was associated with significantly lower blood-alcohol levels and decreased subjective disturbance. While these data suggest the utility of EMG feedback combined with relaxation training for alcoholics, the author's failure to control for sleep occurrence during training and the fact that the design did not allow separation of EMG from progressive muscle relaxation effects make any precise attribution of causality to the specific training procedure quite difficult.

Hartman (1973) discussed a standardized (taped) form of relaxation training which was played for small groups of hospitalized alcoholics. A particular objective of this training program was to enable participants to identify the events which led to anger arousal and then introduce the competing response of relaxation as early in the arousal pattern as possible. Of those alcoholics participating in the group relaxation, 81% completed the entire treatment program while 50% of the participants in group meetings not involving relaxation training did so. This difference is substantial and of possible clinical relevance, but the report did not describe the necessary controls to allow one to conclude that the lessened attrition rate was due solely to relaxation training.

Anderson, Lubetkin, Logan, and Alpert (1973) compared the relative effectiveness of three common methods for inducing relaxation. Thirty hospitalized male alcoholics were matched on demographics and drinking history and assigned to one of three relaxation methods: muscle relaxation, sensory awareness, or a self-relaxation control. The experimental sequence involved an initial 5-minute period during which participants were instructed to lie as quietly as possible; this was followed by an induced arousal phase requiring subjects to view a series of slides depicting alcoholics in varying stages of drinking. Relaxation induction (one 35-minute session) by one of the three methods occurred next and was followed immediately by a second presentation of both the resting and arousal phases. Analyses for simple effects indicated that Jacobsonian relaxation produced significantly greater reductions in resting-phase arousal (heart rate) than sensory awareness, which was significantly more effective than self-relaxation. During the arousal phase, differential relaxation and sensory awareness were equally effective in reducing heart rate, and both were more effective than self-relaxation methods. While the question to which this research was addressed was an important one, it is very doubtful that a single, 35-minute training session in any form of relaxation induction permits a sufficient test of its effectiveness or satisfactorily approximates the parameters involved in its clinical use.

Establishing Alternatives to Drinking

A number of clinician-researchers have proposed that provision of an alternative behavior to drinking as a means of emotional expression might contribute to a decrease in uncontrolled drinking. For example, Martorano (1974) examined the effects of assertion training in an anger-provoking environment on the drinking of four male alcoholic volunteers. The study was divided into three stages: baseline (8 days), experimental period I (12 days), and experimental period II (12 days). Six days of drinking ("wet days") during which alcohol, social interaction, or TV time could be purchased by points previously earned at an operant task or by participation in assertion and nonassertion training were programmed at the end of all three phases. In experimental periods I and II, drinking days were preceeded by 6 training days. During training, the men were placed in situations where they were encouraged to express anger without alcohol through assertive behavior (assertion training) or trained to suppress their anger unless alcohol was present (nonassertion training). Training included a modification of the Scrambled Sentences Test, individual training sessions where role playing, modeling, and coaching were used, and group sessions. Points were delivered contingent on performance of trained responses. Concurrent with training days was a prohibition on drinking ("dry days"). Training was counterbalanced so that two participants received assertion training during experimental period I and the other two men received nonassertion training. Reversal of the training schedule occurred during experimental period II. The data from this study are striking. The men achieved significantly higher blood-alcohol levels following assertion training than they did following nonassertion training. Data from the Adjective Checklist Mood Scale and the MAAC Behavioral Adjustment Scale were analyzed for a comparison of dry versus wet days and assertion versus nonassertion training. When drinking, the men rated themselves as significantly more depressed, vigorous, friendly, and aggressive than when sober. During assertion training, participants rated themselves as significantly more friendly, vigorous, attractive, active, and less tense and aggressive than during the nonassertion training. However, subjective ratings of mood were not confirmed by staff judgments and were not maintained during the wet-day period. Staff rated subjects significantly more negatively following assertion training. While the staff perceived some gains in mood as a result of assertion training, they tended to see the men as more uncommunicative, uncooperative, and less friendly when drinking followed assertion training.

While it is clear that this attempt to modify drinking through assertion training was unsuccessful, the determinants of the present outcomes have yet to be identified. Perhaps alcoholics found assertive behavior more stressful than their typical lifestyle and drank to reduce the tension which assertiveness produced. Another possibility is that assertive behavior was punished by peers and staff, resulting in increased drinking to mollify the effects of punishment. Finally, it may be that the assertion training was too brief or too situation-specific to allow generalization to settings in which access to and use of alcohol was allowed.

Conclusion

Behavior therapies for alcoholism have been liberated from the austerity of their early conceptual foundations. This liberalization has occurred on at least three dimensions which have been described in this chapter: (1) acceptance of controlled drinking as a legitimate treatment goal for some alcoholics, (2) the use of operant environmental contingencies to maintain sobriety in the community; (3) the coordination of multiple procedures to reduce alcohol abuse by establishing new skills thought to lessen the probability of uncontrolled drinking. In addition to the increasing sophistication and comprehensiveness of alcohol treatment programs, these new advancements have contributed to the flexibility with which behavior change methods can be implemented in diverse community settings with a broader range of alcoholics by treatment personnel representing a variety of demographic and training backgrounds.

The ambitiousness of some recent programs (e.g., Hunt & Azrin, 1973) has been reflected in their attempts to use nonprofessionals as active agents, to create support systems (synthetic families, social clubs) directed at promoting social behaviors incompatible with drunkenness, and to sustain community maintenance through post-treatment counselor visits, activity prompting, and environmental structuring. One element of the Hunt and Azrin program which future rehabilitative efforts might wish to emulate was the careful attention paid to *socioeconomic interventions* such as advocatory assistance with job finding, legal problems, transportation facilities, and the acquisition of communication resources such as a TV. In too many reports of behavioral interventions with alcoholics one is left with the uneasy feeling that a supportive socioeconomic milieu was taken for granted rather than intentionally programmed. The replicable relationship between alcoholism and social and economic factors suggests that the most consistently successful treatment programs are ones that will be as committed to social-system changes as they have been to individual-behavioral ones.

One major limitation which behavioral therapies for alcohol abuse have yet to overcome is their inattention to the heterogeneity of alcoholic populations. This deficiency is not specific to behavioral methods but is characteristic of almost all alcohol rehabilitation efforts. To a certain extent, the problem may lie in researchers' tendencies to search for predictive indices in inappropriate or incomplete domains. Personality inventories have been the most frequently employed method of predicting treatment experiences, although the pattern of success is disappointing for even such a basic criterion as the differentiation of completers from dropouts in an alcoholic treatment program (Gross & Nerviano, 1973; Miller, Pokorny, & Hanson, 1968). Gross and Nerviano have concluded that predictions of treatment completion are not possible from a knowledge of personality dimensions alone and have suggested that "a complex of purely situational determinants may indeed explain the dropout phenomena, but a more likely hypothesis is that the patient attrition is a consequence of an interaction between the situation and the personality domains" (p. 515). A more fruitful approach to the matching of client with therapy alternatives might require a careful delineation of a particular alcoholic's historical drinking patterns and responses to previous therapy regimes as well as an assessment of the post-therapy social environment's capacity to support and reinforce the treatment targets which have been selected. The three factors (evidence of past controlled drinking, provision of active social support for controlled drinking, and a request for controlled drinking as a goal) involved in Sobell and Sobell's (1973c) decision to recommend abstinence versus controlled drinking illustrate their emphasis on past behavior in interaction with current environmental resources as a powerful source of outcome variance. Further precision in target selection or outcome prediction could be introduced by consideration of such potential moderator variables as field dependence-independence, internal-external control, or social evaluative anxiety.

As with other social problems such as drug abuse (see Chapter 5), one of the constraining limitations of behavioral therapies for alcoholism has been their disinterest in specifying which method will be most efficacious with varying types of clients. Franks (1970) reaches a similar conclusion in his review of alcohol assessments: "If the alcoholic is to be treated by techniques of behavior modification, then likewise it would seem not unreasonable to try and ferret out matters pertaining to his identification in behavioral terms. At the present time, advances in both the theory and the practice of behavioral assessment lag dismally behind developments in the area of behavior modification" (p. 453).

At this time, the more fundamental shortcoming would appear to be at the theoretical rather than the practical level. At least at the level of assessment practice, behavioral measures of alcoholic drinking have made numerous gains relative to the other two measurement channels of alcohol use—subjective reports and personality measures (P. M. Miller, 1973a). Nathan and Briddell (in press) have summarized three distinct approaches to the behavioral measurement of drinking. Historically, the first of these was the use of alcohol in laboratory settings as a reinforcer to which alcoholics could earn access by engaging in well-defined operant tasks (e.g., Mello & Mendelson, 1965). A second strategy has been to disguise assessments of consumption levels or rates as "taste tests" in which participants are asked to drink an unspecified amount of alcohol and then rate the beverages along some predetermined taste dimensions (Higgins & Marlatt, 1973). Currently the most popular approach is to allow alcoholics free access (within liberal limits) to alcohol in simulated bars or lounges in laboratory contexts which permit time-extended observations of drinking patterns (Sobell & Sobell, 1973c). In addition to the primary advantage of enabling a precise description of drinking parameters, behavioral measures of drinking are more likely to be more sensitive to the pre-post comparisons involved in evaluation of treatment efficacy (P. M. Miller, 1973b).

Associated with these laboratory-based assessments of the drinking response has been the increasing use of archival and unobtrusive data sources for longitudinal follow-up measures of drinking disposition in community settings. Indices related to occupational functioning, physical health, contacts with the criminal justice system, and marital happiness have been monitored in an effort to judge not only adjustment vis-à-vis alcohol use but also to detect changes with respect to overall level of resocialization and community reintegration.

It is heartening to observe that social learning therapists involved in alcoholism treatments are responding actively to the increasing awareness that the extension of treatment effects over time, stimulus settings, and untargeted behaviors requires the intentional programming of particular treatment components (Atthowe, 1973a). There has accumulated in the literature a sizable repertoire of techniques that are purported to facilitate treatment generalization and maintenance, and the incidence of programming these techniques for alcoholics has been reassuringly high, especially in the area of treatment maintenance. In fact, a recent review of generalization-maintenance effects by social learning therapies (Moore & Nietzel, 1975) revealed that in comparison to such target areas as depression, sexual deviation, and childhood/juvenile behavioral problems, treatments of inappropriate consumatory behaviors (which include alcoholism) evidenced substantially more concern for the assessing and programming of generalization and maintenance outcomes.

Among the procedures employed for the promotion of either maintenance or stimulus generalization have been booster or reconditioning sessions (Vogler et al., 1975), post-treatment monitoring and reinforcement (Hunt & Azrin, 1973; Vogler et al., 1975), behavioral prompting (Vogler et al., 1975), goal-to-client matching (Sobell & Sobell, 1973c), programming of peers to continue treatment contingencies (Sulzer, 1965), use of intermittent schedules of reinforcement (Sobell & Sobell, 1973c), fading of contingencies (Wilson et al., 1975), self-administered treatment contingencies (Wilson et al., 1975), and socio-economic interventions to create a more supportive environment (Hunt & Azrin, 1973).

Despite the frequency with which maintenance and generalization procedures have been included in behavioral treatment programs, there is very little empirical data concerning the absolute effectiveness of these methods, their comparative effectiveness, or the differential effectiveness of varying methods applied to specific alcoholic subgroups. Hopefully, this state of affairs will be reversed in the not-too-distant future. Following are four recommendations intended to improve the empirical rigor and clinical sophistication of behavioral research on the generalization and maintenance of therapy effects.

First, researcher-clinicians should include specific treatment components that are predicted to have determinable impact on the durability and/or extensiveness of therapy outcomes. A special priority should be placed on the cultivation and investigation of response generalization procedures, the most neglected aspect of treatment generalization.

Second, researchers could adopt a strategy of initially investigating generalization/maintenance procedures in well-controlled case studies in which the relative strength of different techniques can be examined using reversal or multiple baseline designs. Those techniques which appear from case studies to be of promise could then be investigated more carefully in larger factorial group designs.

Third, journal editors might consider formulation of editorial policies which mandate consideration of generalization or maintenance issues by behavior therapy researchers. Concern with such issues is likely to be engendered by publication contingencies in which assessing and programming of generalization and maintenance effects are rewarded activities.

Finally, it would be useful for researchers to include routinely in the "method" section of their manuscripts a subsection devoted to generalization and maintenance of treatment outcomes. This subsection should include the following elements: (1) careful description of all instruments used to measure generalization and maintenance, (2) sufficient detailing of maintenance/generalization components to allow interlaboratory replication, and (3) theory-based predictions concerning the efficacy of such components. It is hoped that pursuit of these recommendations will result in the accumulation of data that will contribute to the evolution of social learning-based therapies capable of effecting both durable and extensive improvements in alcoholic clients.

Chapter 7
COMMUNITY MENTAL HEALTH

A number of deliberate decisions have contributed to the specific focus of this chapter. The rationale for these decisions will be discussed here because the bases for inclusion and exclusion of material can provide the reader with a brief panorama of community mental health and suggest a framework for both current and future developments of the field.

While behavior therapy techniques are used widely in community mental health centers, have made treatment more effective and efficient (Davison & Neale, 1974), and provide means for serving groups less receptive to traditional verbal psychotherapy (Lorion, 1974), most material on behavior therapy techniques has been excluded. Many books on behavior therapy have appeared recently (e.g., O'Leary & Wilson, 1975; Rimm & Masters, 1974), and a traditional review of such material seems neither necessary nor especially informative.

However, there is a more basic reason for not focusing on behavior therapy. The community mental health movement promised not only to expand direct services (e.g., psychotherapy, counseling) so that more people, particularly the poor, had access to these services but to investigate and employ new methods and perspectives to deal with individual and social problems (Zax & Cowen, 1973). While there have been some important advances in "direct services" (e.g., paraprofessionals, outreach programs, emergency services, and group and behavior therapies), most often these services still have attempted to treat psychologically distressed individuals or groups of individuals. In the present context, this suggests that behavior therapists, while developing new techniques and therapeutic procedures, have not substantially questioned or modified the prevailing social and economic systems for approaching individual and social problems.

Criticisms directed at community mental health programs by "community psychologists" repeatedly have called for an expanded conception of community mental health that would recognize ecological and social system parameters of human problems and the constraints that such conditions place on the effectiveness of traditional service delivery systems (Kelly, 1966). These critics often have outlined conceptual models (public health, ecology, systems theory), interventions ("consultation and education," social action), and research strategies that are appropriate for a more system-oriented and, where possible,

228

preventive approach (Bahn, 1965; Brayfield, 1967; Cowen, 1973; Hersch, 1969; Klein, 1965; G. A. Miller, 1969; Powell & Riley, 1970; Rappaport & Chinsky, 1974; Roe, 1970; Rosenblum, 1968, Sarason, 1972, 1974; Schulberg, 1965; Smith & Hobbs, 1966). However, other critics (Bellack, 1974; Leopold, 1974) have criticized community mental health for becoming too involved in system change and too little involved in direct service.

While not disavowing the need for psychotherapy and counseling services (Hurvitz, 1973), a main purpose of this chapter is the identification of an alternative model of community mental health that stresses community program development, organizational change, and research on the effectiveness of such endeavors as *preferred means of providing mental health services*. Some balance is provided by the detailed presentation of a unique mental health program which uses behavior therapy in direct service work and has a behavioral approach to the management and evaluation of its own organization. In addition, some recent work using pseudo-patients as a consumer-oriented method to assess behaviorally the adequacy of service programs will be presented. Both sections stress the development and evaluation of effective and accountable service systems.

Elaborate accounts of behavioral ward (token economy) programs in mental hospitals also were excluded. The basis for exclusion rested on two premises: (1) much of this material has been reviewed previously (Davison, 1969; Kazdin & Bootzin, 1972) and is selectively presented in Chapter 8, and (2) a conclusion of these reviews is that behavior changes produced in the token economy or other institutional programs generally are not maintained in the community and that the emphasis of such programs should shift from intensive institutionally based treatment to the shaping of behavior changes in the community (Atthowe, 1973a; see also Chapter 8).[1] The usual behavioral hospital program has had the same shortcoming of other hospital programs—insufficient attention to meaningful treatment outside the hospital (Zax & Cowen, 1972).

Some successful nonbehavioral research is emphasized because there has been a backlash against community treatment for marginal people (Atthowe, 1975) and doubt about the future of such programs. Although many communities might be ill prepared for treatment in the "natural environment," most attempts at community treatment have been piecemeal, unsystematic, and unsuccessful (Atthowe, 1975). Currently, it is necessary to present program demonstrations that indicate that the traditional, recalcitrant problem of inadequate community care can be ameliorated, and that successful approaches can be disseminated.

---

[1] In addition, probably the most significant recent changes in hospital admission procedures and care have involved legal decisions (see Chapter 4) and not social-psychological interventions. Ironically, recent legal decisions on the right to treatment might create a situation where hospitals and other institutions are funded liberally and once again become primary settings for the delivery of mental health services.

A number of studies marking the emergence of a behavioral approach to organizational change are presented in detail because previous work in organizational change has been neither experimentally rigorous (Bennis, Benne, & Chin, 1969; Likert & Bowers, 1969; Lichtman & Hunt, 1971; Sashkin, Morris, & Horst, 1973; Seashore & Bowers, 1970) nor consistently effective (Campbell & Dunette, 1968). Effective development and management of community mental health programs and consultation with other systems will depend on the creation of a demonstrably effective technology of oganizational change.

A few studies are described in which behavioral procedures and/or evaluative methodology have been developed for the organization of poor people. While such programs seem somewhat dated in the 1970s (Hersch, 1972), the studies that are presented signal the beginnings of behavioral approaches to social action and community change. They also serve as a reminder of the spirit of some of the earlier efforts in community mental health and such historical antecedents as the war on poverty programs (Zax & Cowen, 1972).

Another section traces the development of a program devised by Risley and his colleagues to provide child care, youth services, and advice on family problems to parents. The framework for these services is particularly significant in that (1) development of each portion of the program was based on a careful analysis of social trends making family life more stressful for diverse strata of society, and (2) the explicit objective of the project was to produce packageable programs that could be widely disseminated. This work provides an excellent example of the frequently discussed but infrequently implemented public health approach to community mental health.

A final section on the combination of behavior analysis with systems theory will be used to synthesize some of the chapter's previous content and point to other program possibilities in the future of community mental health.

Behavioral Community Mental Health

The Huntsville-Madison County Mental Health Center represents a unique attempt to make all aspects of a service center's procedures public, quantifiable, accountable, and based on behavioral-empirical principles and methods. Originally, the center operated from an eclectic orientation, but in 1971 it received an NIMH grant to develop a "totally behavioral mental health system." The initial survival of the center, whose existence was threatened by a number of community individuals and groups, depended in part on the skillful use of behavioral principles including attempts to extinguish verbal and written attacks on the center's methods (Turner, 1975). For example, the term "behavior modification" often provoked extremely hostile responses from community groups. At first, the staff spent much time explaining the meaning of the term, the difference between reinforcement and bribery, etc. These attempts were unsuccessful. The staff next established a response cost procedure providing a fine of $50 for any staff person saying "behavior modification" in public.

While the center has developed many types of clinical programs, only four components of the agency's operations will be detailed here: (1) outpatient services for adults, (2) a program for teaching parents behavioral methods, (3) staff management procedures, and (4) comprehensive evaluation methods.

Rinn and Vernon (1975) have described intake, goal setting, treatment, and follow-up procedures that allow for both process and outcome evaluation. Following a screening interview, the client receives an initial therapy session. First, a short contract is presented to the client which specifies the responsibilities of the client (keep appointments, pay fees, keep records, allow information can be used in research, allow follow-up contacts) and those of the therapist (keep appointments, provide services that have the best chance for effective and efficient treatment, assist in measuring therapy progress, and assure confidentiality). The client is instructed to pinpoint behavioral excesses and deficits and record the frequency and antecedent and consequent events of the target behaviors each week. Baserates are kept on as many as three behaviors; interventions are provided sequentially for different problem behaviors (i.e., a multiple baseline design).

Presentation of the data by the client is required for entry into the next week's session.[2] Using the baserates, client and therapist set quantifiable goals for each problem behavior. The therapist develops a treatment plan for one mutually agreed-upon behavior with the client usually having assignments to complete during the week. Data are collected continually on all targeted behaviors. Treatment continues with a behavioral perspective, and all data collected in therapy sessions are available in a central file.

The quality and integrity of service are assessed by several methods. Pre- and post-training tests evaluate the therapists' verbal competence with different procedures. Case histories are presented prior to and after training, and the therapist must indicate how (s)he would conduct treatment. In vivo evaluations include co-therapy sessions and monitoring of audiotapes. Plans call for videotaping of sessions and feedback to therapists on their performance of specific treatment techniques. Therapists' records are monitored to clarify and quantify their adherence to behavioral procedures and other center policies. Each month, five client files are drawn at random and the therapist's adherence to the previously described procedures are evaluated. Salary increments and other reinforcers are contingent on these evaluations which have revealed an

---

[2]It is not clear what proportion of clients terminate at this point. Further, the validity of this type of self-report may be open to question. For a detailed discussion of the problems of evaluating outpatient services and a presentation of a low-cost evaluation technique, see Schnelle, McNees, Gendrich, and Hannah (1975).

increase in staff conformity to the center's guidelines.

Rinn, Vernon, and Wise (1975) have reported a 3-year evaluation of child-management classes which have been used with over 1,100 parents. Their demonstration provides an excellent example of how evaluation can be used as feedback to modify and improve existing services.

Presenting problems were primarily ones of child management (enuresis, temper tantrums, school attendance). Referrals came from a wide variety of sources. Families were from varied socioeconomic classes, and the average age of the 639 "problem" children was 8.7 years. Approximately 40 persons attended classes, some of which were conducted by doctoral and some masters' level instructors. The course followed a step-by-step outline (instructor behavior was assessed using a time-sampling procedure) and was initiated by the parents signing a contract and paying an enrollment fee of $30. Ten dollars were refundable contingent on class attendance, completed homework assignments, and positive changes in the child's behavior. Admission of parents to subsequent classes was contingent on completion of homework assignments that involved typical behavioral child-management program elements (data collection, development of a program plan). The degree to which behavioral goals was attained also was assessed.

The project's data showed that 79% of homework assignments were completed. Based on a goal attainment measure completed at the end of the class, it was shown that in 92% of the cases, 68-100% goal attainment was achieved. A 6-month follow-up was conducted which involved a random sample of cases for which parents estimated the frequency or duration of the problem behavior. Fifty-four percent of the sample indicated rates in the "much improved" range, while 30% of the cases were in the "moderately improved" category (33-67% goal attainment). In no instance did cases falling into either the moderate or "no improvement" range at treatment termination improve their outcome status at the time of follow-up. While decrements from treatment to follow-up were not a direct function of length of follow-up interval, the results suggested a decline in treatment effects. Other measures indicated that the likelihood of parents seeking additional mental health services for their children was very low at the end of the course and at follow-up points. Consumer satisfaction indices showed the instructors and behavior modification methods received high ratings and that over 80% of the people had recommended the course to others.

Following the guidelines for home observations established by Patterson, Cobb, and Ray (1973), five treatment and three no-treatment families were included in an evaluation in which target behaviors were selected, and home observations were performed before and after the course. Conversion of the pre- and post-course frequency counts for problem behaviors to a goal attainment score revealed a 92% score for the treated families and a 0% score for untreated families.

Masters' and doctoral level instructors attained the same average goal attainment in their classes, suggesting that subprofessional staff could conduct the course with no loss in treatment success. An analysis of the relationship between meeting attendance, goal attainment, and socioeconomic status indicated that lower SES ($5,000 earned annually) attended fewer meetings (3.1) and had a lower median goal attainment score (5%) than a middle-class group of parents (4.9 meetings, 93% goal attainment). It would appear necessary to modify the structure of the course in order to serve lower income patients adequately (Lorion, 1974).

The effects of the monetary contingency were analyzed also. Parents receiving the contingent refund completed about six times more projects and attended more meetings than a comparable group of parents in a noncontingent condition.

As a final evaluation, a cost analysis of the course was performed. Staff time for the 24 classes conducted in 1971-1973 amounted to 240 hours. The individual programming of "failures" or those rquiring additional service after the course (a total of 16% of those taking it) required 414 hours, yielding a total of 654 hours to treat 639 families. It was estimated that 2,594 hours would have been required to treat these families through the usual outpatient services. The total cost for the classes and those requiring additional help was $26,479, while the cost for training the families through outpatient services would have been $77,811.

The utility of systematic program evaluation for program planning was emphasized:

> . . . when it was found that the title of trainer did not affect outcome variables, a marked increase in the use of Master's level psychologists followed. Also the demonstration that financial contingencies affected process variables in a positive manner led to the strengthening of the contingencies. In other words, the ongoing evaluation of the program allowed for the elimination of "superstitious" program elements and the retention of the useful training components. The constant feedback from the program to the planners was invaluable and still continues, aiding in further system refinement. (Rinn et al., 1975, p. 386)

In 1973 the center developed an operant managerial system (Turner & Goodson, 1975) based on the establishment of a contract negotiated through mutual agreement by the supervisor and supervisee which specifies individualized job descriptions, success criteria, and rewards. Key components of the system include: (1) use of staff's baserates for the establishment of performance criteria and goals, (2) behavioral descriptions of all job tasks (3) the ranked importance of job tasks, (4) the use of measurable criteria for success, (5) frequent feedback and supervisor data on job-task behavior, (6) distribution of a manual to all supervisors detailing contract procedures, and (7) clearance of all contracts through a senior administrative staff person to assure consistency in job items and evaluation criteria across service units.

The entire performance evaluation plan is converted to a point system. Points are awarded on meeting performance criteria and the ranked importance of that job task. Points are exchangeable for monetary rewards, special training events, or extra vacation time.

Turner and Pyfrom (1974) have indicated that the center is trying to quantify additional aspects of job performance reflecting the conviction that those aspects of job performance that could not be quantified are associated generally with unreliable ratings and should be excluded from the performance review process. In addition, while monetary and other tangible rewards are given only on a yearly schedule (social reinforcement and feedback is given more frequently), such reinforcers ideally would be dispensed contingently at each pay period.

Essentially the same approach has been used in setting program goals and evaluating the center's service components (Bolin & Kivens, 1974). Every service component (including administration) has a contract between itself and the center. The contract is approved by the director in conjunction with the research coordinator. The research and evaluation unit then collects data for each service and returns the data to each service component every two months. The bimonthly data are used annually for quantitative and narrative performance evaluation of the service components and goal setting for the next year.

An overall appraisal of the Huntsville-Madison center requires attention to the issues of outcome evaluation and dissemination. While the widespread applicability of behavioral methods to community mental health service is impressive, there are important questions about their relative effectiveness compared to other mental health paradigms and the feasibility of disseminating this model to other mental health centers. Turner, the assistant director, has reported (Bolin & Kivens, 1974) that he could find no other mental health centers that maintain similar data, although comparisons are possible on treatment length, goal achievement, persistence of change, and cost per service unit. Other data, such as decline in mental hospital admissions, are beginning to become available (Turner, 1975). The center also is conducting a number of process and outcome studies of specific techniques and services that will provide further data on comparative effectiveness.

The dissemination issue is equally crucial. Turner (1975) and Bolin and Kivens (1974) have stressed that observers of the Huntsville system fail to see that the center evolved from a planned series of successive approximations and shaping of the staff, other agencies, and the community. The complex system that exists today probably could not be duplicated easily or quickly. Other constraints on active dissemination are the necessity for control of employment practices, performance review and reward, the large amount of staff time (about

10%) devoted to evaluation, and the difficulty of finding capable staff leaders totally committed to a comprehensive behavioral system. It is likely that selected portions rather than complete replications of the system will be transferred to other mental health settings. Even this partial dissemination would be a substantial contribution to the field.

It would also seem important for the Huntsville center to demonstrate that the same empirical model can be used to promote changes in other organizations or develop programs that focus more on community development than on therapy-related services. For example, the center could develop a performance contract with another agency that calls for consultant-directed implementation of a behavioral management system. This contract could specify consultation procedures, aspects of the management system to be implemented, expected changes in staff behavior, and service outcomes and remuneration to the Huntsville center contingent on the agency meeting such outcomes.

Use of Pseudo-Patients as an Evaluation Procedure

The recently developed pseudo-patient methodology provides precision, control, and detailed behavioral data on mental health practitioners' behaviors. Coupled with the work from Huntsville-Madison, the pseudo-patient approach could give service providers or consumers a methodology to ensure the development and continuation of effective, accountable service systems.

The use of pseudo-patients involves the planned simulation of problem behaviors or patterns which are presented to many different practitioners thereby allowing a nonreactive evaluation of their methods of assessment and treatment. Another alternative involves presenting different scenarios to the same clinicians and recording their interventions. Important parameters of patient characteristics (sex, SES, etc.), presenting problems, or demeanor (e.g., cooperativeness) could be varied systematically and their effects on manner and quality of service delivery assessed.

Such unobtrusive observational methods have been advocated before (Webb, Campbell, Schwartz, & Sechrest, 1966). Rosenhan (1973) has used psuedo-patients to examine admission practices and staff behavior in mental hospitals. Winkler's (1974) work has extended Rosenhan's by directly manipulating treatment-relevant variables and using the data as feedback to the service agency to facilitate modifications of their practices.

Owen and Winkler (1974) sought to determine the basis upon which Australian physicians presented drugs. A number of research questions were addressed: Did general practitioners openly offer drug prescriptions or did they yield to strong patient requests? If drugs were prescribed, were adequate warnings given? Were referrals to appropriate social agencies made frequently? Would women presenting the same scenario as men receive more drug prescriptions? Would patients be subjected to political influence attempts by practitioners because of controversies between the medical establishment and government about health care policies? The use of pseudo-patients to answer such questions is salient only if some standards of care related to treatment appropriateness and outcome have been established. While psuedo-patients can be used for gathering information on the discrepancies between standards and actual practice, their use is not sufficient to settle most issues related to the codification of appropriate standards.

Five males and five females (ages 29-38, of varied occupations) learned a standardized role in which a mild, situational depression was depicted, a standard personal background was used, and standard responses to typical practitioner questions were programmed. Twenty-five general practitioners selected at random were visited by one male and one female. Outcome data included drug prescriptions, referral notes, warnings concerning drug side-effects, attempts at providing reassurance and counseling, and incidents of political influence. Following completion of these visits, practitioners were sent a questionnaire describing the same history and problem (for a female) and asked to report how they would treat the problem and how adequate they felt in doing so.

The results indicated that the true status of pseudo-patients was not recognized. In 78% of the visits, a pseudo-patient emerged with a drug prescription, and in 90% of these instances the prescription contained at least one psychotropic medication. Yet on 57% of such occurrences, no mention was made by practitioners of possible side effects or related problems such as the danger of alcohol and drug interactions. Reassurance and discussion, liberally defined, occurred in 42% of the visits, and some counseling was provided in 28% of the visits. In 24% of the cases further physical examinations were recommended. Generally no differences on these measures could be attributed to the sex of the pseudo-patient. In 36% of the offices, political pamphlets or signs were on display.

While only 40% of the questionnaires were returned, the practitioners' verbal responses made an interesting contrast to their actual behavior. Practitioners acknowledged that social factors were contributing to "patients" problems and often indicated that social-psychological referrals or interventions would be appropriate.

Even in the absence of patient requests, medication alone was the primary treatment for mild depression actually provided by practitioners. Such prescriptions were obtained in visits whose average time was only 15 minutes. Referrals to more appropriate social agencies were made infrequently despite the physicians' endorsement of such agencies on the mailed questionnaire.

Winkler (1974) has suggested that perceptions are influenced greatly by the role of the perceiver and the environmental context. For example, patients and hospital staff undoubtedly will view the mental hospital milieu differently with each perception being no less valid than the other. However, patients' perceptions often are devalued because any discrepancies with staff persons' perceptions are interpreted as signs of "pathology" with the public stigmatization of the mental patient role further reducing the probability of patients speaking out and/or having their beliefs seem credible. The use of pseudo-patients may be one method to circumvent these problems because an impartial third-party account of the milieu can be provided.

Winkler's preliminary research with mental hospitals differs from Rosenhan's (1973) in a number of ways. First, the pseudo-patients were clinical psychology graduate students with a goal of acquiring a lasting understanding of the patient role. Also, Winkler's pseudo-patients assumed a clearly defined case history rather than a minimal symptom, behaved normally in the hospital, and stayed for only a short time. Similar to a "Nader" approach, the major purpose was:

> . . . to gather information which can be disseminated to the community at large. Public awareness of what pseudo-patients observe in psychiatric hospitals is capable of pressuring hospitals to change more rapidly and more appropriately than they have been, to raise public debate about the need for alternative resources and to assist in developing a more discerning attitude in prospective patients with respect to the way in which the mental health system handles them. (Winkler, 1974, p. 400)

Once admitted, pseudo-patients act normally and take copious notes about hospital procedures, staff behavior, and their own feelings. A detailed, recorded debriefing follows the pseudo-patients' return from the hospital. These data are then returned to the hospital if it requests the information.

A more recent study by Stone, Winkler, and Hewson (1975) showed how this procedure could be used for evaluation, feedback, and program modification when pseudo-patients were sent to the agency with the prior consent of professionals, a probable requirement for research in the United States. The subjects were doctors employed by a family planning association which was interested in developing a sex counseling course. A pseudo-patient, male-female (ages 20-36; n=10) couple presented a standard scenario relevant to this particular clinic and the goals of the counseling course to be evaluated. The presenting problem included a highly reduced libido in women and a history of primary anorgasmia. There were no physical complications, and the women were supposedly taking a birth control pill that could not account for the symptoms. Psychosocial aspects of the problem included limited knowledge about sexual behavior, a puritanical upbringing for the female, poor communication between the couple, unassertiveness, and anxiety associated with sexual behavior. During the consultation, the male remained passive and acted as a second observer.

The design allowed for two groups of doctors with an experimental group which received the training course, and a control group which did not.

Unfortunately, these two groups differed in level of experience with those doctors receiving the course having more experience. The pseudo-patient couple visited one experimental and one control doctor before and after the course was given, yielding a total of four visits by each pseudo-patient couple. Each doctor was seen twice before and twice after the course by two different couples. Pseudo-patients were unaware of the experimental course, the previous performance of the doctor, or order of their visit. The first two visits were completed during a 6-week period prior to the course, and the last two visits occurred over a 4-week period following the course.

The training course involved a 2-day in-service workshop focusing on instruction and role playing in behavioral analysis and behavioral treatment of male and female sexual problems. Dependent measures obtained during debriefing sessions consisted of a consensual response by the couple and included questions relevant to diagnosis (e.g., did the doctor ask about pain during intercourse, use of a contraceptive pill, etc.), treatment (e.g., information, drug prescription, etc.), and ratings of reassurance and doctors' anxiety. The questions had been developed in pilot work with sex therapists in which they noted the types of diagnostic and treatment behaviors relevant to this case history. A follow-up questionnaire assessed the doctors' ability to identify pseudo-patient couples and their degree of certainty about their identification. A system was developed to score proficiency in diagnosis and treatment; in addition, two experienced sex therapists (one male, one female) "blind" to the experimental procedures, independently gave a global rating of the proficiency of the doctors. Interrater reliability for the two therapists was .88, with a correlation of .84 between their rating and the actual proficiency score.

The results showed that the "trained" doctors initially scored higher than the controls on all four measures; however, their performance was not so high as to preclude the need for improvement. No significant differences in pre-post scores could be attributed to the course. Experimental doctors did not change more than controls. Of the 40 pseudo-patient visits, 13 were correctly identified by the doctors, with experimental doctors being more accurate in recognizing the pseudo-patients than the controls. Physician ratings of the effect of recognition on their normal performance varied but were generally high.

The study indicated that the doctors were performing at reasonably high levels prior to the course, and that the training course apparently did not improve their performance. The informed consent procedure, while leading to methodological complications and more reactive observations, did increase the doctors' willingness to receive and use the feedback presented to them. Feedback was presented at an informal party attended by doctors and pseudo-patients.

The research of Winkler and his colleagues represents an intriguing and challenging methodology that allows largely nonreactive, behavioral observations of service delivery personnel in their normal work setting. Such evaluations can be used as an alternative or additional method to assess program effectiveness and provide feedback to personnel involved in behavioral or eclectic community mental health programs. Further research (Martorano & Winett, 1976) can assess the settings and scenarios that are appropriate for pseudo-patient evaluation and the limitations of the procedure when informed consent is required.

Maintenance in the Community and the Dissemination of Community Treatment Models

This section will discuss programs for the maintenance of formerly institutionalized people in the community, a topic which directs our focus toward organizational and system change and the conceptual and technological bases for such change.

Atthowe (1973a) indicated that while several clinically derived procedures (booster treatments, massed treatment, self-control techniques) have been investigated as ways to maintain behavior change, the outcome literature still reports limited success in perpetuating therapeutic gains. Atthowe attributed the existence of this situation to the fact that "we have looked only at the treatment process. We have not taken the next step; we have not attempted to control the eliciting conditions and reinforcers in the person's natural environment which is the maintaining milieu" (p. 35).

He outlined a broad blueprint for change that involved prevention (environmental modification), treatment, and maintenance—a framework he called "behavioral innovation." Atthowe's design involved these important elements:

1. Mental health professionals and all people interested in change must become social planners; changes must be made in the treatment milieu and the social system into which people are released; often such changes will involve the creation of new types of settings (e.g., halfway houses) or extensive change in the community such as the abolishment of restrictive zoning regulations.

2. Knowledge and training relevant to social, practical, and economic systems so as to be able to influence persons in power who possess the resources needed to create change.

3. Comprehensive, egalitarian planning teams that include as members indigenous leaders, political influencers, and trained rehabilitation workers.

4. Behavioral analysis of key behaviors, reinforcers, and techniques necessary for behavioral innovation; by definition of this framework, such

processes apply to the person in need of rehabilitation, significant others, treatment personnel, and social systems that influence the person.

5.   Built-in corrective feedback mechanisms so that ineffective programs can be modified (Harshbarger & Maley, 1974).

6.   Perpetuation of behavior innovation programs by: (a) demonstrating program effectiveness to both program staff and the community; (b) involving professionals and community persons in planning such endeavors and focusing planning on treatment, maintenance and prevention; (c) providing reinforcers for all members of the rehabilitation team; (d) basing program changes on experimental data; (e) maintaining staff skill and enthusiasm through additional training, extension courses, workshops, and time to travel into the community to help maintain patients.

As an example of some of these principles, Atthowe described a Veterans Administration program for chronic patients. The program involved a graduated token economy in which patients earned their way out of the program; relevant, paid, job training within the hospital; transfer to self-help wards in which patients took responsibility for such areas of their life as medication and work in semi-sheltered jobs (house cleaning, gas station attendant, food concessions); small-group meetings to plan a unit-wide move to community apartments and houses, with planning assistance by persons who had made a similar move but were still involved in some of the employment facets of the program; nonprofit ownership or rental of community residences; respectable jobs on the hospital grounds; and membership on the program's board of directors by people capable of influencing hospital and community power structures.

At that time (1973), Atthowe reported that preliminary data indicated a low recidivism rate for program participants. "Operations Re-Entry" was developing as an alternative setting in which ex-patients could move into supervisory positions on and off the hospital grounds. The institutional aspect of the program has been restructured in light of the problems encountered by ex-patients, and day-and-night-care support centers have been established in the community. In addition, the program has been able to continue without any grants or full-time direction from its original developers, thereby demonstrating its own maintenance.

Atthowe's work addressed itself to the often used phrase but rarely enacted treatment philosophy of "continuity of care" (Zax & Specter, 1974). For the most part, mental health care for the chronic patient has consisted of poorly planned cycles of release from the hospital, isolation in family care or boarding homes, and readmission to the hospital for short-term "treatment." Alternatives to this "revolving door policy" must consider several factors which constrain the feasibility of eventual adoption. These constraints involve the following contingencies: (1) community responses to haphazard placement of marginal patients have been hostile and occasionally have provoked legislative attempts to bar ex-patients from neighborhoods (e.g., Long Beach, New York); (2) community resistance is likely to be strongest in periods of high unemployment unless jobs are built into rehabilitation programs; (3) in general the notion of community treatment has been denegrated by the public, although strategies such as Atthowe's have been assessed infrequently; (4) the cost of maintaining a person in an institution is excessive and substantial savings to society can be gained by maintaining people in the community (Atthowe, 1975).

The Elwyn Institute for retarded persons is a private, nonprofit institution founded in 1852 in Philadelphia. It provides another excellent example of a behavioral innovation program. Before 1960, the institute provided only custodial care with no community contact. The arrival of a dynamic superintendent allowed the conversion of Elwyn from a locked institution to an open, community-based treatment-rehabilitation facility (Hospital and Community Psychiatry, 1972).

Currently about 1,000 persons (ages 3 years through adulthood) live on the main campus and about 500 persons are day students. The cost of care is about $6,000 for residents and about $3,000 for day students (1972 figures). The program emphasizes basic training in vocational and social skills. Persons are assessed intensively over a 20-week period by work-sample and other *in vivo* evaluations. Based on these assessments, the trainee is assigned to a contract workshop (jobs are performed for local industries) operated like a factory. From here, the trainee can proceed to more advanced vocational training or use the workshop for long-term employment. Vocational training involves on-the-job experiences in such trades as baker's and carpenter's assistants, cement finisher and bricklayer, cook's assistant, and dental assistant (unfortunately all low-income jobs and an acknowledged problem of the program). While enrolled in job training, the trainees receive both counseling services and help in finding a job.

A variety of living arrangements are available and the trainee may move sequentially through them. The arrangements include living at the institute only at night, moving into a halfway house setting located in a modern apartment building, living in the community for 2 weeks and then returning to the institute for 2 weeks of counseling and additional training, or living entirely in the community. Halfway house locations were chosen specifically because they were close to support facilities such as public transportation, medical facilities, and laundromats. Counselors and social workers are available in the halfway houses and trainees can receive guidance on social skills and personal adjustment problems.

Each apartment is shared by two same-sexed adults, has a private kitchen and bathroom, and is paid for by the trainees. Trainees can stay in the setting as long as they want. However, before they can gain entry, trainees are likely to progress through a quarter-house system that involves living in apartments on campus at night and working in the community during the day. Every trainee living in the halfway house setting has to develop a work skill and learn to deal with simple tasks of daily living such as shopping, cooking, budgeting, and banking (the tasks that institutions typically have performed for their residents). Workshops and classes focus on these tasks and are conducted by the staff and community people. For example, a bank representative might explain financial procedures such as depositing money and checks, writing checks, and obtaining money orders. Role playing is used to practice these as well as job interview and socialization skills. Counselors also will accompany a person on initial shopping trips to provide feedback and advice; electronic hand-held calculators that show each purchase and funds remaining are often given to trainees so that they can more easily stay within a budget while shopping. Sex education and driver education classes are also provided. (Additional skill-building programs for psychiatric residents are analyzed in Chapter 8.)

Initial evaluations of the program have been very favorable. For example, in a 4-year project from 1964-1968, 128 retarded persons (two to 49 years in institutions, $\overline{X}$ = 15 years; IQ scores from 45 to 80) were placed in the community. A follow-up study in 1972 found that 70% of them were employed and working regularly and one was reinstitutionalized. It was found that it cost about $50,000 to rehabilitate 30 trainees. Comparing this one-time cost to the annual cost of about $215,000 involved in maintaining 30 individuals in an institution reveals the substantial cost-benefit of such programs (Atthowe, 1973a, 1975).

Fairweather and his colleagues (Fairweather, 1967; Fairweather, Sanders, Maynard, & Cressler, 1969; Fairweather, Sanders, & Tornatzky, 1974) have provided another excellent example of the development and dissemination of a community treatment program for chronic mental patients. Earlier work (1950s to early 1960s) in the hospital milieu had shown that patients who received either individual or group psychotherapy or lived and worked as groups on wards did no better in terms of community adjustment 18 months after release than those patients who simply worked in the hospital setting. Further, institutional improvement was not related to maintenance in the community, and recidivism rates were high regardless of the treatment approach. It became apparent that a vehicle was needed to lessen the gap between the hospital and the community.

Small, supportive groups of patients were formed in the hospital to meet this problem. These groups focused on both current, daily problems and anticipated problems in the community. The results of this study were partially encouraging. Even the most chronic patients were capable of participating in such groups, the groups showed a good deal of autonomy, and the morale of both the staff and patients increased. However, once the person left the hospital and this support group, he was just as likely to return to the hospital as a participant in a traditional program. Also there was a very strong relationship between people remaining in the community and support received from people they lived with while outside the hospital. Clearly, the support group had to be moved into the community as a unit.

The design of such a treatment model involved the development of a support group on the ward, movement into a converted motel (lodge), initiation of a business (industrial and home cleaning), and reduction of supervision and control by the psychologists and medical staff so that virtually all financial and managerial matters were controlled by the ex-patients, thereby increasing their level of autonomous functioning. A comparison of participants in the lodge program with persons receiving traditional hospital and after-care treatment showed that over a 40-month period persons treated in the lodge program remained in the community about 90% of the time and were employed about 50% of the time. Figures for the traditional-program participants were about 20% for time in the community and 0% for employment. In addition, the lodge program cost only about one-third the amount needed for traditional care. Further, the morale and self-perception of the ex-patients in the lodge program were very positive, and these persons were accepted in their residential area and the business community (Fairweather et al., 1969).

One would expect that such dramatic results would lead to rapid implementation of this treatment innovation by other hospitals and related institutions. This expectation was not validated. Only one other hospital adopted the program at that point.

Researchers often are content to publish their results and enjoy a sense of completion and other rewards. However, Fairweather and his group, disappointed with the failure of hospitals to adopt the program, directly addressed the problems involved in dissemination of their programs.

Fairweather et al. (1974) conducted a national study designed to investigate methods to change organizations so that the lodge program would be adopted by psychiatric hospitals. The "experimental social innovation" methodology (Fairweather, 1967) used to develop and evaluate the treatment model itself was now emphasized in the dissemination phase. Specific parameters of organizations and change procedures to be investigated in the study were derived from the organizational change literature and the researcher's experience with the model (see Fairweather et al., 1974, Chapter 2). Working with 255 psychiatric hospitals across the country, the research design required an equal number of state and federal hospitals in rural and urban settings to be approached about instituting the program at either a high (superintendent, psychiatrist) or low (psychologist, social worker, nurse) level. If interested by the initial contact, hospitals were offered either detailed brochures about the program, a workshop fully describing the program, or a demonstration ward initiated with a consultant's help.

Hospitals still interested in implementing community treatment programs after having received either the brochures, workshop, or demonstration ward, were assigned randomly to either an "action consultant" or "written manual" condition. The action consultant visited the hospital; helped train staff to develop patient groups; found financial support, employment, living arrangements; and helped organize efforts to move the patients into the community. In addition, telephone contact was maintained between the consultant and the hospital. The manual provided written descriptions of these same implementation procedures. Telephone contact also was established with hospitals in this condition.

Throughout the persuasion and adoption phases of the study, it was found that action-oriented approaches were usually necessary to institute actual efforts on the hospital's part to implement the program. Many hospitals were willing to be sent brochures or have workshops presented to them, but such passive procedures were associated rarely with actual efforts to implement the lodge program. Very few hospitals responded positively to the active intervention methods, but those that did were much more likely to attempt to institute the community program. Fairweather et al. suggested that the best persuasion technique would probably be a shaping ("foot in the door") tactic which started with low level, passive interventions (e.g., brochures), secured initial commitments, and then moved sequentially and methodically to more active procedures (workshops, demonstration projects).

A number of factors not associated with adoption of the lodge program are important because they have been discussed widely as significant variables associated with change. These included amount of resources in the hospital, the status level of the person initially contacted at the hospital, the demographic characteristics and social climate of the hospital's locale,[3] and hospital staff attitudes. In general, the results of the study support the notion of an outside, action-oriented consultant instructing, shaping, modeling, and reinforcing a small, cohesive, and committed group of "internal change agents" (with status being unimportant) as an effective vehicle for organizational change.

This study has particular salience for the behavioral community psychologist on a number of accounts. The project reveals that the dissemination process and organizational change can be effected and studied experimentally while at the same time indicating both the type of effort and broad knowledge base needed to institute behavioral innovation programs and the need to advance behavioral research from a demonstration to a dissemination stage of development (Winett, 1976a). There is also a striking similarity between Fairweather's results and the emerging behavioral literature on organizational change and teacher consultation (see Chapter 2). In both areas, active on-site approaches involving information, modeling, feedback, and reinforcement focused on target behaviors have led to

---

[3]This might be true in this research because mental hospitals are "total institutions" apart from the community. In the case of disseminating other programs (e.g., schools, environmental protection) the importance of factors such as social climate may be more important.

replicable change while more passive, inexact, verbal approaches generally have not.

Organizational Change and Staff Development

This section will discuss the behavioral literature that has investigated procedures for the change of organization and staff behavior. The methods used are similar to those described in the section concerning the Huntsville-Madison program and may be considered necessary components in changing any type of mental health program.

Panyan, Boozer, and Morris (1970) concluded that while the staff working with institutionalized persons might be reinforced by the progress made by such persons in skill training or the reduction of severe behavioral disorders, other self-help skills might be acquired so gradually that feedback and reinforcement for the staff is minimal and ineffective. In such a case, staff also would tend to minimize their training efforts. In this study staff first received a 4-week, formal classroom course in operant techniques and then returned to their units in a state institution for the retarded to apply these methods to teaching self-feeding, handwashing, dressing, bathing, and toileting. Staff were assigned specific behaviors to teach two designated residents (the same self-help skills were taught to the second resident once the first resident had mastered the skill). In addition to conducting the training, staff were instructed to keep records on each session. No contingencies were in effect for either conducting the sessions or keeping records. This situation represented a baseline condition which was continued for different lengths of time on each of the four units (a multiple baseline design).

During the feedback condition, each unit received a weekly report that indicated the total possible training sessions for each skill, the actual number of sessions recorded and conducted by each staff person, and the unit percentage of sessions recorded and conducted. This percentage score was rank ordered so that units could compare their performances.

During baseline conditions, staff performance was variable but averaged less than 59% of conducted sessions. The feedback procedure consistently improved staff performance to the 75-100% range. The longer the staff worked after the course without feedback, the more time was required to increase performance to the 75-100% range. Feedback instituted immediately after the course maintained high staff performance for 30 weeks, a rather good indication of the long-term effectiveness of this simple procedure. Panyan et al. (1970) suggested linking salary increments, vacations and holiday, or work-shift preferences to the performance-feedback system.

Pomerleau, Bobrove, and Smith (1973) extended this work in several important ways: a number of information, feedback and incentive procedures with psychiatric aides were investigated; reinforcement to the aide was contingent on patient improvement; and the focus was not only on a single response but improvement on a range of psychiatrically relevant behaviors.

Nine aides and an average of 23 patients in the behavioral treatment program of the Temple University Unit of Philadelphia State Hospital participated. The patients presented severe behavioral disorders but were without organic complications. The program was a locked-ward token system that emphasized social interactions among patients and also attempted to reduce the frequency of behaviors that had resulted in institutionalization. Aides were assigned one or more patients with the tasks of developing a relationship with the patients, completing specific behavioral programs with them, and maintaining the token economy system.

Patient behavior was assessed with a previously validated rating instrument which was completed twice a week by a psychiatric technician and a nurse. The instrument tapped patient appearance and demeanor, verbal behavior, and adaptation to ward routine. A patient's weekly score was the average of the two ratings. Ratings were compared to the previous week's ratings to derive a behavior change score. A weekly performance score for an aide consisted of the average of the change score of their assigned patients.

After these procedures were routinized, the following conditions, each lasting about 4 weeks, were enacted: (1) a $20 award which was given to the "most cooperative aide," the aide who helped fellow workers with their patients (the award was not contingent on patient improvement, and the improvement of assigned patients was not announced); (2) feedback in which the aides were ranked on the basis of their residents' improvement; (3) an award of $10 to the aides on each tour of duty whose patients showed the most improvement ("aides of the week") plus a $20 award to the "most cooperative aide"; (4) replications of this previous procedure but with $20 and $30 for "aides of the week"; (5) a replication of the $20 "aides of the week" and "most cooperative aide" awards but with program consultation between aides and a professional staff person; (6) a supervisory condition in which *in vivo* instruction and feedback from professional staff were given to the aides along with the daily consultation (monetary awards for winners of the aides' contests also were continued). Feedback on patient performance was included as part of all incentive conditions. These data showed that some patient improvement was associated with the initial feedback procedure and the initial introduction of the $20 aides-of-the-week award; marked improvement in patient behavior was evidenced under the $30 awards, but reintroduction of the $20 award was associated with a return to baseline levels. Patient improvement was affected only slightly by the consultation and supervisory conditions. Complete termination of all aspects of the program (including many aspects of the basic token economy) following these experimental conditions led to decrements of patient ratings below baseline levels.

The results suggested the importance of feedback and incentives and to a lesser extent supervision for staff management and concomitant patient behavior change. Additional studies on potent reinforcers other than money and systems that do not require aides to compete against one another are needed. In this regard, Pomerleau et al. have indicated some of the potential research and service delivery problems associated with cash awards:

> After the cash incentive conditions were put into effect, several aides began to hint that cessation of awards for research purposes might be met by a refusal to work. The original procedure called for the presentation of cash awards in increasing amounts (giving the aides time to acquire appropriate skills before competing for larger awards), followed by several conditions in which no award or a $20 award was given. The deterioration in the behavior of patients and in the morale of the aides when the cash awards was decreased from $30 to $20, however, suggested that termination of awards might produce a major disruption of service to the patients. For this reason, in the third phase cash awards were continued at the same level and a new independent variable, supervision, was introduced. (Pomerleau et al., 1973, p. 389)*

Pommer and Streedbeck (1974) have reported similar work with house parents of a facility for children with severe problems. House parents in this program were assigned specific tasks (e.g., toilet training) with the children. Procedures intended to increase the percentage of these tasks completed by the staff included public notices, a list of the jobs to be done, job slips which were redeemable for one dollar each, and a combination of these procedures. The combined procedures proved to be the most successful managerial procedure with over 90% of the tasks completed compared to about 40% during baseline, about 75% for public notices, and about 85% for the job slips alone.

A more recent study by Quilitch (1975) in an institution for the retarded has extended the previously noted work in a number of ways. He identified one of the key problems in institutions as the unsystematic staff performance of potentially effective procedures. In other words, there is often a deficit in managerial technology. The development and evaluation of managerial systems would be essential for programmatically disseminating much of the behavioral technology discussed in this book. In this study, several standard managerial procedures (memos, in-service training, feedback) were experimentally analyzed. The dependent measure involved a simplified observational system of patient behavior, a system that could be operationalized easily by on-line staff in many settings.

---

*Pomerleau, O. F., Bobrove, P. H., and Smith, R. H. Rewarding psychiatric aides for the behavioral improvement of assigned patients. *Journal of Applied Behavior Analysis*, 1973, *6*, 383-390.

The major target problem was the chronic inactivity of the residents, 95 mentally retarded persons, living within four wards of the Nevada Mental Health Institute. Such behavior is a general problem of institutionalized retarded persons and is incompatible with the development of behaviors essential for either good health or a satisfactory adjustment in the community. The program was staffed by an adequate number of nurses, mental health technicians, and volunteers who had access to materials and books on the implementation of therapeutic activities with the residents.

The dependent measure was the Planned Activity Check Evaluation designed for group-care facilities. The wards were observed for 4 minutes at four random times between 9 and 11 a.m. The observer first counted the number of residents that were present; on a second tour, the number of active (doing a chore, reading or writing, conversing, using recreational materials) residents were recorded. The figures were summed, yielding a proportion of active residents to total residents present. Reliability data, in part collected by minimally trained observers, revealed high interrater agreement.

Experimental procedures designed to increase the activity of the residents included: (1) an official *memo* from the Chief Administrator stressing the importance of daily activities for the residents and suggesting they be carried out on each ward between 9 and 11 a.m.; (2) an instructional *workshop* on how to lead recreational activities; the workshop featured talks, film slides, and discussions on the importance of engaging residents in activities; (3) a *scheduling and feedback* procedure which involved specifying the recreational activities to be conducted and the technicians responsible for leading the activities as well as a poster and graph identifying the activity leader and the average number of residents participating in activities.

The results showed that after the memo and workshops only about 4-6% of the residents were active. The scheduling and feedback system raised the percent-active residents to 25-30%. To determine whether the memo and workshop conditions were necessary antecedents to the successful implementation of the scheduling and feedback procedure, two wards implemented this later condition immediately after a baseline condition. The percentage of active residents increased from baseline levels of about 10% to about 45% during the scheduling and feedback condition, indicating that the memos and workshops were not necessary prior conditions.

Quilitch also used two procedures to "socially validate" these changes. Seventy-five staff persons and five parents of the residents of the Nevada facility were given written descriptions of the recreational activities in which the staff was intended to engage the residents. When these persons were asked if the activities would be beneficial for the residents, all of them responded affirmatively.

Two staff persons from each of the wards were asked to rate the proportion of residents engaged in activities (1 = "none engaged" to 10 = "all engaged") before and after the scheduling and feedback procedure. "Before" ratings averaged 2.2 while "after" ratings averaged 9.0. Thus, many people judged the activities to be worthwhile, and people in a position to judge change indicated a large increase in the percentage of residents participating in activities.

Iwata, Bailey, Brown, Foshee, and Alpern (1975) have demonstrated how behavioral management programs can be made more cost-effective. A weekly lottery was instituted in which staff could win the opportunity to rearrange their work schedules if they met designated performance criteria in their work with multiply handicapped retarded persons. Though changes in staff behavior were not dramatic, sufficient staff improvement was evident so that the loss of the lottery winner on a given work day did not hinder overall staff performance.

In summary, these studies provide demonstrations that experimental analysis and behavioral principles can be used to develop effective management systems and change mental health organizations. Perhaps in the next few years, such methodology will be extended to the evaluation of such widely discussed procedures as flexible work hours and worker control of salaries, production, and other working conditions.

Another important aspect of organizational changes involves development of staff competence. Gardner (1972) observed that little attention had been directed at assessing effective methods to teach behavior modification techniques. In this study, 20 female attendants enrolled in an in-service program for new employees were matched on demographic variables, nursing skills, attitudes, and knowledge about retardation, and were randomly assigned to one of two groups. One group received eight 1-hour lectures presenting behavior modification principles (reinforcement, shaping, and stimulus control) in everyday language. The other group was enrolled first in six 1-hour role-playing sessions in which behavior modification techniques were demonstrated and then role-played by the participants with feedback provided by a technician. Each group then received the form of training not previously administered.

Two dependent measures were used. One was a skill test involving the ratings of trainees' role-played behavior modification procedures. This measure had been shown to correlate with actual performance with retarded children. Another measure tapped the trainees' verbal understanding of behavioral techniques. Tests were administered before the programs started, after the first training segment (role playing versus lectures), and after the total program was completed. In this way, the effects of individual components and their order of presentation were assessed.

The results indicated that on the skill test those trainees who received role playing first significantly outscored trainees who received the lecture series first. After both groups had received both types of training, scores were equivalent. Similar results were found for verbal knowledge of behavior principles except that the trainees who initially received the lectures outscored those who participated initially in role-playing sessions. Scores of the two groups were about the same after completion of both phases of training. The results suggest that although neither sequence was preferable, both verbal and skill components need to be present in the optimal training program.

Gardner concluded that New Careers trainees (low income, high unemployment, inner-city residents) scored about the same as regular trainees on initial and post-tests. However, Gardner warned that though the program imparted new knowledge and skills, its "prescriptive" and mechanistic nature tended to discourage participation in such training by the brightest attendants. This finding suggests that changes must be made in the format of behavioral training programs to attract a variety of persons.

Paul and his associates (Paul & McInnis, 1974; Paul, McInnis, & Mariotto, 1973) as part of their larger comparative social learning versus milieu study have investigated various methods of training mental health technicians. In one of the few studies that relates paraprofessional training to actual job performance, Paul and McInnis (1974) found that for a group of predominantly female technicians (n=42) a sequential program in which classroom instruction preceded on-the-job training led to better academic performance than an integrated program which featured classroom instruction combined with clinical observations performed by experienced technicians. However, the integrated approach was related to better on-the-job performance. On-the-job training involved shaping procedures in which the trainee observed a supervisor performing a specific task and then practiced the task under conditions of total, minimal, and then no supervision. Data on staff performance were collected by observers who recorded all staff behavior that was functionally related to residents' behavior. A "goodness" of performance score was derived from these observations based on the amount of staff-resident interaction and included rate and extent of programmatic errors. Those receiving the integrated approach scored better on this measure (higher interactions and fewer errors).

Neither group showed performance decrements when supervision was faded, and both groups scored very well on the performance measure. However, within both groups, academic performance was found to be significantly related to the quality of the on-the-floor performance, suggesting that paraprofessional training programs should include some "academic" component. This also confirms Gardner's finding concerning the reluctance of bright individuals to be involved in behavioral training programs. Based on these data, Paul and McInnis (1974) recommended that technician training should focus on job-related behavior rather than a general work orientation, concrete functions rather than abstract theory, modeling and feedback rather than totally didactic presentations, and specific programs that focus on staff and resident behaviors in designated settings.

It is highly probable that in the next several years behaviorists increasingly will devote their energy to paraprofessional training (Zax & Specter, 1974). For example, a technology needs to be developed that can teach line-staff how to translate problem areas into programs with explicit procedures and tasks. One method might involve writing training manuals understandable by a range of paraprofessional staff. The efficacy of such manuals coupled with other procedures could be tested by observing on-the-job performance before and after exposure to the manuals. Manuals associated with high performance also could provide a mechanism for program dissemination.

The research on organizational change and staff training and development is still in its infancy. However, it is already apparent that principles that have been shown to influence behavior in other settings, such as schools (see Chapter 2) are just as applicable in mental health settings and that relatively passive approaches (e.g., workshops, memos, lectures) are relatively ineffective in changing work behaviors or teaching new skills. As this research continues, it should be possible to begin developing effective, specific, and replicable methods for assessing and remedying organizational difficulties (Petrock, 1975).

Community Organization

Several recent behavioral studies have focused on developing settings to improve poor communities. These studies also illustrate an alternative mode of service delivery to the reliance on outpatient psychotherapy. L. K. Miller and O. Miller (1970) have claimed that:

poor persons are increasingly rejecting approaches to poverty based on changing their behavior to conform to existing institutions. They are demanding that existing institutions be changed and even that new institutions be invented ... Part of this more complete approach has focused on creating new organizations composed and governed exclusively for poor persons and directed toward planning and executing programs for their own benefit. (p. 57)

Self-help, "grassroot" organizations that have been developed must be capable of attracting and maintaining the participation of poor persons if they are to be potent forces in creating the social changes which they desire. However, most of these groups have had as their focus longer range goals (e.g., educational or governmental changes) where immediate benefit is usually absent or difficult to identify. In light of data presented by Miller and Miller (1970) on the relatively low rate of participation by poor people in such voluntary organizations, a strategy for immediately reinforcing participation would appear to be an important development.

Following a behavioral paradigm, Miller and Miller identified attendance at meetings as a behavior which was crucial to other organization behaviors and could be observed and reinforced readily. The study participants were recipients of Aid to Families with Dependent Children (ADC). Two self-help groups held monthly meetings which focused on individual and welfare-related problems (allowances, prompt receipt of welfare checks) and community affairs affecting group members; strategies for dealing with problems were devised through group discussion.

Two procedures were investigated. In one condition, all ADC recipients were informed by mail of meetings intended to establish self-help groups. In another condition, the same recipients were informed by mail of such meetings as well as the fact that persons could collect two free Christmas toys and other items and services (e.g., furniture, clothing, assistance with problems, birth control information) for attending the meetings. An A-B-A-B design was used to examine the effectiveness of the reinforcement procedures.

The data showed the importance of the reinforcers in influencing attendance. Without reinforcement, an average of three people attended meetings; with reinforcement average attendance was about 15 persons. Members also tended to continue attendance at meetings more during the reinforcement than the nonreinforcement phase. "Generalization" data revealed that presidents of the self-help groups attended many more meetings of civic groups and social action organizations after joining the self-help groups. While only 20% of the eligible ADC recipients attended meetings, attendance was maintained well in those persons who experienced the reinforcement system. Thus, a crucial problem for attracting more persons is one of reinforcer sampling (Ayllon & Azrin, 1968). Further, the potential exists for defining and reinforcing other important self-help group behaviors that either solve personal problems or have impact on the community. The use of supplementary reinforcers could keep the group oriented to longer range problems when immediate reinforcement is not forthcoming.

Briscoe, Hoffman, and Bailey (1975) have observed that many federal programs in the 1960s and 1970s required the "maximum feasible participation" of low-income persons in decision-making roles in programs and agencies. Based on a number of reports, Briscoe et al. concluded that such participation was mostly ineffective. As with self-help groups, it is apparently insufficient to simply outline a participation modality; important requisite behaviors must be established and maintained. One possible reason for the ineffectiveness of low-income persons in such activities as policy board meetings is the lack of familiarity with formal group decision-making processes. Typically, programs and agencies have provided very little training in such procedures.

The purpose of this study was to demonstrate methods for teaching low-income members of a community board specific problem-solving skills. The participants were elected representatives (three men and six women) to a self-help, community continuing educational project sponsored by a university. Ages ranged from 15 to 67, and all nine participants had very low incomes. The focus of the project was to identify and solve community problems (e.g., finding and distributing new sources of welfare and medical care) and manage the $20,000 budget to fund these efforts. Participants were paid $4.00 to attend each of the 18 meetings held during the study. Meetings were held in a school located in this rural black community; all meetings were audio- and videotaped.

Early work with this group indicated a good deal of unsystematic discussion, decision making, and planning. Several attempts were made to remedy this situation but were unsuccessful. Further analysis indicated three crucial steps for effective problem solving: (1) identification and isolation of the problem under discussion; (2) explication and evaluation of alternative solutions; (3) selection of a solution and specifications of plans to implement the solution. The technique for establishing these skills involved teaching the board members how to use key statements as introductions to the components of problem solving described above. Every board member was taught this strategy.

Dependent measures consisted of key statements that were used to identify problems ("The main problem is . . ..."), solve problems ("Another solution is . . . "), and decide on a course of action ("How will it be done?"). Observers viewing the videotapes recorded the frequency of these types of key statements for each person and for each agenda under discussion.

Training in problem-solving skills initially consisted of written definitions, instructions, demonstrations, and written responses for each person. This approach proved to be unsuccessful. Individual training sessions then were held with seven of the board members. These sessions preceded the meetings and lasted for 30 minutes. Training consisted of practicing the use of key statements in simple and then more complex situations. The training package contained fading, shaping, prompting, modeling, role playing, and social reinforcement elements.

Data were collected for each person from 1 week to 2 months after the training. The study used a multiple baseline design across skills and subjects. Groups and individual data generally showed that increases in the use of the key statements were associated only with training. In some cases completion of training was associated with a decline in the use of the statements. Two persons who received no training did not show any changes in their use of key statements.

Briscoe et al. (1975) suggested that in terms of increased maintenance, future studies should examine using different sorts of statements that might be reinforced, more intensive training and monitoring of meetings, and extrinsic reinforcement for problem-solving behaviors. They also concluded that it is important to see whether such training assists a group in successfully fulfilling both its short- and long-term objectives.

Reiss, Piotrowski, and Bailey (1976) investigated methods to encourage low-income persons to use dental services. They pointed out that most efforts to prevent and control dental disease and other dental problems have entailed educational campaigns in schools, clinics, or the media. Participation in such programs is low (about 20%), and programs infrequently change dental care behaviors. Reiss et al. suggested that programs should focus on actual dental health behavior such as having a parent bring his (her) child to a dental clinic.

Children (n=180) from a rural public school were screened for dental problems by a public health dentist and hygienist. Then children were placed in one of four categories that reflected need for dental care. Fifty-one children who fell into the two most severe categories served as participants in the study and were assigned in blocks (matched for sex, grade, race, and SES) to one of three experimental conditions.

In the "note only" condition, parents received a single notification on the school's letterhead informing them of the outcome of the screening. The nature of the child's dental problem, possible health and school effects of the condition, and a specific recommendation to seek dental care were included in the note. To assure that parents received the note, a coupon that was redeemable in a school-operated store was attached to the note's envelope. A parent had to sign the coupon in order for the child to redeem it.

In the "multiple notification" condition, parents first received a note identical to the one described above. After 3 weeks, a school staff person (usually the child's teacher) called the parent, and 3 weeks later a dental hygienist conducted a home visit. The call and home visit generally conveyed the same information as the note.

In the "$5 incentive condition," a "dental coupon" was included with the original note. The coupon was redeemable if the parent made a dental appointment, took the child for an examination, obtained the dentist's signature on the coupon, and returned it in the stamped, addressed envelope that was provided.

The dependent measure consisted of records of visits to a public health dental clinic or private dental offices. In addition, data were kept on the number of minutes spent by school staff on the telephone, and total mileage and time spent by the dental hygienist in the home visits.

In the "note only" condition only 22% of the children visited a dentist compared to 70% for both the incentive and multiple notification procedures. The cost of each procedure was calculated for each student in each group and for each participating student. In the "note only" condition, the cost for each student was $0.14 and for each participating student $0.63. For the multiple notification procedure, the respective costs were $7.13 and $10.38.

The $5 incentive condition (with a cost of $5.30 for each participant) provided an equally effective procedure but at a lower cost. However, while the note condition resulted in only 20% participation, it was inexpensive, easy to administer, and could therefore be widely used. It was also unclear what the efficacious components or their most effective ordering were in the multiple notification procedure, and whether the incentive procedure used in this study would maintain dental contact.

Pierce and Risley (1974b) have demonstrated the utility of behavioral principles and methodology in developing a special setting for poor people. A recreational program was established in the Juniper Gardens Community Center which was used by all area youths aged 7-13 years. A problem in attracting new members was not remedied by advertising the program. A procedure then was instituted wherein any current member of the program who brought a new member to the center could enter the center with the new member one hour before the regularly scheduled opening time on another recreation day.

This procedure was effective in increasing new membership. During the experimental procedure, attendance averaged 5.0 persons per day compared to .9 per day when no additional recreation time was offered. Further, 58% of the new members were enrolled during the membership drives, which accounted for only 20% of the study's time.

Pierce and Risley also discussed the high degree of destruction and vandalism occurring in urban recreation areas that frequently leads to the termination of programs. In this study, a response cost procedure was used in a recreation program intended primarily for black teenagers. Rule violations (smoking at proscribed times, trash on the floor, property damage) resulted in advancing the closing time of the center by a specific number of minutes dependent on the number and kinds of rules broken. The center was checked every 15 minutes, after which violations and associated penalties were posted. The use of a multiple baseline design (by type of rule violation) showed that instituting the procedure resulted in a very quick and consistent reduction in violations.

In another study (Pierce & Risley, 1974a) Neighborhood Youth Corps aides working in a recreational program were found to be performing very few specified job tasks. This presented a crucial problem to the maintenance of the program and the continued employment of these indigenous aides who were involved in the program not only to earn money but to learn some employment skills. Several procedures were attempted, including giving the aides detailed job descriptions and feedback on their completion of tasks and threatening to fire them for failure to complete their responsibilities. These procedures did not increase completed tasks beyond the 50% level. However, a procedure in which wages were made contingent on number of completed tasks rather than number of hours present resulted in completion of almost 100% of required duties. While it could be argued that this procedure represented a return to piecework, such methods are probably preferable to firing the aides which would have precluded their opportunity to have successful and meaningful job experiences.

The studies reviewed in this section reveal the potential usefulness of behavior change procedures in creating, maintaining, and expanding community organizations and service programs. Individual and social change involve not only the creation of new settings or the alteration of present ones (Sarason, 1972) but also the development and maintenance of behaviors appropriate to these settings.

The development, design, and operation of community settings reflect the prevailing social and economic conditions of our society, and the fact that change at the societal level may be necessary for the survival and continuation of new or modified settings. Salient issues here include the instability of funding sources tied to particular political administrations, the constant high level of unemployment that seems to be a by-product of our economic system, credentials required for some types of employment, career ladder opportunities, style of service delivery, fee structure, and geographic location. In some cases (e.g., the welfare system) self-help groups seem relegated to minimal impact unless they become oriented to larger scale organization directed at the total revamping of social service systems.

An Example of a Public Health Approach to Community Mental Health

Recent work by Clark and Risley (Clark & Risley, 1974; Risley, Clark, & Cataldo, in press) has exemplified (1) a synthesis of behavioral and public health approaches to the secondary prevention of family problems and (2) an alternative to the reliance on the individual therapy model that focuses on the remediation of neglected or severe disorders. The rationale for movement toward the public health model involves the perceived importance of preventive interventions:

> Increasingly the focus of applied behavioral research is turning away from finding solutions to severe, unusual problems and toward investigating ways of helping normal people deal with troublesome everyday situations. For this work to have its maximum social impact, we must look further than the immediate problems people bring to us. We must try to predict and prepare for the types of problems that can be expected to trouble families in the future. Our first step must therefore be to take a close look at significant societal trends that have the effect of placing additional pressure on families. (Risley et al., in press, p. 1)

A number of recent trends are likely to have an important impact on families: (1) While there has been a steady decrease in the birthrates, two deviations from this downward trend have led to an unusual situation. The marked drop in the birthrate in the 1920s and the post World War II "baby-boom" have created a society that has a disproportionately high number of dependent children and young adults but a relatively low proportion of productive and responsible adults (ages 40-55); (2) although the birthrate per family is low, significant reductions in the overall birthrate will not occur because a large proportion of children and young adults will soon be of child-bearing age, and therefore children will be distributed over a larger number of families with *inexperienced* parents; (3) a much larger proportion of women (and mothers) are working outside the home. The data suggest this trend will continue and that there will be an expanded need for various forms of child care (Winett, Moffatt, & Fuchs, 1975) and youth supervision; (4) young families with children are increasingly geographically mobile with most moves by young families being from urban to suburban areas. Families living in the suburbs frequently find themselves in neighborhoods with similar young families who are also inexperienced parents. In addition, such mobility has led to the demise of the extended family and a strong network of friends, both of which have been frequent sources of child-care and child-rearing advice.

Solutions are needed that can be widely disseminated to families with two inexperienced parents who are working and living in environments that offer minimal support for raising their children. The current dimensions of this work are directed at: (1) the development and evaluation of child-care centers with well-specified and efficient child-care routines, delineation of staff assignments to promote quality child care, and promotion of social and educational interactions. The procedures developed from these and other studies have been described in training manuals intended for nonprofessional staff. The manuals have been associated with a high level of staff performance of the routines; (2) the development of pre-adolescent programs in "survival training" (academic and job-related skills) and adolescent "safe passage" programs intended to provide an alternative to "the streets" or troubled peers. The present focus of these child-care and youth programs is the development, marketing, and further evaluation of software packages with specified quality control procedures usable by state licensing and other agencies to monitor the extant programs; (3) the development of advice-giving systems that will provide information on child rearing to parents.

While parent training programs, family counseling centers, high school parenting-family preparation courses, and a popular literature on parental effectiveness are available in many communities, such approaches usually are intended to provide people with a theoretical framework or set of principles to deal with serious problems. These forms of child-rearing advice are most appropriate for well-educated parents or parents desperate for help. Effective ways have not been found to give many families advice on everyday problems, information which was once provided by the extended family and friends. Preliminary work conducted at the Johnny Cake Child Study Center suggested that many child-rearing problems revolve around a fairly small number of specific times and places in the daily life of a family (e.g., sibling arguments during the morning "rush hour"; disruptive behavior in public settings). Additional research indicated that solutions to such problems could be presented in the form of advice that could be transmitted through the media to large numbers of parents.

The development of this system involves a sequence in which networks of families first are interviewed and observed to identify some situationally specific problems and determine what advice is needed to alleviate these problems. The effectiveness of the advice is then field evaluated using the network of families to ensure that the problems were perceived as problems by the participants and that the advice was acceptable, readily understood, and usable. Procedures have been designed to provide straightforward, specific advice intended to improve the children's behavior and enhance family interactions. "We need to guard against developing advice which provides parents with quiet, docile kids, when what parents are looking for are ways in which the limited time the family has together can be more pleasant and significant for all members of the family" (Risley et al., in press, p. 24).

One example of a situation for which advice is being developed is shopping trips. Parents usually are absorbed in their shopping with children merely "tagging along" or engaging in annoying minor mischief. Through interviews and observations, it was confirmed that parents frequently encountered this problem, were interested in finding a way to manage their children better while shopping, and also felt that the children might be given a chance to make a purchase if they were well behaved. Advice concerning this problem was developed by having a number of families attempt the solution; these families were observed when the advice was being used and when it was not in use. After revision, a second set of families was recruited. The best solution involved specifying the rules of acceptable shopping behavior and giving each child 50 cents to spend at the end of the trip. For each rule infraction, a nickel of the allowance was subtracted but could be redeemed on a future trip if the child behaved in accord with parental guidelines.

Initial evaluations showed that the procedure reduced distracting behavior of the children of two families on shopping trips. However, one problem was that the children also curtailed much of their conversation with their parents, thus limiting potentially enjoyable and educational interactions. An enhancement procedure was introduced in which the parent talked to the child about shopping, noted what they were looking for and where the item might be found, had the children look at different brands, compared prices and quality, discussed credit cards, and so on. It was found that this addition to the original solution resulted in a series of interesting and educational interactions while distracting behaviors remained infrequent.

The next proposed stage in this model involves packaging the advice. Steps include: identifying the particular audience (e.g., single parents) for the advice; identifying how (TV, magazines, radio) and when to reach the audience; and determining the best form (educational TV programs, pamphlets, short TV spots) for the advice to take. A crucial step at this stage would involve similar testing, feedback, revision, and retesting procedures as in stage one until a package was identified which could alleviate specific problems for many families.

In the dissemination stage, advice will be presented over the designated media with feedback and reinforcement built into the system using information obtained from surveys, interviews, and, if possible, family interviews. This three-stage system assures the development, packaging, and dissemination of parental advice that is quality controlled and empirically derived.

This public health model emphasizing social trends influencing many normal families and the experimental development of advice to alleviate familial problems represents an important early secondary prevention framework to be followed in community mental health. Depending upon the nature and concerns of the target population, different centers might focus on different kinds of advice. Examples might include information and assistance concerning problems associated with unemployment, old age, or changes from traditional sex roles to more egalitarian ones.

While such a model involves an expanded direct service approach, concomitant primary prevention efforts could focus on changes in social and economic structures that contribute to the development of such problems. For example, problems in child care and supervision might be reduced by more flexible work hours, career-related, part-time employment, and subsidies to families with young children whose parents choose to work part time. Such programs are already being tried in countries such as Sweden.

Behavior Analysis and Systems Analysis

In an extremely important book which emerged from a 1973 conference at West Virginia University, Harshbarger and Maley (1974) presented a series of papers focusing primarily on the design of accountable, effective, and "health" oriented service delivery systems. While systems analysis and behavioral analysis follow different problem-solving pathways (systems analysis: deductive-conceptual; behavioral analysis: inductive-empirical), they are essentially complementary strategies. A problem-solving approach for system and organizational change is needed that relies on "a careful preliminary analysis, concrete goal specifications, a behavioral design which includes specification, observation, and consequation; reasonable implementation strategies; continual evaluation; and procedures which lead to a constant recycling through the entire process" (Harshbarger & Maley, 1974; p. 318). At the same time, the behavior analyst needs an approach that provides reliable data concerning the best focus of organization interventions and the most effective mobilization of resources or information in a system. Likewise, behavioral interventions will have minimal impact unless social policy is made to support such interventions. Behaviorists must become aware of and plan for correlated changes produced in a social system by interventions at any given point in the system (Willems, 1974).

The previous discussion of Atthowe's article provides a good example of the convergence between behavioral and systems analysis. A holistic analysis of mental hospital admission, "treatment," and release procedures indicated that high recidivism rates were related to the lack of community-based treatment and other (social, economic) support systems for the ex-patient. While behavioral principles and technology provided the conceptual and evaluation tools for Atthowe's "innovation" model, social policy changes such as community zoning guidelines, employment contracts, and community and professional attitudes toward marginal people must be modified to translate a treatment plan into a reality.

Harshbarger and Maley (1974) also discussed the need for accountability in service delivery systems. While a number of procedures were presented to arrive at a "cost/benefit ratio," the development of an accounting system requires that treatment procedures, problem behaviors, and objectives be clearly specified and that data be kept on treatment outcomes and the costs of achieving them. An example of such an approach was provided by the prior discussion of the Huntsville-Madison Community Mental Health Center. The need for empirical validation of treatments is likely to increase in the 1970s as fiscal resources for mental health are modified, and service centers are required to justify expenditures for given treatments. In addition, such accounting systems can publicize the expenses associated with treatment outcomes, thereby fostering better planning and less arbitrary funding decisions.

The conference participants consensually endorsed the importance of training paraprofessional and indigenous workers. It was noted that these mental health personnel are more likely to be effective using specific, easily conceptualized types of interventions. Another identified need was the development of integrated, multiservice agencies that treat the person as a total organism and provide rehabilitative, preventive, and growth-oriented services by using both person-oriented and system/community change strategies (Cowen, 1973). Further, such centers must develop programs that are based on an analysis of present and future social trends (e.g., the nature of the work force, age distribution of the population). A good example of such an approach is represented by the development of Risley's research on child- and youth-care centers and advice giving to parents.

Many of the papers in Harshbarger and Maley's book stressed the need for interdisciplinary training and conceptual models so as to provide a knowledge base and framework that would allow the mental health professional to understand and influence the social, political, and economic structures of our country.

Conclusion

This chapter presented a highly selective version of community mental health where services are evaluated by providers and consumers, marginal people not only survive but prosper in communities that accept them, organizations and their staffs are responsible and changeable, community organization is not unfashionable, and preventive programs are based on careful analyses of systems, communities, and social trends. The selection of this material was motivated not by a desire to bemoan the discrepancy between this work and the reality of current community mental health but to emphasize the present and future potential of soundly conceptualized, empirically based programs.

While this work is considerably removed from the traditional reliance on outpatient psychotherapy as the main component of community mental health, it would be fruitful to discuss briefly some current developments in psychology and related fields that might form a basis for a community mental health or a community psychology that is even more ambitious than the material presented in this chapter.

Often when psychologists note "constraints" on the effectiveness of psychological interventions, they are acknowledging the host of environmental influences that are major factors in creating psychological problems. These factors usually have not been defined, studied, or changed by psychologists. However, some recent work suggests that such influences are now being addressed.

Murrell (1973) has defined community psychology as the study and change of systems and presented a conceptual scheme for describing and modifying various organizational structures. Although Murrell's theoretical basis is derived from social psychology rather than behavior modification, his stance is in many ways consistent with that of Harshbarger and Maley (1974). Likewise, Willems' (1974) recent attempt to provide behaviorists with an eco-system framework indicates the strong need to provide system-level conceptualizations and interventions.

In somewhat different contexts, Bronfenbrenner (1974) and Krasner and Ullmann (1973) have outlined broad "ecological" or "social influence" models that attempt to systematize the gamut of social factors affecting human behavior. Bronfenbrenner has presented a position which synthesizes four concepts stressed in this section: prevention, a systems-ecological perspective, a public health model, and social experimentation. His ecological model focuses on systems affecting children, families, and enduring child-family environments and examines the effects of such influences as employment practices (e.g., part-time, career-oriented work) on family interactions and the use of day-care centers. In social analyses, macro-system variables (income, neighborhood characteristics, employment) are considered often as unmodifiable characteristics of the environment. However, Bronfenbrenner has advocated that such variables be treated as manipulable, independent variables and that social policy questions be addressed by social experimentation on these types of influences. Important parallel research emphasizes concern for the impact of the physical environment on behavior (Ittelson, Proshansky, Rivlin, & Winkel, 1974), the construction of "humane" environments (Sommer, 1974; Chapter 11), and experimental analysis of the effects of economic variables on consumer behavior (Winkler, Battalio, Kagel, Fisher, Miles, Basmann, & Krasner, 1975). While such research can ensure social scientists' contributions to social policy making, it also can advance psychology's relevance to national priorities by aiding its understanding of optimal environments for human development.

This framework may provide the basis for the evolution of a community mental health that resembles closely the principles of what might be termed "social ecology" (Moos & Insel, 1974). A component of this evolution involves the demonstration that problems for which psychologists traditionally have not claimed an expertise can be conceptualized and modified from the perspective of social ecology. For example, the problem of energy conservation is being addressed by examining issues such as price controls, tax incentives for the adoption of pro-environmental policies, and family living habits (see Chapter 11). While few psychologists would advocate the use of family therapy for households that overuse fuel, few would actively consider interventions that rely on economic contingencies to be sufficiently "psychological" to justify their professional participation.

In the same vein, typical psychological interventions may be inappropriate for ameliorating complex social problems facing many young families (inadequate child care, interpersonal isolation associated with geographic mobility). But there are identifiable alternatives that may enhance family life. These include flexible work hours, career-oriented, part-time employment for either or both parents, subsidized family incomes for parents in part-time occupations, subsidized child-care centers, and more liberal child-care allowances. Varieties of planned communities that provide for employment, diversity in living arrangements, child care, education, medical and social services, shopping and recreation, all within a contained geographical area, are being developed and occasionally carefully evaluated (Krasner & Ullmann, 1973; Zax & Specter, 1974). The psychologist possessing a knowledge base in a number of disciplines could propose, develop, and evaluate reforms for social problems unique to a particular community or indicative of the country as a whole. This type of broad, empirically based social planning could become the "community mental health" of the future.

Chapter 8
SOCIAL SKILLS TRAINING FOR PSYCHIATRIC RESIDENTS

The total resident population in public mental hospitals has consistently decreased since 1955 (Paul, 1969b). This encouraging trend has been attributed primarily to four changes in the hospital system: an introduction of psychoactive drugs (MacDonald & Tobias, 1976; Tobias & MacDonald, 1974), a return to the "moral treatment" philosophy including open-doors (Paul, 1969b), hospital unit decentralization (Gilligan, 1965; Ullmann, 1967), and an increased focus on the community (Bellak, 1964). The decrease resulting from these changes has been interpreted by many analysts as an index of increased hospital effectiveness for more recent institutional programs. Close analysis of the trend, however, indicates that this apparent increase in efficiency affects less than one-third of all institutional resident beds (Paul, 1969b). More than two-thirds of the persons currently listed on public institutional roles have remained untouched by institutional policy changes; they face less than a one in 15 chance of ever attaining release with subsequent successful adjustments to the communities (Paul, 1969b).

Characteristics describing this untouched segment of institutional populations have been the focus of a great deal of research. Their most important pre-hospitalization characteristic is the presence of withdrawn, inadequate interpersonal adjustment (Paul, 1969b). The most critical within-hospital characteristic is length of hospital stay, with longer stays associated with a smaller chance of successful post-release adaptation (Lehrman, 1961). And the most important post-hospitalization characteristics associated with unsuccessful continued community residence are the lack of employment, the lack of social participation, bizarre behavior, and presenting management problems to supporting families (Paul, 1969b).

In general, excluding the economic characteristic of post-hospital unemployment, persons not helped by hospitalization are singularly characterized by a demonstrable absence of social skills (Gripp & Magaro, 1974; Hersen & Eisler, 1976). In this context, "social skills" refers both to the performance of that set of complex interpersonal behaviors that may reasonably be expected to result in social reinforcement as well as the abstention from performing behaviors that may reasonably be expected to result in interpersonal punishment or withdrawal (Libet & Lewinsohn, 1973; MacDonald, 1975b). While there is considerable evidence that persons admitted to mental institutions are deficient in social skills to begin with (Paul, 1969b), there is overwhelming evidence that hospital settings as they are usually structured—with few consistent opportunities or encouragement for social skills development and with conditions highly conducive to social withdrawal and emotional apathy—precipitate even greater social performance-skill deficiencies than were originally present (Zusman, 1966).

Tremendous advances have been made this past decade in the technology of changing apathy-fostering elements of institutional environments (Kazdin, 1975a). However, even "progressive" programs in the majority of settings continue to be designed toward the inadvertent end of facilitating adjustment within the institution (cf. Atthowe, 1973b). A more appropriate end would be ultimate institutional release and subsequent successful adjustment to post-institutional placements. The failure to incorporate this more appropriate end has attracted recent attention and has prompted more than one criticism of applied behavior modification (Bornstein et al., 1975); it can be expected to prompt more. The response to this criticism seems fairly clear: socially acceptable treatment procedures should be applied within institutions to foster socially acceptable ends—namely, pro-social behaviors appropriate for extra-institutional environments.

Quite recently, social learning researchers have afforded increased efforts toward developing treatment programs for promoting pro-social interpersonal skills (MacDonald, Lindquist, Kramer, McGrath, & Rhyne, 1975; Twentyman & McFall, 1975). Most of this work has been directed toward developing a set of specific social skills known as "assertion," a term referring to "the open expression of preferences, through words or actions, in a manner causing others to take them into account" (MacDonald, 1974a). Moreover, the persons included in these studies have been drawn primarily from college populations. However, a portion of this work has involved direct applications of the procedures derived within this focused context to broader social skills problems with more severely deficient populations.

Three research strategies have been employed. The first has been an examination of the effects of behavioral treatment packages or programs involving more than one presumably active intervention element, generally in comparison with the effects of no-treatment or an attention-placebo control (Paul, 1969a). The second has been an exploration of the effects of a specific behavioral treatment in isolation, again generally in comparison with the effects of no-treatment or an attention-placebo control (Paul, 1969a). The final strategy has involved the comparative effectiveness of two or more behavioral treatments pitted against one another, often with appropriate auxiliary control conditions.

Behavioral Treatment Packages

The work of Galassi, Galassi, and Litz (1974) is illustrative of the first research strategy. These investigators were interested in documenting the effects of multiple-component treatments as they are ordinarily applied in counseling settings; they focused on increasing that subset of social skills termed assertion in a sample of 32 college students. Treatment consisted of eight training sessions with videotape modeling, behavior rehearsal, video, peer, and trainer performance feedback, bibliotherapy, intersession task assignments, trainer exhortation, and peer group support. Training included learning a series of assertion responses appropriate for a given situation rather than a single response; in addition, training covered several different types of assertion rather than the more specific target of refusing unreasonable requests (cf. McFall & Lillesand, 1971; McFall & Marston, 1970; McFall & Twentyman, 1973). Session format followed a specified sequence: discussions about the rationale for assertion training, related assigned readings, and preceding intersession task assignments, followed by viewings of assertion model videotapes, followed by behavior rehearsal in dyads with feedback. In comparison with a no-treatment control group, treated participants evidenced significant improvements in assertion skills as measured by several self-report inventories and an enacted role-play assessment device (Galassi et al., 1974).

While their research strategy deliberately sacrificed the ability to separate relative contributions of specific treatment elements, these investigators were careful to capture the spirit of thorough intervention realism in their programmed procedures (MacDonald, 1975a). Treatment was appropriately comprehensive. Perhaps because of their success in accomplishing their end of replicating thoroughness in treatment, the Galassi study documented the maintained effectiveness of their procedure at a 1-year follow-up. Locating all 32 of the original sample, they found significant differences on a well-validated self-report measure of assertion. With the 20 members of the original sample agreeing to participate in the enacted role-play assessment device (nine experimental subjects and 11 controls), there were significant differences favoring the experimental group (Galassi, Kostka, & Galassi, 1975).

Rathus (1972, 1973) followed a similar research strategy for evaluating the utility of a behavioral treatment package; his comparison was against a no-treatment control group as well as an attention-placebo control. In the most recent study, Rathus (1973) selected 78 single, undergraduate women from his own psychology course who stated an interest in becoming more outgoing or less fearful in social situations. Volunteers for his program were exempted from an alternative class requirement. Rathus (1973) assigned the participants to one of three experimental conditions: an assertion-training procedure (n = 28), an attention-placebo condition (n = 25), or a no-treatment control group (n = 25). Both contact conditions met for 1 hour a week over a period of 7 weeks.

Members of the assertion-training group were given a rationale for the effectiveness of the procedure, exposure to videotape models discussing assertion and reconstructing assertion situations, and the between session assignment of engaging in and recording 20 instances of assertive behavior. Training focused on nine discrete skills: assertive talk, or demanding rights; feeling talk, or the spontaneous expression of likes and dislikes; greeting talk, or outgoing interaction initiation; active and passive disagreement; questioning authority figures' motives; talking about oneself; agreeing with compliments directed toward oneself; avoiding any justification of one's stated opinions; and looking people in the eye. Members of the attention-placebo group watched films of women undergoing systematic desensitization for an equal amount of treatment time and had a parallel between-session assignment of listing the reasons for and origins of their fear. Supportive results for the comparative effectiveness of Rathus' procedure were found with both a written and a verbal self-report measure; assertion scores for members given the behavioral treatment package were significantly greater than scores for members of either the attention-placebo or the no-treatment controls. Kirschner (1975) replicated these effects and reported evidence suggesting that the level of assertion modeled by the therapist in his or her implementation of the training program was of more than negligible importance.

Twentyman and McFall (1975) again employed the research strategy of comparing the effects of a behavioral training package against a no-treatment control and again worked with college students. Their treatment target was a somewhat broader set of social skills, however, and involved increasing the dating skills level of shy males. Twentyman and McFall (1975) selected 30 college men who reported general incompetence in handling specific dating situations and who had dated less than one time during the preceding month. Sixteen of these men were assigned to an assessment-only experimental condition, while 15 of them received three weekly, individual training sessions. During the first of these sessions, telephone skills were the focus; during the second session, a set of standard face-to-face encounters with college women was the target. During the final session, training was directed toward handling individually specified difficult heterosexual situations. The intervention procedures for each session included modeling, coaching, covert and overt rehearsal, and, quite innovatively, a programmed between-session assignment to be completed with a cooperating female confederate who was designated to the subject as such. There were significant effects following treatment indicating the value of the treatment package as compared with a no-contract control on a variety of self-report and enacted role-play behavioral measures.

In one of the earliest applications of this treatment package research strategy with psychiatric populations, Lomont, Gilner, Spector, and Skinner (1969) examined the effectiveness of a social skills-training program as compared with an insight-only control. They selected 12 psychiatric patients who were judged to be socially anxious, to evidence no organic brain pathology, to display no psychotic thought disorder, and to have an IQ score of 80 or more. Half of their samples was randomly assigned to one of the two treatment conditions. Members of both groups met 5 days a week for 90 minutes per day over a period of 6 weeks. The insight-only group was well conducted: treatment procedures conformed very closely to the components considered important in analytic therapy and included reflection, confrontation, and interpretation, among others. The skills-training program involved a creative combination of procedures: participants initially used scripts to enact specified social situations; over time, the scripts were faded out with the substitution of therapist coaching and feedback; ultimately, therapist coaching was also eliminated and practiced situation contexts were varied to provoke participant response innovation. In light of the care with which these investigators designed and implemented their treatment conditions, it is unfortunate that their work preceded the popularity of behavioral assessment procedures (MacDonald, 1974a). They employed dependent variables generally insensitive to treatment effects (MacDonald, 1974c), the Minnesota Multiphasic Personality Inventory and the Interpersonal Checklist. Nevertheless, their results did yield tentative support for the superiority of skills training over insight only for their treatment participants.

Bloomfield (1973) reported a preliminary investigation of the effectiveness of group-assertion training with outpatient schizophrenics. He worked with eight males and females, all of whom had been previously hospitalized for a period of at least 2 years. Treatment consisted of hourly sessions once a week; session format included an identification of individual response targets, a discussion of the disadvai.tages resulting from remaining unassertive and the potential advantages of behaving more assertively, a conceptual distinction between assertion and aggression, and behavior rehearsal with coaching modeling, and feedback. Bloomfield (1973) reports that his procedure was apparently effective, although he neither included a comparative control group nor collected data to evaluate the effects of his program. His report may be considered, then, only a multiple case study (Paul, 1969a); it has value, however, because of the network of prior studies demonstrating more objectively the effectiveness of the procedures he employed and because of the nature of his target population, none of whom was rehospitalized during the year of the study.

Gutride, Goldstein, and Hunter (1973) implemented a design similar to the one employed earlier by Lomont et al. (1969) using a behavioral treatment package including different elements than those employed by the Lomont study and with more tenable measurement devices. Gutride and his colleagues selected 87 psychiatric inpatients, 57 of whom had been hospitalized continuously for at least 1 year. They compared the effects of three treatment conditions for increasing rates of ward social interaction: structured learning therapy consisting of modeling, behavior rehearsal, and social reinforcement versus traditional psychotherapy and a custodial treatment control. Active treatments were implemented in tri-weekly group sessions over a period of 4 weeks. The effects of their program were evaluated on a variety of staff-rated scales and observation inventories; while the results were not unambiguous, comparative differences indicated significant effects for both behavioral intervention and psychotherapy, with only a slight and statistically nonsignificant superiority for the structured learning therapy.

In the most thorough investigation following a package evaluation design strategy, Goldsmith and McFall evaluated the effects of a carefully developed interpersonal skills-training program with psychiatric inpatients. Recognizing that "the content of a skill-training program is at least as critical to its ultimate success as the training methods it employs" (Goldsmith & McFall, 1975, p. 51), these investigators included two phases in their research program.

The first phase involved identifying the critical content legitimately incorporated into a skills-training program via a modified behavioral assessment strategy (MacDonald, 1974a, 1975a). Sixteen psychiatric outpatients, selected because they reported experiencing affective and performance difficulties in initiating and sustaining interactions with strangers, were interviewed individually for 1 hour. During the interview, the outpatients described in detail specific examples of situations they had encountered which had presented them with difficulties; in each case, the most critical moment of each encountered situation was also identified. Fifty-five distinct problematic situations were extracted from this interview information. The general interpersonal contexts of these situations were dating, making friends, having job interviews, relating to authorities, relating to service personnel, and interacting with people perceived as more intelligent, more attractive, or demographically different from them; the most frequently identified critical moments within these contexts were initiating or terminating the interactions, making personal disclosures, handling conversational silences, responding to rejection, and behaving assertively. The 55 situations were subjected to an item-analysis procedure using ratings from an inpatient population (n = 20), and 32 of the items met two of the following three criteria: they were perceived as difficult to handle by 80% or more of the inpatient sample, they were perceived to be situations in which 20% or more of the sample anticipated being both uncomfortable and incompetent in the situation should they encounter it, and they were judged to be personally relevant by 25% or more of the rating inpatients. Responses for each of the situations were generated by eight professional staff members; a second panel of judges evaluated the degree of effectiveness of each response generated for the several situations and specified the rationales underlying their evaluations. Criteria extracted from these rationales formed the basis for both the response scoring procedures when the situations were employed as an assessment device and the coaching content when the situations were employed as stimuli in the skill-training procedure.

The second phase of Goldsmith and McFall's (1975) study involved the evaluation of the effectiveness of a skill-training package as compared with attention-placebo and assessment-only controls. Thirty-six male psychiatric inpatients were randomly assigned to one of three conditions. Those 12 inpatients exposed to skill training received three 1-hour individual training sessions within 1 week. During this time, each of 11 situations drawn from the original item pool was the focus of 15 minutes of training; the final 15 minutes were devoted to a general review. During training, behavior rehearsal, modeling, coaching, recorded response replay, and corrective feedback were employed as techniques; a typical training sequence involved listening to the recorded situation, receiving instructions about the principles of an effective response in such a situation, hearing a pre-recorded effective modeled response, hearing a review of effective response principles and a statement of the likely response consequences for an effective response, rehearsing a response in reaction to the replayed situational stimulus, evaluating the effectiveness of the rehearsed response and hearing trainer evaluation of the response, and repeating the rehearsal-evaluation sequence until effective responses had been rehearsed for two consecutive trials. The 12 inpatients exposed to the attention-placebo treatment also received three 1-hour individual sessions during 1 week; session time was devoted to playing the 11 training situations and encouraging participants to explore their feelings about each situation and achieve insight into why they reacted as they did. Assessment-only subjects were pre- and post-tested concurrently with members of the other experimental conditions. On the self-report measure of skill based on the originally identified 55 critical situations, gains for skills-training subjects were significantly greater than gains for members of the assessment-only control but not the attention-placebo control. With two enacted role-play measures, skills-training scores were significantly greater than scores for members of both control conditions.

Unqualified conclusions from many of the studies reviewed thus far are unwarranted in light of frequent therapist by treatment confounds (e.g., Lomont et al., 1969) or failures to separate effects due to specific treatments from effects due to treatment per se (e.g., Twentyman & McFall, 1975). However, the number of independent studies suggesting the utility of skill-training packages, some of which have been appropriately controlled (e.g., Gutride et al., 1973), is encouraging. Extrapolating from these results, Foy, Eisler, and Pinkston (1975) reported an interesting and innovative clinical application of several of the investigated procedures; their report is useful both as an example of applying empirically tenable procedures in a clinical context and as an example of design strategies to increase the empirical contribution of case histories.

The client described in the Foy et al. (1975) report was a 56-year-old male psychiatric inpatient. This person presented a history of "behaviorally comply-ing with what he felt were unreasonable demands from others until he released anger in a verbally abusive and often assaultive manner" (Foy et al., 1975, p. 1).

His current hospitalization was precipitated by one of these explosive assaults. Conceptualizing the problem as the person's deficiency in behaving assertively rather than either inappropriately submissively or aggressively (MacDonald, 1975b), these authors investigated the remedial effectiveness of behavior rehearsal, modeling, and instructions. Four behaviors were identified as contributing to the client's assertion skill deficiency in a baseline assessment session: frequent hostile comments, frequent irrelevant statements, frequent compliance, and infrequent requests for different behavior from the other person. Modeling and behavior rehearsal were introduced simultaneously for all four behaviors, but an instructional component was introduced sequentially for each behavior and therefore constituted a modified multiple baseline design (Kazdin, 1975a). Changes over time for each behavior (see Fig. 8-1) were dramatic. For each component except irrelevant comments, instructions seemed to produce increased effects over behavior rehearsal and modeling alone. Quite importantly, effects were maintained after training not only while the patient remained in the hospital, but also at four testings conducted at various intervals during the 6 months following the patient's release. Self-report data from the client suggested that his experimentally documented skill level change had affected beneficially his interaction with significant others: his relationships with his work supervisors had improved and he was getting along better with his son.

Single Intervention Elements

The second major design strategy for examining social skills programs—that of investigating single intervention elements in isolation—has been the least popular. Its infrequent use does not grow out of any lack of scientific integrity, provided appropriate control groups are included. The strategy's disfavor seems to be attributable to two factors. First, skills training in actuality generally involves several treatment elements in combination so that more practical value is derived from examining that package as it ordinarily occurs rather than any single element. Second, the information derived from demonstrating the effectiveness of any single technique is not as great as the information derived from comparing the relative effectiveness of that single technique or technique package to other treatment procedures; this latter consideration gives rise to the popularity of comparative outcome studies (Paul, 1969a), although this second strategy is optimally efficient for establishing the value of a novel procedure.

The second design strategy does characterize several studies that have appeared, however; one of them is extremely provocative. Using a multiple-baseline design, Eisler, Hersen, and Miller (1974) demonstrated that instructions coupled with feedback were effective in increasing assertion skill behavioral components with two male psychiatric inpatients. Wagner (1968), with a very

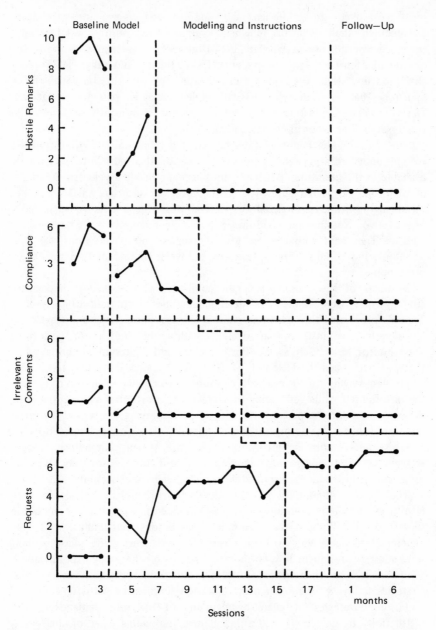

Fig. 8-1. Target assertive behaviors during the four phases. (From Foy, O. W., Eisler, R. M., and Pinkston, S. Modeled assertion in a case of explosive rages. *Journal of Behavior Therapy and Experimental Psychiatry*, 1975, 6, 135-138. Reprinted by permission of Pergamon Press.)

271

well-controlled group design and sophisticated assessment procedures, documented that behavior rehearsal coupled with positive reinforcement increased assertion, or as Wagner (1968) termed it, expressions of anger, with nonorganic, female psychiatric patients. Eisler, Hersen, and Miller (1973) found that modeling alone was effective in increasing five of eight component verbal and nonverbal assertion behaviors with male psychiatric patients. Wallace and Davis (1974) demonstrated that reinforcement significantly increased the conversational behavior of chronic patient dyads.

The work of Meichenbaum (Meichenbaum & Cameron, 1973) falls into the second design strategy and represents some of the most intriguing results available in the literature. Meichenbaum selected 10 male psychiatric inpatients, all of whom had been diagnosed schizophrenic; their mean age was 36, and their mean length of time hospitalized was 15.5 months. The patients were assigned to one of two experimental conditions: a training program or a yoked-practice control. Treatment contact time for members of both conditions was eight 45-minute individual sessions spread over a 3-week period; total treatment time was 6 hours.

Members of the training program condition were trained in a cognitive strategy—they were trained, as Meichenbaum put it, to talk to themselves. Training progressed through three phases. The first phase focused on developing an adaptive, self-instructional strategy within the context of performing sensorimotor tasks such as the Porteus Maze and digit symbol. Initially, the therapist performed the task and, while doing so, modeled "talking to himself" or problem-solving for the patient. The subject was then encouraged to perform the task himself while verbalizing the modeled cognitive strategy; eventually the subject was trained to perform the task while employing the cognitive strategy subvocally—hence the term "talking to himself." The strategy modeled by the therapist and eventually incorporated by the patient emphasized coping: recognizing failure and responding adaptively to it; the phrases "pay attention, listen, repeat instructions, disregard distraction" were fundamental.

The second training phase extended self-instructional practice to more cognitively demanding and interpersonally evaluated tasks such as the similarities subtest of the Wechsler scale, common associations to stimulus words, and coherent interviews with no bizarre verbalizations. During this phase, patients were additionally taught how to monitor their own behavior and spontaneously self-instruct. The training procedure was the same: therapist modeling of strategies followed by subject overt imitation terminating with subject covert imitation. Strategies included restatements of the task demands, general instructions to go slowly and think before responding, uses of imagery to facilitate abstract problem solving, and delivery of self-rewarding statements. The final training phase concentrated on teaching the patient to become sensitive to interpersonal cues from others which indicated that his behavior was either bizarre, incoherent, or irrelevant. The patient was trained to regard these cues as signals to evaluate his own behavior and to initiate the self-instructions "be relevant, be coherent, make oneself understood." In addition, he was taught interpersonal strategies for redirecting an interaction he had discovered to be misdirected: "It's not clear; let me try again."

The yoked controls received amounts of task practice (without strategy training) and amounts of social reinforcement equal to that of their experimental counterparts. Comparative analyses for the two groups indicated a consistent picture of superior performance results for the trained subjects on a variety of attentional, conceptual, and language tasks. This superiority was maintained at a 3-week follow-up and was evident on interpersonal tasks not included in the training procedure as well as sensorimotor and interpersonal tasks that were.

The importance of Meichenbaum's (Meichenbaum & Cameron, 1973) work cannot be overlooked. By training general interpersonal strategies through sequential tasks and hierarchical strategy complexity, he was successful in raising schizophrenic performance levels in highly abstract social interactions. This work deserves to be regarded as more than a demonstration of the effectiveness of specific technique; it provides a general paradigm with demonstrable but unexplored potential and consequently presents a fruitful area for further research.

Comparative Studies

Comparative outcome design strategies (Paul, 1969a) have dominated the field of social skills-training research. As a consequence, some information about the relative contributions of discrete intervention elements or treatment packages is available. However, most of this work has been done with college populations, and there is reason to believe that the magnitude and direction of differences found with college students—populations typically highly verbal and motivated—may not be directly paralleled with psychiatric patients (cf., Glickman, Plutchik, & Landau, 1973; Paden, Himelstein, & Paul, 1974). Consequently, design replications with institutionalized populations would provide valuable information stimulating both better treatment and future research.

McFall and Marston (1970), in one of the earliest comparative studies of assertion skill training, evaluated the relative effects of behavior rehearsal with and without trainer feedback against attention-placebo and no-contact controls. College subjects role-played responses to audiotaped situational stimuli which had been carefully identified as relevant situations presenting the subject with an opportunity to refuse an unreasonable request. Rehearsal-with-feedback subjects were given information about the degree of assertion exhibited in their responses, while rehearsal-without feedback subjects were not. Results on a variety of self-report measures and enacted role-play assessment tests indicated that both behavior rehearsal conditions were significantly more effective than either the attention-placebo or the no-contact control conditions; however, there were no significant differences between degree of effectiveness with the two rehearsal conditions.

In a later study (McFall & Lillesand, 1971), McFall compared the effects of one treatment package—overt behavior rehearsal, modeling, and coaching—with the effects of a second treatment package—covert behavior rehearsal, modeling, and coaching. The essential difference between the two training procedures was that with the first, college student subjects rehearsed out loud their reactions to audiotaped stimuli, while with the second, they "talked to themselves." Again, there were significant effects in the target response of degree of assertion in refusing unreasonable requests for both training conditions as compared with a no-treatment control on a variety of self-report and enacted role-play measures; and, again, there were no significant differences between the two experimental treatments.

Longin and Rooney (1973) employed a similar design with psychiatric inpatients. They selected 35 women, hospitalized for a mean of 11 years, all of whom were designated as ready for discharge. Subjects were assigned to one of four treatment conditions: assertion training with overt rehearsal, assertion training with covert rehearsal, a test-only control group housed in the same ward with members of the training conditions, and a test-only control group housed in a more traditional ward. Training consisted of four weekly individual sessions lasting between 15 and 20 minutes apiece. Both training conditions followed a similar sequence: participants were given an introductory rationale about the value of assertive behavior, exposed to eight situational stimuli and two female models reacting with assertion to those situations, coached about the characteristics of an appropriately assertive response, and presented with an opportunity to rehearse their reaction to the situation; overt rehearsal condition subjects rehearsed their reactions out loud, while covert rehearsal condition subjects were instructed to do so silently. Treatment effects were evaluated with a 16-item enacted role-play assessment device. Both training conditions were significantly more effective than both controls in increasing assertion skills; moreover, the overt rehearsal procedure was significantly more effective than was covert rehearsal.

Programmed interactions, or interventions consisting of prearranged social contacts, may be considered a form of behavior rehearsal (Arkowitz, 1973). While the content of these sequences is not specified, the situational context itself increases the likelihood that some beneficial behavior rehearsal will naturally occur. Following hypotheses to this effect generated by a supportive case study (Clark & Arkowitz, 1974) and a similarly supportive preliminary investigation, Christensen, Arkowitz, and Anderson (1975) systematically evaluated the effects of "practice dates" for dating skills in college students.

Three experimental conditions were compared: practice dates with subsequent written feedback originating from the dating partner and delivered by the therapist versus practice dates with no feedback versus a no-contact control. Both contact conditions were exposed to six practice dates. Following treatment, several behavioral and self-report measures indicated significant gains for the contact conditions as compared with the no-contact control. Consistent with the earlier work of McFall and Marston (1970), the differential effects of receiving or not receiving explicit feedback were not significant.

Weinman, Gelbart, Wallace, and Post (1972) examined the effects of programmed interactions for unassertive and withdrawn inpatients. They selected 63 diagnosed schizophrenics, all of whom had been hospitalized for at least 1 year; the mean number of years hospitalized was 11.7. Subjects were assigned to one of three treatment conditions. The first was socioenvironmental therapy, which consisted of five weekly group activities requiring social interaction and several weekly informal activities to encourage additional social contact; staff were trained to prompt and support patient social interactions during both the formal and the informal activities. The effect of this treatment was compared with standard systematic desensitization and relaxation therapies on an enacted role-play assessment device. The arranged interactions were found to be significantly more effective than the other conditions for raising performance levels with the chronic inpatients.

O'Brien and Azrin (1973), developing a conceptually similar strategy from a different theoretical position, applied a quasi-arranged interaction procedure to psychiatric residents. Observing that patient-family visits were extremely infrequent, these investigators initiated a program termed "interaction-priming" with their subjects. The procedure involved sending invitations to patients' families for visits with the patient and providing transportation for the patients to their families' homes, analogous to prearranging an interaction in the work of Arkowitz and his colleagues (Christenson et al., 1975); moreover, subsequent to each visit, patients were given feedback about how to be more reinforcing to their families by an accompanying observer. While the design O'Brien and Azrin (1973) employed does not permit strong conclusions, and while no direct assessment of interaction skill level was included, their results are encouraging: the mean pre-treatment level of visitation was zero minutes per week; following intervention, the mean weekly level of visitation jumped to nearly 2 hours.

Behavior rehearsal, both formally and informally structured, has been one of the most popular strategies for influencing interpersonal skills levels; modeling has been another. Young, Rimm, and Kennedy (1973), working with college students, investigated the relative effects of modeling alone versus modeling with verbal reinforcement, compared with both attention-placebo and test-only controls. Forty volunteer subjects were assigned to one of the four conditions. Treatment consisted of two 30-minute individual sessions. Members of the attention-placebo condition explored the histories of their lack of assertion during this time, while members of the active treatment conditions were exposed to models behaving assertively in 12 different situations and imitated their performances. Persons assigned to the modeling-with-reinforcement condition were praised for appropriate imitations of the models. While differential effects from the manipulations were not overwhelming, there was support for the superiority of both modeling conditions over both controls on an enacted role-play measurement device. There were no significant differences between the modeling conditions.

Goldstein, Martens, Hubben, vanBelle, Schaaf, Wiersma, and Goedhart (1973), noting that characteristics of the model and modeling display are known to influence the technique's effectiveness in laboratory work, reported a series of three investigations examining the effects of altering model and display characteristics. Their target behavior was termed independence, but the content of those materials operationalizing the term was highly similar to what is more generally known as assertion.

In the first investigation, 90 male and female psychiatric outpatients, classified neither as psychotic nor organic, were assigned to one of three conditions: independence modeling, dependence modeling, or a no-modeling control. Following pre-treatment assessment, all subjects listened to 30 audiotaped two-person interactions in which a stimulus person instigated either frustration or a threat to the independence of the target person. Members of the control group were provided with cards listing one independent and one dependent response alternative for each encounter. Their task was simply to respond with one of the alternatives. Members of the independent modeling condition heard a rewarded model respond independently for a randomly selected 20 of the training stimuli and were reinforced for selecting the independent response alternative for the other 10 stimuli. Members of the dependent modeling condition were exposed to the same stimuli except that the responses modeled and reinforced were the dependent ones.

Results from this first investigation were fascinating. On a well-constructed enacted role-play assessment device, there was a significant increase in independence for both men and women in the independence-modeling condition as compared with the no-model controls. The dependence-modeling condition, however, was effective in significantly increasing dependence as compared with controls only for the female subjects in the study.

In their second investigation (Goldstein et al., 1973), these researchers were interested in extrapolating from the laboratory result that modeling is more effective when the observer has been given the set to view the model as warm or attractive. They worked with 60 male and female psychiatric outpatients similar demographically to those included in their first study. Following a procedure similar to the one employed before, they demonstrated that structuring of the model as an interpersonally cold individual produced significantly less modeling than was evidenced for either no structuring or structuring of the model as interpersonally warm.

The third study investigated the effects of modeling and instructions in a two-by-two factorial design. Instructions involved prompting the person that it was good to be independent, explaining that "this means that if someone gets in an unpleasant situation, such as being accused of something he did not do, he should not pipe down, but should stand up for his rights" (Goldstein et al., 1973, p. 39), and providing two examples of independent responses. Modeling involved the presentation of audiotaped independent models as implemented in the prior work.

Fifty-four male psychiatric inpatients, all diagnosed schizophrenic and all hospitalized for at least 8 years, were assigned to one of the four conditions: modeling and instructions, modeling only, instructions only, or a materials exposure control. All three experimental groups increased their levels of independence significantly more than the materials-exposure control; however, there were no significant differences between results with the experimental groups.

Goldstein et al. (1973) interpret their results as demonstrating that instructions only are as effective as modeling displays. This conclusion must be accepted as tentative, however, for two reasons. First, statistics as an analytical tool provides techniques for only two alternatives: proving an alternative hypothesis or accepting the null one. While the null hypothesis can and in many instances must be accepted, it can never be deductively proved. Second, the instructional condition provided in the study included in it two modeling sequences. As a consequence, the contrast between instructions and modeling was not pure.

In a more controlled study, Hersen, Eisler, Miller, Johnson, and Pinkston (1973) evaluated the relative effects of practice, instructions, and modeling on several verbal and nonverbal components of assertive behavior. These investigators selected 50 male psychiatric inpatients who reported low levels of assertion on the Wolpe-Lazarus self-report scale. The mean age of their sample was 44.9; 15 of the participants had been diagnosed alcoholics, 21 were diagnosed neurotic, and the remaining 14 were labeled psychotics in remission. Ten residents were randomly assigned to one of the five experimental conditions. Members of the test-only control were exposed only to pre-treatment and post-treatment assessment sessions. Members of all other conditions were exposed to five different assertion situations four times during a period of 3 days. During these exposures, subjects in the practice-control condition merely responded to the stimuli. Subjects in the instructions-only condition received focused instructions on specific behaviors to monitor during their exposure-rehearsal sequences. Subjects in the modeling-only condition received exposures both to the assertion situations and to a similar model demonstrating an assertive reaction to the situation prior to their rehearsal. Subjects in the modeling-plus-instructions condition received exposure to the situations, exposure to the assertive model's reaction, and focused instructions on specific behaviors to monitor. Pre- and post-treatment differences on component behaviors during an enacted role-play assessment device strongly suggested that the modeling-plus-instructions procedure was the most powerful overall. Practice alone was relatively inert, while instructions-only affected the specific component of loudness most strongly, and modeling-only was the most powerful procedure for the specific component of compliance content. Over three of the other components, however, including duration of reply, affect, and overall assertiveness, modeling-plus-instructions was clearly superior to all other treatment conditions.

Kazdin (1974b) has developed an innovative form of modeling which has not yet been implemented with psychiatric populations; his results suggest, however, that it should be. Noting that live, filmed, and audiotaped models had all been applied successfully to assertion training, Kazdin (1974b) suspected that a more easily arranged form of modeling might be similarly effective. The type of modeling he employed he termed covert modeling, a procedure wherein "subjects imagine a covert model who engages in those behaviors the subject wishes to develop" (Kazdin, 1974b, p. 240). Furthermore, extrapolating from laboratory work with traditional modeling as Goldstein et al. (1973) had in their research, Kazdin reasoned that the consequences of the behavior that accrue to the covert model would influence covert modeling's effects just as overt model behavior consequences have been shown to influence overt modeling effects. His design, then, included an experimental group incorporating successively greater amounts of the covert modeling sequence: specification of the situational context, model response, and subsequent consequences for the model. In addition, a test-only control group was included.

Treatment for all contact conditions consisted of four sessions. During the first session, each subject was given a rationale for the appropriate procedure and exposed to five covert scenes. Sessions two, three, and four each provided exposures to 10 difference scenes. For the context-only condition, scene exposure involved only visualizing the situational context for which assertion would be appropriate, a procedure analogous but not equivalent to standard systematic desensitization. For the covert modeling condition, subjects visualized the appropriate situational contexts as well as a similar-to-themselves model reacting to the situations in an assertive manner; subjects were instructed in the specific behaviors comprising the model's reaction prior to visualizing it. For covert modeling-with-reinforcement subjects, visualization instructions included both the situational contexts and the model's specific reactions as well as a description of consequences following the model's response.

Kazdin's (1974b) dependent variables included four self-report scales, an enacted role-play test, and two follow-up measures. His results indicated that both covert modeling conditions were significantly more effective than either the context-only or test-only controls with his college student sample. There were no clear differences between the two covert modeling conditions, although there were trends indicating a slight superiority for covert modeling with reinforcement.

Kazdin's (1974b) technique is relatively new and has not yet had time to generate replications with similar target problems. The care with which his study was executed, however, affords a considerable level of product (Paul, 1969a) to his results. The implications of having an effective technique in which persons can cognitively construct nonpresent stimuli are clear for populations located in an environment different than the environment for which they are being trained; as such, the potential benefits of covert modeling for psychiatric inpatients deserves experimental attention.

A variety of comparative studies with college student samples that demonstrate the superiority of various combinations of skill-training intervention elements over nonspecific treatments have appeared. MacDonald et al. (1975) documented the effectiveness of behavior rehearsal with modeling and coaching in increasing dating skills with nondating college males; no additional benefits were derived from including between-session task assignments with the skills-training procedure. McFall and Twentyman (1973) found that covert rehearsal with coaching was more effective than modeling alone and was not increased in effectiveness by the addition of modeling in raising college student assertion skills; moreover, covert and overt rehearsal were not differentially effective. Gormally, Hill, Otis, and Rainey (1975) demonstrated that instructions, modeling, behavior rehearsal, and feedback were significantly more effective than a nonspecific treatment control in increasing assertion skills; differences between subjects given feedback verbally in comparison with subjects given feedback by videotape were not significant. The results of these studies and others (Bander, Steinke, Allen, & Mosher, 1975; Curran, 1975; Friedman, 1969; Gambrill, 1973; Hedquist & Weinhold, 1970; McGovern, Arkowitz, & Gilmore, 1975; Melnick, 1973; Rathus, 1972) provide sufficient support for the general effectiveness of direct skills-training procedures in increasing social performance levels with college students. For applications of these interventions with psychiatric populations, three tasks remain. First, investigations identifying the specific interpersonal skills requisite for successful community adaptation should be conducted. While it is reasonable to assume that assertion and dating skills will be among these interpersonal skills identified, it is equally reasonable to assume that additional skills such as same-sex conversational strategies, group interaction skills, and interaction styles for noninvolving situations will also be important. Second, intervention procedures maximally effective and efficient for engendering these skills with psychiatric populations should be investigated. Given the heterogeneity of persons falling into the general category of psychiatric patient, design strategies should focus on including patient types, calibrated on standardized, behavior-relevant dimensions as an additional factor. Finally, techniques for incorporating demonstrably useful procedures into the ongoing treatment regimen of existing institutions should be developed.

Treatment Milieu

Regardless of the effectiveness of skills-training procedures, they will be of limited utility if they are embedded in a hospital context that discourages out of session those very skills taught during skills-training periods (Paul, 1969b; Zusman, 1966). Such hospital structures additionally contribute to the deterioration of social skills originally present at admission in a subset of patients (Paul, 1969b; Zusman, 1966). When designed to be supportive of social interactions, token economy programs have been effective in at least maintaining interaction skill levels already present in patients.

Shaefer and Martin (1966) assigned 40 chronic female inpatients to one of two groups: those selectively reinforced for more involved social behaviors versus those not so reinforced. They found a significant improvement in interaction levels for members of the reinforcement condition as compared with members of the nonreinforced group. Atthowe and Krasner (1968), with the express purpose of reducing apathy and fostering more socially involved behavior, dispensed selective token reinforcement to 32 inpatients for attending group activities. Their manipulation was not only effective in significantly increasing scores on a behavior rating scale indexing increased social responsiveness, it also precipitated an increase in the frequency of patient use of overnight, day, and accompanied passes. Work in token economies appearing since these reports generally supports the conclusion that appropriately designed contingencies are effective in raising levels of social interactions (cf. Gorham, Green, Caldwell, & Bartlett, 1970; Gripp & Magaro, 1971, 1974; Kale, Kaye, Wheelan, & Hopkins, 1969; Shean & Zeidberg, 1971; Steffy, Hart, Craw, Torney, & Marlett, 1969). It is important to recognize that the crucial element accounting for their success is not in the delivery of tokens; these programs work because they reflect an interaction-supportive environmental design. Naturally occurring reinforcers, when monitored and contingently delivered by staff, can have similar effects (Robertshaw, Kelly, & Hicbert, 1973; Rostow & Smith, 1975). Even aspects of the environment such as furniture arrangement in the ward have been shown to exert powerful control over the amount of social interaction observed among inpatients (Holahan, 1972). Behaviors are maintained in environments only if they are reinforced (Ullmann & Krasner, 1975). To perpetuate adaptive social skills either originally present in admitted patients or engendered through skills training in deficient ones, hospital environments must be designed to encourage them uniformly. And in reaction to Bornstein, Bugge, and Davol's (1975) reminder, the environmental design of the hospital must be scrutinized to insure that the interaction skills it fosters are ones adaptive for functioning in the extra-institutional community rather than an idiosyncratic community existing only within the bounds of the institution (additional discussion of the effects of environmental redesign is presented in Chapter 11).

While careful environmental design can maintain present skills and strengthen incipient ones, it cannot engender complex skills not available in the person's repertoire (Kazdin, 1973b). Where elements of those complex skills are available to the person, the skills-training strategies previously described, such as behavior rehearsal and modeling, can be expected to be effective. Where elements of those complex skills are not apparently available, however, more extensive intervention is a prerequisite for such strategies. Thomson, Fraser, and McDougall (1974) worked with two near-mute, withdrawn schizophrenic inpatients. With a procedure involving asking direct questions and following those direct questions with prompts for speech paired with consumable reinforcement for correct responding, these investigators were successful in producing an increase in frequencies of verbalization. Stahl, Thomson, Leitenberg, and Hasazi (1974), working with psychiatric patients previously unresponsive to social praise, established praise as an effective reinforcer by repeatedly pairing it with token delivery. Regrettably little attention has been afforded to developing such fundamental interaction elements with psychiatric patients, although effective procedures have been developed for other populations such as persons classified as mentally retarded. Kazdin and Erickson (1975) used a reinforcement procedure to shape instruction-following in severely retarded women. Rubin and Stolz (1974) established self-referent speech in a retarded adolescent with operant procedures. Williams, Martin, McDonald, Hardy, and Lambert (1975) adapted the "backscratch contingency" (Powers & Powers, 1971), a procedure wherein one member of an assigned pair was reinforced when the other person performed appropriately, to increase social responsiveness with retarded children.

Two factors have probably discouraged the application of similarly effective procedures to psychiatric patients for developing behavior elements fundamental to complex social skills. First, the belief in a physiological cause and cure for profound schizophrenia still lingers (Ullmann & Krasner, 1975) and dictates that training efforts would be futile. Second, the time investment required to instigate first basic skills such as verbalizing and attending to others, followed by intermediate skills such as conversing coherently and assertively, is enormous. With more than half the patients currently residing in public hospitals destined to spend the rest of their lives there, however, it would appear that the patients, at least, have time.

Implicit Social Skills

While social skills training with most populations, including college students, psychiatric patients, and persons diagnosed as mentally retarded, has emphasized communicational social skills, there are additional personal characteristics that exert powerful controls over the amount of positive reinforcement one will obtain from his or her social environment. Appearance is one of them (Clore, 1974). Glickman et al. (1973) reported data to suggest that the contingent delivery of either social reinforcement or access to lunch was effective for increasing frequencies of combing hair and washing faces in eight diagnosed psychotics; not surprisingly, contingent access to meals was a more powerful manipulation. As part of a token economy program designed specifically to prepare patients for eventual community residence, Heap, Boblitt, Moore, and Hord (1970) demonstrated that contingent token delivery could effectively maintain shaving, bathing, combing hair, brushing teeth, and dressing appropriately in hospital males. Lloyd and Garlington (1968) demonstrated similar effects with hair combing, neatness, cleanliness of clothing, and quality of facial makeup in hospital females.

Effective social functioning requires both the performance of behaviors likely to result in social reinforcement and the nonperformance of behaviors likely to result in social punishment or withdrawal. While in many instances the establishment of pro-social, effective skills will result in a decrease or disappearance of unusual, disapproved behaviors (cf. Meichenbaum & Cameron, 1973), there is evidence to suggest that sometimes the frequency of unusual behaviors is so high as to prohibit a successful overlay of more adaptive skills. Under these circumstances, procedures must be included to suppress or eliminate those behaviors resulting in social punishment. Wincz, Leitenberg, and Agras (1972) employed feedback and token reinforcement contingent on non-delusional speech to reduce the frequency of delusional statements with 10 diagnosed chronic paranoid schizophrenics. Feedback alone was effective for decreasing the behavior with about half the sample; feedback with reinforcement was effective with an additional one-third. Anderson and Alpert (1974) reported effects with an analogous procedure applied clinically with a 26-year-old male.

Haynes and Geddy (1973), noting that psychotic hallucinatory behavior (defined as verbal responses independent of external environmental stimuli) was incompatible with adequate social functioning and responsiveness to environmental stimuli, reported a single-subject design in which 10 minutes of contingent timeout was apparently effective in reducing the frequency of hallucinations with a 45-year-old male schizophrenic hospitalized for 22 years. Cayner and Kiland (1974) reported similar effects for a 5-minute contingent timeout procedure with replications; their procedure was effective for both reducing delusions and suppressing assaultive outbursts. Winkler (1970) incorporated a response cost or "fine" procedure contingent on the occurrence of violent and noisy behavior with members of his token economy. The manipulation was effective in reducing both noise and violence on the ward.

Especially because the last several procedures discussed involve manipulations related to punishment, a point raised in an earlier context warrants reiteration here. The larger goal of treatment procedures must be remembered: establishing those skills required by society for adaptive social functioning. If quasi-punitive methods are employed for the end of making patients more adapted to the hospital environment, those methods are unjustified. For such an end, the method loses its status as treatment, a term reserved for procedures applied *in order to cure*. Within the context of an overall program designed to equip a recipient for effective community functioning, and with evidence that non-punitive procedures are ineffective, quasi-punitive methods of documented utility are not only treatments with legitimacy, they are ultimately humane.

The directions for social skills training with psychiatric patients are clear. Hospital environments should be designed to maintain existent community-adaptive skills and strengthen incipient ones. Training programs for establishing complex skills and, if necessary, fundamental elements of those skills should be incorporated. Procedures for insuring the eventual maintenance of those skills without artificial environmental supports should be included (cf. Jones & Kazdin, 1975; Patterson & Reid, 1973), and transitions from the institution to the community should be facilitated. (The necessity for external, environmental modifications for chronic psychiatric residents is explored more completely in Chapter 7.) With the exception of one published descriptive report (Spence, Cohen, & Kowalski, 1975), no professionally reported programs with such comprehensive planning have appeared. The utility of social skills training in its broadened sense for the plight of psychiatric patients as well as other social problems presented in this volume such as juvenile delinquency (Lewis, Kifer, Green, Roosa, & Phillips, 1973), drug addiction (Callner & Ross, 1973), and marital discord (Eisler, Miller, Hersen, & Alford, 1974; Fensterheim, 1972) is empirically tenable. The limits of skills training remain to be found.

Chapter 9
AGING

The nursing home with its variants, geriatric units in state and federal hospitals, has evolved as this country's primary service facility for persons over the age of 65 (Morris, 1967). In large measure, contemporary cultural acceptance of nursing homes as legitimate treatment centers has been fostered by the widely held assumption that nursing homes provide adequate and necessary medical care for aging Americans (MacDonald, 1973). Recent federal investigations, conducted by a special Senate subcommittee on long-term care, however, have noted the fact that there is a service crisis throughout American geriatric centers. Once thought to be the panacea for growing old, institutions for the aging were termed in their report "the most troubled, and troublesome, component of our entire health care system" (Moss, 1974, p. iii).

This Senate subcommittee charge was not made lightly. It represented a thoughtful conclusion based on evidence from intensive national investigations, and it followed from the documentation of a considerable number of alarming facts. Their inquiries revealed, for instance, that patient abuse, including cruelty, negligence, callousness, and unnecessary regimentation, is a common occurrence in geriatric facilities (Moss, 1974). Moreover, geriatric facilities were found to be both physically and medically unsafe: in 1974, one out of every five nursing homes reported fires, tragedies resulting in 538 deaths; food poisoning and virulent infections are frequently discovered in the wake of widespread failures to maintain hygiene standards (Moss, 1974).

The appalling conditions in nursing homes reported by Moss and his Senate colleagues are neither new nor recently discovered. As early as 1960, the United States Subcommittee on the Problems of the Aged and Aging labeled the lack of medical care and restorative services the number one issue in the nursing home field (Braverman, 1970). In 1963, the President's Council on Aging (1963) reported that there were serious deficits in facility medical provisions and hygiene precautions, that 60% of all licensed nursing homes failed to meet minimal standards of safety and building maintenance, and that 50% of those institutions claiming skilled nursing care did not have a registered professional nurse on staff. In 1970, The Associated Press released a series of articles documenting the following conditions: one-seventh of all drugs given to nursing home residents are given incorrectly; most drugs are administered for the purpose of making patients easier to handle; the average food expenditure per patient was less than one dollar per day; the average amount of physician care per patient was 2.5 minutes per week (Pryon, 1970). In 1971, Ralph Nader reported numerous observations of widespread substandard practices (Nader, 1971). And in 1972, Tomlinson documented the following conclusions: patient care is primarily the responsibility of poorly trained and underpaid aides and orderlies; violence against patients erupts shockingly often; poor hygiene precautions have resulted in such tragedies as 25 deaths from a single incident of salmonella food poisoning (Tomlinson, 1972).

In search of the cause for these shocking conditions, critics frequently point accusing fingers at the nursing home industry itself. It is not entirely inaccurate to do so, since 77% of this country's nursing homes are operated for profit often inflated by illegal supplier kickbacks (Moss, 1974), and since nursing home industry representatives have actively obstructed federal attempts to legislate facility standards (Moss, 1974). However, faults within the nursing home system provide far from a complete explanation for the "treatment" that has evolved. A legitimate analysis of the nursing home problem cannot stop with a description of the industry's characteristics; it must question why the industry was allowed to develop in the fashion that it has. The answer to this question reaches far beyond individual or even collective facilities or profiteers; it stretches into the very fabric of this country's cultural and economic structure (MacDonald, 1973).

Around the turn of the century, growing old in America was a matter of individual pride. Becoming older meant becoming wiser, and reaching the age of 65 had no negative implications for one's employment status or general social role (United States Congress, 1965). With the rise of the industrial and technological revolution, however, "the responsibilities formerly allotted to older people became irrelevant in a mechanized economic system and a fast-changing society" (White House Conference on Aging, 1971, p. 16). And because the prestige of the aging in any culture is universally dependent on the number of important societal functions the aging perform (Simmons, 1964), rapid advances in technology resulting in the evaporation of their function, coupled with society's faiiure to provide valued, alternative social roles, resulted in a concomitant rapid decline in the status of the aging (Clemente & Summers, 1973). Exclusion from employment became a matter of course (MacDonald, 1973), and this institutionalized unemployment brought both poverty and rolelessness along in its wake (United States Congress, 1965).

Conditions have only deteriorated in the half century since the cycle began. Today, more than 15% of this nation's poverty problem involves the aging 10% of the population (United States Congress, 1965). The impact of this financial status has several deleterious effects, not the least of which is the degradation and induced insecurity befalling any impoverished member of a generally affluent society (Kalish, 1971; Spreitzer & Snyder, 1974). While monies for emergency medical care are provided by federal funding, preventive health and dental care for the aging become financially prohibitive at the very time when those services are most needed (MacDonald, 1973). Recreational activities, critical for the maintenance of emotional well-being (DeCarlo, 1974; Schonfield, 1973a, 1973b), are unattainable because of their cost (Brotman, 1968); as a consequence, by and large the aging do not participate in enjoyable events (Lewinsohn & MacPhillamy, 1974). Limited financial resources also result in inexpensive and nutritionally inadequate dietary patterns (Caird, Judge, & Macleod, 1975; Robinson, 1969), habits definitively linked to cognitive dysfunctioning (Lowenthal, 1975). Transportation cannot be afforded, so that needed services based in distant locations become inaccessible (Cutler, 1972); moreover, such constricted mobility has demonstrably negative psychological effects (Cutler, 1975; Libow, 1973; K. J. Smith & Lipman, 1972).

The economic aspects of institutionalized unemployment in and of themselves are damaging enough. However, these effects are visible, and legislated attempts have been made, generally unsuccessfully, to remediate them (MacDonald, 1973). The invisible effects of the social practice of conferring a role change on the person reaching 65, symbolized by institutionalized retirement, are far more difficult to overcome. By removing a central social role without providing a valued alternative, forced retirement initiates an overwhelmingly negative self-image (Lehr & Dreher, 1969; Thompson, 1973). The role which is provided for the aging—that of being sick and useless—produces an internalized sense of incompetence (Kuypers & Bengston, 1973) and is the most negative role provided for any minority (Palmore & Manton, 1973). With no valued social function, and as an economically dependent group, the aging perceive themselves and are perceived by others as a socially superfluous category of people (MacDonald, 1973). It is within this social context that nursing homes and geriatric units began to develop; over time, they flourished as warehouses of people waiting to die (Hudson, 1970).

The problem with aging, then, does not reside solely in the functioning of geriatric facilities. It is a social problem, one that touches all individuals personally as they reach the age when society and they themselves begin to think of themselves as old and useless. Not surprisingly, the most common psychological problem affecting the aging is depression (Feigenbaum, 1974); but that problem is not a problem emanating from the aging person. It is, instead, a rational reaction to the overwhelmingly depressing situation in which most aging persons find themselves:

> After I reached the senior citizen bracket, I had to move in with my daughter and several grandchildren. . . . I felt more and more in the way. . . . Finally, I found a small apartment and moved. I have no transportation, but I have a closet of my own, a cupboard for my dishes

and groceries, plenty of peace and quiet. . . . I spend every penny I have every month just to survive, but I have no plans to move. (Gaitz & Scott, 1975, p. 50)

Just as critics have sought to assign the source of the aging's problems to a single cause—nursing homes—they have looked to a single profession—medicine—for the solution. Again, there is some basis for this conclusion in fact: while aging is not itself a disease (Boyd & Oakes, 1969), it is a period of life during which there is a heightened susceptibility to various disease processes (United States Department of Health, Education, and Welfare, 1970) and during which preventive care becomes of increased importance (Boyd & Oakes, 1969). However, most physicians dislike working with the aging (Field, 1970; Reichel, 1973), have received training that stressed the futility of treating this population (Hazell, 1960), have only minimal motivation toward curing them (Boyd & Oakes, 1969), and engage in few preventive procedures (Barrow, 1971). Partially as a function of programs in medical schools, which generally do not include courses in geriatrics (Reichel, 1973), physicians' negative attitudes toward treating the aging are both abiding and consequential. Efforts to train physicians to have more positive attitudes toward the aging have been uniformly unsuccessful (Cicchetti, Fletcher, Lerner, & Colemen, 1973). Moreover, their belief in the hopelessness of this group has prevented their consultation with psychiatric and psychological colleagues, even in those instances when they would have done so had the problem involved a younger person (Garetz & Garetz, 1973; Ginsburg & Goldstein, 1974). As believers in the cultural misconception that aging and illness are synonymous (Barrow, 1971), physicians are quick to categorize any person over 65 as beyond help:

Recently I became ill in a strange city and went to a hospital. A doctor took one look at me, and without a question or a test pronounced me hopelessly senile. (Gaitz & Scott, 1975, p. 50)

There is neither a single solution nor a single cause for the problems of the aging. Aging is a social problem with multiple causes. An effective solution will be found only in multiple changes at a variety of societal levels. Fortunately, there have been promising initial steps.

Home Services

As a guiding formulation, Robert Kahn, in á recent overview, stressed the importance of employing the "Principle of Least Intervention" with the aging (Kahn, 1975). In effect, this formulation implies that effective help should be provided when it is needed, but that no more help than is needed should be given. In this context, help refers to various types of assistances—medical, psychological, economic, and environmental among them. With these elaborations, Kahn's principle should be a guiding dictum in working with the aging, in part because the number of people in need of help is too great to justify providing superfluous assistance to any subset, and in part because it is by retaining as much functional independence as possible that this group can best be encouraged to continue as part of society's mainstream.

It is desirable to encourage continued community residence rather than insititutionalization, a form of total care, for the aging. This statement is supported not only by data documenting deleterious effects resulting from institutionalization (MacDonald, 1973), but also by the aging's stated preference. Eight in 10 community-dwelling elderly report that they would prefer to continue living in their own homes (Shanas, 1962). Moreover, the majority of the elderly presently in institutions state that they would prefer community living (Gottesman & Bourestom, 1974; Tomlinson, 1972).

It is often thought that once institutionalized, an aging person cannot resume community residence successfully. Evidence indicates, however, that the institutionalized aging *can* successfully return to their communities with minimal home assistance (Macleod, 1970). Home assistance takes the form of trained helpers who travel to the person's home and provide various maintenance services; it is the most commonly recognized need for all community-dwelling aging (Gold, 1972).

Berg, Atlas, and Zeiger (1974) reported the outcome of their home-assistance program. Among the services provided were cleaning, home maintenance, laundry, shopping, and food preparation. In evaluating their program, Berg and his colleagues suggested that the primary reason for its success was their willingness to respond to the stated needs of their serviced population. Several of the services they ultimately provided, such as food preparation, were not ones they initially intended to provide when planning the program. As the program evolved, however, they were recognized as needed and subsequently included in the service complement.

The vast importance of assistance with home maintenance tasks cannot be underemphasized; to date, however, only the Berg et al. (1974) program has been reported. The absence of other similar programs cannot be attributed to a lack of need; it is much more a function of a lack of money. Home assistance, while a documented general necessity for community-dwelling aging (Gold, 1972) is not federally funded.

Home health service is a second very major assistance need. Many community-dwelling elderly suffer from one or more chronic but treatable health problems (Burvill, 1970). The complexity of the health-care system (Harris, 1975; Poe, 1975) and the difficulties of arranging transportation to medical centers (Bell & Olsen, 1974; Cutler, 1972), however, serve to discourage the aging from seeking medical treatment.

Bell (1975) reports an exemplary program responding to home health service needs. Using a converted school bus, he developed a fully equipped mobile medical center. This center served both screening and service delivery functions. In 15 minutes, by progressing through the unit's several examining room and laboratory compartments, each person received the following: medical history recording and evaluation; vision, blood pressure, temperature, vital capacity, and heart rate checks; and blood and urine analyses. When warranted, prescriptions were given and referrals were made. Nearly 3,000 persons were serviced during the unit's first 6 months of operation, and 12.8% of them were referred for further testing or treatment.

The Bell (1975) program is designed for rural areas. An equally effective and more carefully evaluated program was reported by Moss and Lavery (1974) for an urban community with a more concentrated population. Their delivery system was comprised of a network of local, storefront offices scattered throughout the community. Each office served as the headquarters for physician-nurse teams who made house calls to nearby homes. After evaluating health needs, these teams made referrals when warranted to an in-community, cooperating hospital; quite notably, referrals which were made were followed through to completion. The system's effectiveness for the community was evaluated after a year of operation; Moss and Lavery's (1974) strategy of service delivery resulted in nearly every aging person's receipt of necessary medical services for the duration of the project.

Home health services are funded by Medicare (Butler, 1969). Despite this assistance and their intuitive and empirical effectiveness, however, they are not readily available. Only one aging person in six resides in a location where home services are provided; not surprisingly, they are concentrated in the country's urban areas (Butler, 1969).

Home psychological services are not funded by federal assistance programs. In part because of this absence of funding, and in part because of psychology's general failure as a profession to attend to the needs of the aging (MacDonald, 1973), few home delivery programs have been developed. Leonard and Kelly (1975) describe the only professionally reported program to date. Their service accepted referrals, primarily from general practitioners recognizing a need, and subsequently sent a physician-nurse team to the referred person's home. Once there, the team evaluated the person's needs and made appropriate referrals to available community agencies. Unfortunately, staff resource limitations precluded follow-through on the completion of the referrals, and no data were collected in support of the usefulness of the program. (Leonard & Kelly, 1975). The report does make a contribution, however, by suggesting a service content not previously considered.

Home maintenance, health, and psychological services fill a tremendous need, in that they either bring necessary services to the aging or facilitate the aging's access to the services. At present, however, they share two major disadvantages which detract from their utility. First, more often than not, they focus on the delivery of a single service. While one service is certainly better than none, it is obvious from the host of problems simultaneously facing the aging—medical, psychological, economic—that on a broad scale, coordinated multiservice programs would be more beneficial. The second major shortcoming was implied in the descriptions of home services presently provided: more often than not the aging person is left to his or her own resources to complete a prescribed referral, and follow-through on the part of the referring service is infrequent. Parameters on the number of referrals completed are not available, but estimates suggest that the number is quite low (Harris, 1975). Again, multiple service agencies with coordinated services would provide a solution.

Multiservice Centers

Multiservice centers for senior citizens may fall into one of two categories: they may evolve out of existing community mental health facilities or they may be independently established. Both types of centers have been described. Gurian and Scherl (1972) reported on the functioning of a unit developed within an existing community mental health center. At its inception, the unit had five objectives: to provide comprehensive mental health services to the aging both directly as well as indirectly through consultation with other care-givers; to develop and implement training programs for persons involved with the aging; to create a base for community organization and action by the aging themselves; to develop methods and instruments for evaluating the effectiveness of the unit's programs; and to engage in research specific to the mental health needs of the aging population. After 2 years of functioning, the unit had achieved some of its objectives. Unit members had consulted with several nursing homes. They had consulted with local physicians in an effort to upgrade the quality of hospital care. They had established a schedule for home visits to aging community residents. Finally, they had provided in-service training for staffs from several local nursing homes. The program did seem to be beneficial; however, no formal evaluative research was conducted.

The discrepancy between Gurian and Scherl's (1972) unit objectives at inception and achieved functions over time was unfortunately quite large. Such a discrepancy is more often the case than the exception with centers serving multiple populations (Estes, 1974). This observation suggests that board effectiveness requires complete commitment to the aging; Santore and Diamond (1974) describe a center of this sort.

Santore and Diamond's (1974) program was notable in that it sprang from an assessment of the community's needs and responded to changes in need as they developed. The index signaling a need for developing the center was a noted discrepancy between the proportion of persons over 65 served by an existing community mental health facility and the proportion of persons over 65 living in that facility's catchment area: 3.5% and 10%, respectively. In response to that index, the existing center contacted an indigenous group already interested in the aging—the clergy. Together they established a base of operation for the geriatric agency. Consistent with the philosophy of working through members of the population to be served, the agency planners hired a woman over 60 to function as center organizer. They recruited and trained eight aides, also over 60, who were paid during the training period. The trained staff functioned in a storefront center. Among the services they provided were transportation to medical facilities, senior citizens clubs, Sunday dinner programs, a crafts shop, a drop-in center, and an emergency medical cadre. They were influential in encouraging the nearby relocation of several auxiliary services, including homemaker and food stamp distribution centers. During its first 6 months of operation, more than 500 aging individuals had been directly served. The program seemed to be successful in part because its political activism was low-keyed and limited to times of necessity; political involvements occurred only as ultimate responses to visible needs. Other similar centers with political activism as an explicit objective apart from any demonstrably present need have not been successful (Blonsky, 1974).

It is difficult to compare the gains made by Santore and Diamond's (1974) program with those made by Gurian and Scherl's (1972). Santore and Diamond (1974) focused on indirect services; Gurian and Scherl (1972) concentrated on direct service delivery. Asking which emphasis was more beneficial obscures the fact that neither type of intervention alone can be ultimately successful; lasting impact demands comprehensive interventions on multiple levels (MacDonald, 1973). As novelties in the American service delivery system, such comprehensive programs have not yet had time to develop; but England, a country whose commitment to servicing the aging precedes this country's by about a decade, provides an instructive example of what can emerge.

Robinson (1969) describes one British "geriatric community center," a facility established exclusively to serve the aging. The center's program operates with coordinated service levels, so that persons falling anywhere on the spectrum of degree of needed assistance can be maintained. The first level is an outreach screening program: registered nurses with a year's graduate training in social work make an annual home visit to every elderly person in the center's catchment area. The visit serves two functions: prevention and remediation. Preventive services include diet, financial, and safety counseling. The remedial services include psychological and medical evaluations with appropriate, follow-through referrals to psychologists and physicians. The second service level is supportive services, and a myriad of them are provided and coordinated: home nursing, home helpers, night sitters, laundry services, welfare food, speech therapy, occupational therapy, ambulation and transportation aids, volunteer social services, meals on wheels, and a visiting library. Each of these supportive services was established in response to a need estimate based on reports from the first-level outreach nurses. The third level involves a cooperative program operating within a community hospital. This level coordinates in-hospital treatment. In addition to comprehensive quality medical care, the unit provides for its inpatients' rehabilitative, occupational, recreational, and milieu therapies. Programs designed to maintain staff interest in treatment, including regular case conferences and regular extramural service training, are provided. There are also inpatient treatment safeguards: regular review and reassessments of long-term patients are included to prevent staff neglect, family contact and family counseling is provided to prevent family neglect, and regular follow-up visits after discharge are programmed to prevent community neglect.

Robinson's (1969) program, financed entirely by the local community, provides a paradigm for geriatric intervention. Its multilevel structure provides a vehicle for implementing Kahn's (1975) Principle of Least Intervention. Services are both comprehensive and multidisciplinary. Programs are established in response to evaluated need and coordinated once they are established. The financial base forces professional accountability to the serviced population.

Only one addition should be made to Robinson's (1969) program in applying its structure in this country. As an area of great cultural diversity, the United States possesses a heterogeneous aging population (Maddox, 1963; Maddox & Douglass, 1974). Facilities suitable and appealing to one subset of the aging population may very well be unsuitable for another (Rosenzweig, 1975). Before services are provided, then, both population needs (Sears, 1974) and effective styles of service delivery (Rappaport & Chinsky, 1974) must be evaluated, and a most important source of information for the evaluative process—which is all too often overlooked—is the stated need and preferred style expressed by the group to be served (Erwin, 1974; Lewis, 1975).

Day-Care Centers

Recent federal funding has encouraged the proliferation of day-care programs, services intended to provide an alternative to multiservice centers that was both viable and economically expedient (Matlack, 1975; Rao, 1971; Shore, 1974). Day-care programs specifically servicing the aging, a relatively new concept in the American service delivery system, first appeared in England in 1958 (Mehta & Mack, 1975). Though consistently successful and popular in Great Britain, there were fewer than 20 such programs in the United States through early 1974 (Mehta & Mack, 1975). In conception, day-care programs were designed to provide a broad spectrum of treatment services in a fixed location; participants were to be transported to the program each day and returned to their homes each evening (Irvine, 1974). In actuality, however, there are wide variations in the types of programs offered, with most centers supplying only one or two services (cf. Grauer, Betts, Birnbom, 1973; Lorenze, Hamill, & Oliver, 1974; Oster & Kibat, 1975; Reingold, Wolk, & Schwartz, 1971; Silver, 1970). Those centers that do supply multiple services (Mehta & Mack, 1975; J. W. Wilson, 1973) appear to be nothing more than daytime duplications of existing institutional facilities; they report, in fact, that the majority of their program participants are transferred directly to nursing homes (Mehta & Mack, 1975). While originally intended to provide alternatives to institutionalization (Arie, 1975), day-care programs appear to be developing into mere extensions of traditional nursing homes.

Institutional Treatment

Because the United States has not yet successfully developed progressive, comprehensive programs such as the coordinated multiservice center described by Robinson (1969), and because minimally supportive services are not widely available (Butler, 1969), analysts have concluded that older Americans who need assistance are presented with only two alternatives: remaining in the community unassisted or moving to a total-care institution (Matlack, 1975). It is, in fact, true that institutional residence has been by far the most common "treatment" provided (Moss, 1974). In light of recent indisputable evidence that long-term care facilities have generally failed as a system (Moss, 1974) and convincing evidence that such facilities are harmful to persons living there (MacDonald, 1973; Markson, Levitz, & Gognalons-Caillard, 1973; Prock, 1969), some analysts have taken the position that long-term facilities should be eliminated (Shore, 1974). While this position is understandable, one cannot overlook the fact that there are aging persons who do need total care (Burvill, 1970; Shanas, 1973; Sherwood, Morris, & Barnhart, 1975; Shore, 1974). Moreover, until alternative services are more readily available, there will continue to be displaced persons who must go to institutions for partial care (Gottesman & Bourestom, 1974; Rosin, 1970; Stevens, 1970). The challenge then becomes much more demanding than simple obliteration of existing facilities; programs of demonstrable or anticipated treatment effectiveness must be incorporated into facilities as they are.

Three general types of therapies have been suggested for facility-wide programs to improve resident functioning: reality orientation or remotivation therapy (Barnes, 1974; Gubrium & Ksander, 1975; Remnet, 1974), milieu therapy or therapeutic communities (Goldstein, 1971; Grauer, 1971), and sheltered workshops (Finkestein & Rosenberg, 1974). Reality orientation, by far the most popular (Birkett & Boltuch, 1973), is generally conducted in daily classroom sessions by facility aides and attendants. Sessions are structured to foster group discussions about concrete topics and to reorient confused residents toward aspects of reality such as the day of the week, date, and location. Milieu therapy is designed to transform the entire facility into a treatment unit by organizing a patient governing body that determines as much of the institution's policy as possible. Sheltered workshops provide structured, task-oriented sessions during which residents construct various products, usually for manufacturing companies; residents are paid for their work.

Although each of these therapies has been asserted as beneficial, little empirical evidence supports these claims. MacDonald and Settin (in press) examined some issues by comparing the effects of reality orientation and a modified sheltered workshop program against a no-treatment control. Thirty residents of a prorpietary nursing home were assigned randomly to one of the three experimental conditions. Treatments were applied in group settings, and each of the two facility staff members led one group in each condition. Residents assigned to reality orientation met for 15 hour-long sessions over a period of 5 weeks. During each meeting, they discussed a different concrete topic and a current article from a local newspaper. Residents assigned to the modified sheltered workshop program met for an equal period of time. During each meeting, members of the workshop program constructed gifts for a nearby school for exceptional children. The results of this study indicated that participation in the workshop program produced a significant increase in life satisfaction as compared with both reality orientation and the no-contact control. There were indications that reality orientation resulted in a substantial reduction in life satisfaction, although the shift was not statistically significant ($p < .10$). Other investigators have reported that reality orientation is beneficial (Barnes, 1974; Birkett & Boltuch, 1973), however, and more intensive investigation of the issue is in order.

As early as 1966 (Cautela, 1966; Kastenbaum, 1968), empirically oriented clinical psychologists were suggesting the potential utility of behavior modification for treating the aging. Since that time, several studies have appeared demonstrating that treatments based on behavioral principles are, in fact, effective. Investigations with groups have focused on three major areas: exercise, activity, and social interaction. A variety of targets has been explored in the context of single-subject designs.

Promoting exercise has been an especially popular focus and a worthwhile one, since the usual inactivity fostered by total-care institutions results in muscular atrophy and general physical deterioration (Quilitch, 1974). In an incomplete single-subject design, Libb and Clements (1969) established baserates of exercising on a bicycle exerciser for institutional geriatric patients, all with a diagnosis of chronic brain syndrome. After baseline, Libb and Clements (1969) reinforced increased exerciser activity with marbles later exchangeable for consumable reinforcers. This manipulation was apparently responsible for nearly doubling activity levels on the exerciser with three of the four men studied.

In a more controlled study, Stamford (1972) evaluated the physiological effects of increased exercise with 17 men in a geriatric unit of a state hospital. After screening the men to insure that their medical histories and current functioning did not contraindicate their inclusion in the program, Stamford (1972) assessed the heart rates and blood pressures of all participants and assigned them at random to either experimental or control conditions. The men in the experimental condition were encouraged to exercise by environmental structuring (specifying a time and place). The exercise program involved walking on a treadmill for a progressively longer period of time to a maximum of 20 minutes; sessions were held 5 days a week for a period of 12 weeks. At the end of the program, men who had exercised showed significant beneficial training effects when compared with nonexercising controls: decreased heart rates and systolic blood pressure during exercise and decreased heart rates while at rest (Stamford, 1972).

Similar physiological benefits from exercise for groups of aging men and women have been reported by Adams and deVries (1973), Frekany and Leslie (1975), Stamford (1973), and Powell (1974). Powell's work goes beyond the findings of the other studies, however, and deserves special attention. Working with 30 screened geriatric mental patients, Powell compared the effects of three experimental conditions: light exercise for an hour a day 5 days per week, social therapy consisting of talk and games for an equivalent amount of time, and a no-contact control group. After 12 weeks of treatment, members of the exercise group showed significant improvements in two tests of cognitive ability. No other changes were significant.

The benefits of increasing the time geriatric patients spend in goal-directed activity have long been known (Reichenfeld, Csapo, Carriere, & Gardner, 1973). Without activity programs, the institutionalized aging spend most of their waking hours just waiting for meals and bedtime (Turner, 1967). Quilitch (1975) has reported an exploratory study investigating levels of activity. Working with 43 male and female geriatric patients, all designated "psychiatrically impaired," he demonstrated that the amount of time spent in purposeful activity on the ward could be quadrupled by simply providing an activity opportunity. Purposeful activity was defined as reading, writing, talking, listening, using recreational materials, or doing a chore. The activity provided was bingo, a generally popular game with geriatric patients. Refreshments and prizes were given during the activity period. Quilitch's (1975) work represents a clear example of the notion of environmental design (Krasner & Ullmann, 1973); from this perspective, the problem of patient inactivity was not due to the patients, but was due to changeworthy properties of the environment.

In a series of carefully executed studies, McClannahan and Risley (1973, 1974a, 1974b, 1974c) have demonstrated this same major point. In their first study (McClannahan & Risley, 1973), they documented that active use of a nursing home's lobby area was more than doubled by providing a department store shop in that area. In their second study (McClannahan & Risley, 1974a), they demonstrated that providing recreational materials to generally inactive nursing home residents dramatically increased the amount of time they spent in purposeful activity; this study was especially important in that the subjects included were all severely disoriented and represented a group of persons not ordinarily addressed by psychological treatment research. Their third study documented the effects of publicizing upcoming events to increase event attendance (McClannahan & Risley, 1974b). The final study investigated the importance of two program elements—prizes and snacks—for encouraging activity attendance. Both prizes and snacks were found to increase attendance, but prizes showed an overwhelming effect, while the increase due to snacks was moderate (McClennahan & Risley, 1974c).

Dunn and Strang (1970) provide a creative suggestion for incorporating these findings into existing institutional settings. They propose the appointment of "ward hostess," a paid staff member excused from nursing responsibilities and charged with the responsibility of "stimulating and coordinating group and individual activity in long-term patients" (Dunn & Strang, 1970, p. 268). In a sense, providing a ward hostess is analogous to providing a structured opportunity for activities, provided he or she has resources and is effective. One would expect, then, an increase in activities following the person's introduction; and, in fact, such an increase was noted by Dunn and Strang.

Social interaction has been the focus of the final cluster of group investigations. The general infrequency with which geriatric patients converse among themselves was once thought to be an index of "disengagement," an inherent aspect of increasing age (Brown, 1974). Recent investigations have demonstrated this observed social withdrawal, however, to be a function of environmental factors discouraging interaction (Hoyer, Mishara, & Reidel, in press). MacDonald (in press) selected three aging men designated by ward staff as socially isolated and withdrawn. With a single-subject design, she demonstrated that baserates of verbalization could be significantly increased by providing conversational topics and socially reinforcing responses to those topics. In addition, there were strong indications that increasing the rate of verbalization led to increased enjoyment of the sessions for the experimental participants (MacDonald, in press). Mueller and Atlas (1972) and Hoyer, Kafer, Simpson, and Hoyer (1974) demonstrated similar effects with similar populations using material reinforcement.

Three studies have appeared investigating ward-wide rates of social interaction. Sommer and Ross (1958) found that simply rearranging the lobby furniture so that chairs faced each other more than doubled the rate of between-resident conversation. Silverstone and Winter (1975) reported that integrating formerly sex-segregated wards increased rates of social interaction and elicited improved grooming and manners with the male patients. Mishara and Kastenbaum (1974) reported that serving wine in the evenings both increased social interactions during serving times and decreased barbiturate medications requested for insomnia. Conflicting results reported by Burrill, McCourt, and Cutler (1974), however, suggest that it is the social context surrounding the alcohol rather than the alcohol itself which serves as a social facilitator.

Surprisingly, few programs have directly addressed improving affect. Two studies have appeared, however, both of which reported success. Power and McCaroon (1975) describe the effects of half-hour, weekly individual contact with staff members as treatments for depression. Participants in the study were primarily bedridden or confined to wheelchairs. Treatment progressed through several phases: establishing familiarity, shaping patient involvement with the staff member, and prompting patient relationships with other patients. After both a 15-week treatment period and a 6-week follow-up period, participants receiving treatment were rated as better adjusted and less depressed than members of a control group. Arthur, Donnan, and Lair (1973) provided college-age companions for a group of institutionalized aging. The program consisted of 90 minutes of weekly visits for a period of 10 weeks. At the end of treatment, there was a significant improvement in patient morale for persons with companions compared to noncompanioned controls. At a 6-week follow-up, there were indications that the program's effects were more persistent if the companionship had been with several different people rather than the same person.

Because of the wide variation in types of persons residing in geriatric facilities (Maddox, 1963), successful individualized treatments for specific target problems are extremely useful as sources for both direct information and indirect extrapolation to analogous targets. MacDonald and Butler (1974) reported on the effectiveness of a prompting-reinforcing sequence for encouraging walking in physically competent residents who had not walked during the previous 6 months. Geiger and Johnson (1974) employed a similar procedure to improve the amount of food consumed by previously undereating patients. Fowler, Fordyce, and Berni (1969) increased toleration of elevation on a tilt-table with contingent staff attention. Brody, Kleban, Lawton, and Moss (1974) and Colthart (1974) have reported impressive success using highly individualized programs for each ward member.

Only one persistent problem has met with little success: the treatment of incontinence (Collins & Plaska, 1975; Pollock & Liberman, 1974). The reasons for failure are, as yet, unclear; they may be related to physiological malfunctions, environmental constraints, urinary tract infections, or medicinal side effects. Only one thing is clear: the failure of training programs with this problem is not due to the population's inability to learn (Ankus & Quarrington, 1972).

By and large, then, programs developed following Cautela (1966) and Kastenbaum's (1968) suggestions have been highly successful. Unfortunately, however, the treatments developed have enjoyed limited application. Quilitch

(1975) and Hickey and Spinetta (1974) have noted that a major problem exists in bridging the gap between procedures known to be effective and procedures known to be applied. While these authors addressed their comments to institutional treatment, the observation is equally descriptive of service delivery to the aging in all its dimensions.

The overall direction in which American geriatric service delivery programs are developing is still inadequate. In large part, all programs share two major assumptions: that becoming older is a personal problem and that treatment requires either changing the person to resemble a younger individual or patronizing the person as long as she or he lives. But, examined more closely, growing older in America is a social problem. It exists because of our collective failure to assign worth to any social role made available for the aging. It exists because of our collective hesitation to modify the environment to accommodate the aging's needs (Chapanis, 1974; Grauer, Betts, & Birnbom, 1973; Tucker, Combs, & Woolrich, 1975). It exists because, until very recently, no one really cared.

As with a number of social problems including substance abuse, delinquency, crime, and social ineffectiveness, the present chapter illustrates a prevailing objective of behavioral community psychologists—namely, the development of community and individual competencies. Although behavior modification historically has emphasized the expansion of response repertoires as an intervention goal, the present volume stresses two additional requirements for an effective behavioral community psychology. First, more attention needs to be directed at maintaining and generalizing the newly developed, fragile competencies which our interventions instigate. In other words, one goal of such efforts would be the "stabilization" of skills as described in the present volume's Foreword. Second, competencies need to be stabilized at a community as well as an individual level. Throughout the preceding chapters, this theme has been exemplified by developments such as the use of nonprofessionals, the provision of community-based alternatives to institutionalization, the mobilization of community contingencies to encourage constructional skills, and the recommendation that communities increase their tolerance for the behavioral diversity which their members display. Hopefully, future behavioral research on the problems of the aging will be typified by an increasing attention to these two programmatic requirements.

Chapter 10
UNEMPLOYMENT

Analysts of the urban crisis, which dramatically erupted in the late 1960s, have identified unemployment as a major cause of contemporary social strain (National Citizens' Committee for Community Relations and the Community Relations Service of the United States Department of Justice, 1967; Report of the National Advisory Commission on Civil Disorders, 1968). At the individual level, unemployment signifies uselessness and engenders a sense of chaos especially for American males, who have no well-defined social role other than employed worker; unemployment has been implicated as a primary cause of both aggression and mental illness (Work in America: Report of a Special Task Force to the Secretary of Health, Education, and Welfare, 1973). At the societal level, unemployment has been linked to a variety of unfortunate effects: poverty (Ferguson, 1971), higher crime rates (Johnson, 1964), increased incidence of alcoholism (Plant, 1967), and more frequent institutionalization (Hollingshead & Redlich, 1958). Whether examined from the perspective of the individual or society, and whether measured by economic and material loss or by human waste and suffering, the cost of unemployment is enormously high (McCarthy, 1965); its pervasive effects led to its designation as America's major mental health problem in 1975 (Proshansky, 1975).

Prior to the recent economic crisis, unemployment was estimated to affect about 5% of the American labor force (Okun, 1965). This figure, compiled by the Labor Department, included only those persons out of work who were actively seeking employment at the time; it excluded those most significantly affected—the hard-core unemployed and persons chronically out of work who were not actively job searching (Ferguson, 1971). Because of this omission, the Labor Department's estimate provides a conservative and inaccurate assessment of the magnitude of the unemployment problem; more accurate estimates are not, however, available (Ferguson, 1971).

While unemployment is detrimental to any person, its effects are most pronounced with this group of unknown proportions—the hard-core unemployed. These persons tend to be young, untrained, and uneducated; they are primarily black (Ferguson, 1971). There is little normative pressure within the group's subculture to seek employment (Feldman, 1974), in part because

299

members of the group do not believe that being unemployed has more personal disadvantages than does being employed (Feldman, 1973).

This subcultural belief in the personal futility of employment has been construed by many as both irrational and indicative of a host of underlying negative personal characteristics (Triandis, Feldman, Weldon, & Harvey, 1974). In large measure, however, the belief is a valid one. Discrimination in hiring and promotion policies continue (Ferguson, 1971); more often than not, the effect of civil rights legislation on industry has been to make discrimination less visible, but not less real (Arvey & Mussio, 1974; Boehm, 1972). As a consequence of discrimination in hiring, there is little encouragement to seek out employment. For those who do seek and find employment, more often than not their assigned jobs are underpaid and under abrasive social and physical working conditions (Bloom & Barry, 1967; Richards & Jaffee, 1972). Discriminatory promotion policies make it unlikely that their job status will ever change, so that these working conditions function to discourage continued employment (Argyle, 1972). While working, members of this group have daily exposure to non-black workers in better—and, for them, unattainable—positions; over time, this exposure increases both job and life dissatisfaction to an extremely high level (Hulin, 1966). For those who continue working despite these conditions, job security is marginal because, as unskilled and consequently easily replaced workers, they are the first group to be eliminated in times of company cutbacks (Killingsworth, 1965). Sooner or later, most return to the group of unemployed.

The effects of this cyclical work-nonworker status are telling on the individual (McCarthy, 1965). On family life, the effects are of paramount proportions. During periods of unemployment, there is an exaggerated family instability resulting from increased rates of moving to locations with potentially better job opportunities (Bass & Alexander, 1972). Also during unemployment, there is a husband-wife role reversal for which males are poorly prepared (McCarthy, 1965). During periods of unemployment, there is heightened stress-produced familial aggression (McCarthy, 1965).

The characteristics of children from these families remain a matter of debate, but there is general agreement that early on they learn the necessity for sheer survival (Goodale, 1973) and the reality of extremely limited job opportunities (Schwartz & Henderson, 1964). In many instances, these children drop out of school before finishing—perhaps to help support their families, or perhaps because they are exposed to the same sorts of abrasive conditions at school that their fathers are at work; their drop-out status places them in the pool, then, of unskilled laborers. In some instances, the children turn to delinquency as a means to resolve the dilemma of surviving in the face of limited employment opportunities (McCarthy, 1965). In most instances, these children are not exposed to and therefore do not learn the interpersonal skills (Himes, 1968) or attitudes (Paine, Deutsch, & Smith, 1967) necessary to favorably impress potential employers. Their subsequent lack of adequate income, clothing, general education, and specific vocational skills makes it virtually impossible for them to ever escape their cultural legacy (Goodale, 1973). In time, it becomes their children's heritage.

Macro-economic Contributors

The phenomena described thus far analyze contributors to repeated unemployment at an individual or small group level. Macro-economic conditions are additional contributors. The federal unemployment compensation system, essentially unchanged since its inception during the 1930s, structurally encourages both employers and employees to behave in ways that inflate levels of unemployment (Feldstein, 1973; Ley, 1966). Moreover, federal fiscal policies, designed to protect the stability of the dollar, have relied to a large extent on deliberate increases of unemployment to control inflation rather than alternative but equally effective price control techniques (Ferguson, 1971; Okun, 1965).

The established American economic structure includes four distinct types of unemployment, all of which affect the hard-core unemployed more harshly than any other group. Cyclical unemployment, due primarily to consumer demand-industry supply vicissitudes, and seasonal unemployment, arising from production dependencies on temporal parameters, could both be reduced by proper federal coordination (Feldstein, 1973). Transitional or fictional unemployment arises from temporary mismatches between labor skill demands and labor skill supplies and appears to be virtually unavoidable in any dynamic economic system. It is the fourth type—structural unemployment—however, which has produced the greatest difficulty for the hard-core unemployed. Structural unemployment, depicted symbolically in Fig. 10-1, refers to joblessness which results from permanent and pervasive changes in an economy's fabric (Wolfbein, 1965). Automation rendered such an effect in the American economy (Killingsworth, 1965) by increasing the demand for highly skilled workers and decreasing the demand for workers with little or no training, the category most applicable to the hard-core unemployed. As automation progresses, then, the already inadequate job market for primarily untrained hard-core unemployed may be expected to become even smaller.

Federal Manpower Programs

Partially in response to high rates of unemployment (Sewell, 1971) and partially in response to increased sensitivities to civil rights concerns (American Enterprise Institute for Public Policy Research, 1970), Congress enacted a series of bills to counteract the effects of structural unemployment. The initial legislation in the series was the Manpower Development and Training Act of

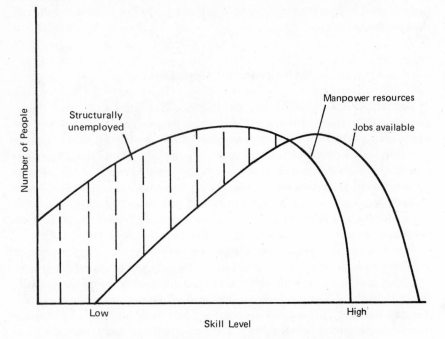

Fig. 10-1. A hypothetical plot of structural unemployment

1962 (Sewell, 1971). This legislation emphasized the training and rapid placement of persons presently unemployed; it had three purposes: vocational education, basic education, and job creation (American Enterprise Institute for Public Policy Research, 1970). As the program developed, however, the use of traditional trainee selection criteria, such as aptitude and general intelligence tests, resulted in an applicant rejection rate of 64% (Sewell, 1971). Consequently, the program reached only the cream of the unemployed crop, those who were between the ages of 25 and 45 and who had completed high school, persons described subsequently as probably not in actual need of such an intervention (Becker, Haber, & Levitan, 1965).

In 1966, the Manpower Program was redirected with additional legislation specifying that 65% of all trainees must be drawn from "disadvantaged" populations—the young, minorities, uneducated, rural, hard-core unemployed, and the aging; it further specified that training was to be primarily on-the-job rather than in the classroom, since the latter modality was effective only with educated middle-class participants.

In 1968, following the linking of unemployment with civil unrest, private enterprise joined in the effort and established a program called Job Opportunities in the Business Sector with an implementation agency named the

National Alliance of Businessmen (Goodale, 1973). In the last several years, then, aggressive recruiting and hiring policies have become fashionable in both the public and private business domains (National Citizens' Committee for Community Relations and the Community Relations Service of the United States Department of Justice, 1967). Unfortunately, as general economic conditions have declined, such programs have become less prevalent (Kirkpatrick, 1973); paradoxically, this is the time when they are needed most.

Evaluations of early manpower programs indicated three general trends. First, on-the-job training was more effective than general educational training and oral presentations of information were more effective than written presentations (Petty, 1974). Second, job-relevant training was more beneficial than general educational training (Gordon, Arvey, Daffron, & Umberger, 1974). And, finally, training programs were generally effective in increasing the incidence of successful job attainment over baserates of the target group's employment (Sewell, 1971), although not to a level equivalent to that of persons in the ordinary labor force (Triandis et al., 1974). Broad-scale studies of program effects on germane criteria other than hiring, such as level of income and length of employment subsequent to hiring, however, were generally overlooked.

Sewell (1971), in the interest of extending these results, conducted the first careful analysis of broad-scale manpower training program effects on previously ignored criteria. He studied the Manpower Improvement through Community Effort program, an experimental and demonstration project designed to help the rural poor. Based in several poverty pocket counties in North Carolina, the project worked with a population of several hundred persons conforming closely to the characteristics of the hard-core unemployed: 88% of the group were non-white, 75% had not completed high school, and 77% were male. Training which was primarily on-the-job, included clerical, sales, mechanical, service worker, nurse's aide, and building tradesman skills; counseling was provided for any personal problem which arose during training. Sewell (1971) found that completion of the program was associated with substantial increases in average weekly earnings at the time of his evaluation—16 months following training. Moreover, he replicated the findings of other investigators demonstrating the superiority of on-the-job rather than classroom training procedures.

Magnum and Robson (1973) conducted a similar archival study in evaluating the effects of programs based in Boston, Denver, San Francisco, and Oakland. Using statistical analyses not quite so powerful as Sewell's (1971), they examined the effects of English (language), clerical, automobile repair, machine repair, construction, and drafting skills training on several hundred trainees recruited under the revised Manpower Training and Development Program criteria. In general, training appeared to be beneficial; its effects were more pronounced, however, in those communities with employers and unions receptive to its goals.

By late 1973, 24 studies of the recruiting, hiring, and training of the hard-core unemployed had appeared (Goodman, Salipant, & Paransky, 1973). In examining these reports, most of which were not available in the public domain, Goodman et al. (1973) concluded that while manpower programs have demonstrable effects on initial rates of hiring, they seem to have had no consistent impact on job continuation or performance. The inconsistency of their conclusions with the results of Sewell (1971) appears to arise from something other than sampling error; Goodman et al. (1973) concluded that while manpower programs were not lastingly effective in general, under specified conditions they did produce demonstrable effects. Rural residence, a characteristic of Sewell's (1971) sample, was one of those conditions; being married, being a woman, or being over 21 were others (Goodman et al., 1973). The implication of these findings is that asking the question "is manpower training effective?" reflects a naivete analogous to that embedded in the question "is psychotherapy effective?" from two decades ago (Paul, 1969a). The task becomes one of identifying which programs are effective for which populations in which placement settings.

Refined Studies of Unemployment

Very few experimental studies addressing these clarified questions have appeared, in large measure because psychology as a profession has ignored the problems of the unemployed (Tiffany, Cowan, & Tiffany, 1970) and focused on more management-oriented questions such as optimal selection and production procedures (cf., Argyle, 1972; *Journal of Applied Psychology*, 1960-1975). Some studies addressing aspects of the dilemmas of the hard-core unemployed are available, however, and a literature of correlational studies implying promising directions has arisen.

The first step in reducing unemployment is getting jobs. O'Connor and Rappaport (1970), recognizing the importance of this step, worked with six black men recruited from a local branch of the Opportunities Industrialization Center. The six men were representative of many hard-core unemployed: they ranged in age from 21 to 30 and had either graduated from high school only after being placed in special classes for "slow learners" or been unemployed for 10 years or just been released from prison. The target jobs for these men were positions as child-care aides in residential cottages for the retarded and emotionally disturbed. Acquiring these jobs depended on two factors: passing a Civil Service Examination and successfully completing a job interview. O'Connor and Rappaport (1970) prepared programmed materials to educate the men in those areas requisite for the examination. Training of these materials was provided during 12 hourly sessions coupled with between-session practice; participants were paid during training. To transmit interviewee skills, O'Connor and Rappaport (1970) employed modeling and role playing with feedback during mock interview sessions. Their program was effective for successfully employing four of the six participating men.

Most employers endorsing affirmative action programs have recognized that standardized tests such as Civil Service examinations systematically discriminate against the hard-core unemployed (Boehm, 1972) and have replaced them with personal interviews in their selection process (National Citizens' Committee for Community Relations, 1967). However, prospective employees must still make a favorable impression in their personal interviews. Since members of the subculture are unfamiliar with the requisite skills for creating a favorable impression (Himes, 1968) training in job interview skills becomes extremely important.

Barbee and Keil (1973) recognized that the hard-core unemployed typically appear passive and unspontaneous in personal interviews and that they generally display poor language skills. These investigators selected 64 trainees, all of whom were involved in job skill-training programs in one of three local manpower agencies. They assigned the trainees to one of three experimental conditions: interview skills training (n = 24), videotape feedback (n = 21), or a test-retest control (n = 19). Subjects in all conditions completed an application form for a position advertised in the newspaper and enacted a 10-minute job interview for that position. Members of the interview skills-training condition subsequently viewed a videotape of their performance and identified, with the aid of a trainer, deficient behaviors in self-presentation. During the remainder of their 30-minute session, they rehearsed more appropriate behaviors with both coaching and feedback from their trainers. Members of the videotape feedback condition merely watched replays of their interview during their 30-minute period; neither instructions nor feedback-coaching were supplied. On post-testing, which was a live enactment of the pre-test interview, members of the skills-training condition showed significant improvements over both videotape feedback and test-retest controls on the dependent variables of rated presentation of self and acceptability as an employee; the control groups were not significantly different.

Azrin, Flores, and Kaplan (1975) employed a systems approach to getting a job and provided training in all aspects involved in locating employment. They worked with a group of 120 persons comprised of individual's responding to a newspaper notice about the program as well as individuals referred by the state employment agency or personnel departments in several local firms. All participants wanted full-time employment, were not currently employed full-time, and were not receiving unemployment compensation; their mean age was 25.5, mean months of employment during the past year was 5.5, and mean years of education was 14. While the characteristics of this sample are clearly different than those of the hard-core unemployed, the procedure is applicable to the target problem.

Subjects were matched on an index of probable employability made up of age, sex, race, education, marital status, desired position and salary level, number of dependents, and current financial resources; members of each matched pair were randomly assigned to either a counseling or a control condition. Counseling consisted of daily group meetings designed to make job seeking a group rather than an individual concern. The program was multifaceted and included strategies for identifying job leads, pursuing job leads, and successfully conducting interviews. Participants continued attending meetings until they were employed. Results from the study indicated significant effects: the median number of days preceding employment was 14 for members of the counseling group as compared with 53 for persons in the control condition; after three months, 92% of the counseling subjects were employed as compared with 60% of the controls.

Rosen and Turner (1971), directing their attention toward maintaining employment following selection, investigated the relative effectiveness of two job orientation programs with the hard-core unemployed. They selected 49 black men from welfare roles, day-labor lines, and supportive community agencies, assigned them to low-skill jobs in a cooperating industry, and exposed them to one of two experimental conditions. The first condition was a university-affiliated quasi-therapy group led by a white clinical psychologist. The second was a company job-oriented group led by the industry's personnel director. Both groups met 14 times over a period of 12 weeks. The content of the quasi-therapy group was fairly traditional with discussions focusing on feelings and personal concerns. The content of the job-oriented group included job-related information and discussions of individual and shared job problems. While Rosen and Turner's (1971) results on their dependent variables of absenteeism, turnover, and supervisory ratings at 6 months were not unequivocal, the pattern suggested general effectiveness for both programs with the job-oriented sessions showing superiority over the quasi-therapy condition. On supervisory ratings, persons exposed to the company group were scored above those in the university group, although the difference was not significant. On turnover, the rates of the hard-core unemployed were not different than those of other workers in the company; although the university group's turnover was significantly higher than either the company group or the company's ordinary turnover baserate. Absences with the hard-core unemployed were significantly higher than the company's baserate with non-hard-core workers; however, absences for members of the company group of hard-core unemployed were significantly lower than absences for the university group members. The authors conclude from their results that "if hard-core unemployed are given extensive orientation training, particularly if such training is job oriented in content and directed by company personnel, and if company standards regarding absenteeism are loosened during the early employment period, the hard core will turn out to be as stable a work force as men hired via normal hiring channels" (Rosen & Turner, 1971, p. 300).

V. E. O'Leary (1972), also interested in employment maintenance following selection, investigated the effectiveness of orientation training in job problem solving with the hard-core unemployed. She studied 72 black women meeting Manpower criteria who had been hired by a major Midwestern utility firm. All of the women had completed an 8-week skill-training program in basic education and occupational training prior to their inclusion in the study. O'Leary assigned half of the women to her active treatment condition consisting of twelve weekly, 1-hour group meetings; the remainder of the women served as test-retest controls. During initial group meetings, participants role-played solutions to job problem situations anticipated on the basis of pre-employment interviews; during later meetings, role-played situations were based on actual problems encountered on the job. O'Leary's (1972) dependent variables were turnover and a variety of self-report measures. Her general results were not especially encouraging: orientation training apparently had no effect on reducing turnover. Because of her care in locating all of her sample at post-testing, however, her across-condition comparisons between those who maintained employment and those who terminated provided valuable data. She found two differences of special importance. First, those women who reported greater increments in self-concept, as measured by pre-post changes in semantic differential ratings, were the women most likely to terminate employment. O'Leary (1972) interprets this finding as indicating that greater appreciation of self reduced the perceived attractiveness of the low-paying, repetitious job the women had been assigned. Her second finding was equally important: at post-testing, her subjects were asked to report whom they had consulted most frequently when troubled by a problem at work. Across conditions, women who continued employment were significantly more likely to report talking with their supervisors; women who terminated were significantly more likely to report talking with their familes or friends.

Friedlander and Greenberg (1971) obtained data in support of conclusions dovetailing with O'Leary's (1972) second finding. Like O'Leary (1972) and Rosen and Turner (1971), these investigators were interested in the effects of programmatic interventions on job maintenance with the hard core unemployed. They studied the effects of a Manpower training and Development program on nearly 500 persons selected in accord with Manpower program criteria. The program package was similar to that employed in most Manpower centers and included individual and group training in human relations, job orientation, money management, grooming and personal hygiene, and use of mass transit. The characteristic distinguishing this study from earlier ones evaluating Manpower programs was the inclusion of dependent variables related to the work environment itself; earlier studies had monitored only characteristics of the workers or the training programs (Goodman et al., 1973).

Friedlander and Greenberg (1971) collected a massive amount of data. In addition to demographic variables, trainee characteristics such as attitudes toward work and attitudes toward unemployment were assessed at three points:

prior to training, prior to employment, and 3 months following placement. Work environment dimensions (including new worker treatment, peer support, and supervisor support) were assessed 3 months following placement. Program effectiveness criteria of job retention, work effectiveness (based on supervisor ratings of competence, congeniality, effort, and reliability), and work behavior (based on supervisor ratings of smartness, friendliness, and conscientiousness) were also measured 3 months following placement.

A number of results emerged. Neither demographic variables nor attitudes toward work were related to any of the effectiveness criteria. Moreover the training program itself had no demonstrable behavioral or attitudinal effects. While on most dimensions supervisor ratings for the hard-core unemployed were about the mean of their ratings for all company employees, these ratings were either unrelated or inversely related to job retention. The most revealing finding was that the most reliable predictor of both work effectiveness and job retention was the trainee's rating of his work climate supportiveness; without exception, the trainee perceived his work climate as dramatically less supportive than did his supervisor.

Friedlander and Greenberg (1971) concluded that the social structure of work organizations is strongly related to and in some instances actually causes the problem of continued unemployment. In supportive work climates, trainees feel encouraged to consult with their supervisors and are more likely to both remain on the job and perform well while there, a conclusion similar to O'Leary's (1972) result. In nonsupportive climates, workers react either by increasing their frequency of lateness or absences or they quit.

This conclusion is of paramount importance. It suggests that neither characteristics of the worker, such as attitudes toward work, nor characteristics of training programs are as central to maintaining employment following placement as are characteristics of the work environment itself. A variety of laboratory studies suggest that for the black worker, especially if that black worker is a woman (MacDonald, 1974b; Reid, 1975), the typical work climate is generally one fostering failure and encouraging retreat. Katz and Cohen (1962) found that white peers consistently criticize the performance of black partners, even when their performance level is equivalent to that of their white critics. Katz, Goldston, and Benjamin (1958, studying biracial work teams, found that whites dominate all conversations and that both whites and blacks direct most of their conversations toward white workers. More recently, Richards and Jaffee (1972) found evidence for racial bias in peer ratings and concluded, on the basis of objective criteria, that "white subordinates behave differently when supervised by blacks, and that some of these behaviors impeded the effectiveness of the black supervisors" (p. 240). When blacks are supervised by whites, the supportiveness of the supervisory relationship is a critical factor (Beatty, 1974; L. M. Davidson, 1973; Triandis & Malpass, 1971); data suggest, however, that these relationships are typically nonsupportive (Morgan, Blonsky, & Rosen,

1970).

In light of these findings, it is not surprising that nearly half of the 400,000 hard-core unemployed recruited between 1968 and 1972 by the National Alliance of Businessmen quit their jobs during the first 6 months of employment (Goodale, 1973). Moreover, the observation that the average black in industry is more concerned with injustices being perpetrated against him than the average white (Slocum & Strawser, 1972) becomes a comment about environments rather than individuals.

Manpower programs, then, are not enough. Their aims of identifying the hard-core unemployed and locating job opportunities are necessary; in and of themselves, however, they are not sufficient. Structural changes on a variety of levels are necessary to address the real issues of chronic unemployment.

On the national level, macroeconomic strategies must be revised to reduce our economy's dependency on unemployment as a tactic for controlling inflation (Ferguson, 1971). The unemployment compensation system should be restructured to avoid encouraging high rates of unemployment (Feldstein, 1973). Manpower location, training, and placement programs must be continued despite our present general economic distress as remedies for structural unemployment, but the content of the training programs should be altered to include system negotiation skills (Magnum & Robson, 1973) and placement should focus more on matching individuals with desirable jobs (Schoenfeldt, 1974). Moreover, programs should be expanded to include job problem counseling, job skill coaching, and requisite supportive services following placement (Magnum & Robson, 1973).

At the industrial level, the recent reawakening of interest in humanizing the work social climate (Argyle, 1972; Robens, 1970; Tchobanian, 1975) should be encouraged. While this trend is important for all workers, it is especially important for maintaining employment with the hard-core unemployed; consequently, special attention should be afforded to their needs. Supervisors should be trained in supportive skills and job problem counseling (Orr, 1973; *Report of the National Advisory Commission on Civil Disorders*, 1968). Merit raise systems awarded on the basis of objective criteria and more open transfers should be provided (Hulin, 1968). Environmental design programs, effective for maintaining worker satisfaction as well as productivity, should be explored and developed (cf. Adam, 1972; Pedalino & Gamboa, 1974; Sielaft, 1974).

At this point, psychology's contribution to the plight of the unemployed has been virtually nonexistent. The failure of the profession to offer solutions may have been due, more than anything else, to a prior lack of understanding of the work climate impact on perpetuating unemployment and the only recent professional shift toward seriously attending to environmental variables (Krasner & Ullmann, 1973). Whatever the reasons, however, psychology is now in a position to develop programs that accomplish two ends: maintaining industrial production at a profitable level and effectively incorporating the hard-core unemployed into the labor force.

Chapter 11
ENVIRONMENTAL PROBLEMS

Population growth . . . environmental degradation . . . and human relations crises . . . face man today. He must solve these problems if he is to survive in a livable environment. He must also find ways of aiding society to adopt the solutions found. Such problem-solving action requires basic social change. The underlying challenge to society is to create the changes needed to solve survival problems as they occur. If man is to survive, he must find mechanisms for creating the needed changes in his living patterns, in his interpersonal relationships and his social institutions. (Fairweather, 1972, p. 1)

The research topics of this chapter include litter control, recycling, energy conservation, transportation, architectural design, and population change. Fairweather's introductory quote emphasized the urgency of finding solutions to these problems and also accentuated the somewhat ironic but increasingly recognized view that the amelioration of conditions which degrade the environment may have more to do with maintaining and improving the quality of our life and "mental health" than much of the current work conducted under the rubric of mental health. These topics are clearly distinct from the more typical concerns of most psychologists and reflect a broadening of behavior modification and psychology that is a major theme of the current volume.

This chapter has been limited largely to the recent behavior modification literature. A number of factors influenced this final structure. First, the environmental movement in psychology and related disciplines is burgeoning, and at least two comprehensive environmental psychology texts (Ittelson et al., 1974; Proshansky, Ittelson, & Rivlin, 1970) review nonbehavioral approaches. Second, environmental research from an applied behavioral perspective is recent and relatively circumscribed thereby allowing a complete review of it. Third, the "open field" methodology typical of many of the reviewed studies is an especially appropriate model for the investigation and remediation of environmental problems at a community level (the explicit, eventual goal of most of these studies). While this methodology is not without its problems, its integration of empiricism with a responsible activism is an identifying ingredient of behavioral community psychology.

The behavior analytic approach is quite different from other research strategies used more prevalently in environmental psychology. For example, Hayes and Cone (in press,a) have suggested that:

> The dominant orientation of the environmental literature . . . can best be termed "reactive" . . . This approach is characterized by (a) a concern with either the reactions to a given environmental situation (e.g. attitudes or out migration as a function of pollution density) or with variables and behavior relevant to the situation, (b) a concern with "understanding" the situation as it exists, and not in demonstrating understanding by control of behavior in the situation, (c) a high degree of reliance on intervening variables and hypothetical constructs, and (d) a general lack of applied experimental work, relying instead on observation, theoretical and correlational approaches.
>
> Ironically, research from a reactive orientation on environmentally destructive behaviors can only continue so long as the destructive behaviors themselves continue. Sole reliance on reactively oriented research could lead to the anomalous effect of inadvertently contributing to the continuation of environmental degradation . . .
>
> . . . research from an applied behavior analytic orientation . . . in the study of man/environment relations . . . seeks to determine how environmentally relevant behaviors, both protective and destructive, are initiated, maintained, or altered. (p. 1)*

While these comments suggest the advantages of the behavioral approach, the framework of this chapter also emphasizes diversified methodologies and conceptualizations. In environmental protection, a new and growing field, the goal should not be isolation—i.e., the development of "schools" (Kazdin, 1975b)—but rather the cross fertilization of multiple perspectives. Therefore, this chapter's selective focus on behavioral work should not be construed as a rejection of other methods. Our intention is to document the view that behavioral principles and the process of behavioral analysis can make a unique and important contribution to the understanding and solution of environmental problems, particularly when combined with prior and concomitant data from other methods (e.g., surveys on consumer preferences) (Nietzel & Winett, in press) and other disciplines (e.g., economics, engineering, architecture, urban planning, and political science).

---

*Hayes, S. C. and Cone, J. D. Reducing residential electrical energy use: Payments information and feedback. *Journal of Applied Behavior Analysis*, in press.

Littering

Littering has received the most attention of the environmentally related problems. This is probably because in comparison to energy conservation, transportation, and recycling, litter control is less controversial and involves a more discrete set of behaviors and solutions. The quantity of work can be attributed to the pioneering efforts of a group at the University of Washington, which stimulated much of the subsequent research. Studies of litter reduction generally have focused on antecedents that deter littering or consequences that promote litter removal.

Antecedents

Studies that have focused on the prevention of littering by investigating antecedent events are less well known than studies that have reinforced litter removal.[1] While the results are not as powerful as those from litter removal studies, the procedures investigated are inexpensive and require limited person power or surveillance.

Marler (1970) gave campers entering a National Forest leaflets that emphasized either the fact that litter removal could prevent injuries or that litter could cause injuries to them. A "neutral" leaflet only stated possible dangers from littering. Ratings of campsite cleanliness indicated that the leaflet stressing potential personal injury was the most effective of the leaflets. However, the data reveals that about 40% of the campers never read the leaflets and that control (no leaflet) campers answered more questions correctly on a quiz about littering than campers in the leaflet conditions. These data render the findings concerning the effectiveness of one of the leaflets questionable and suggest that messages and prompts must be delivered in forms that are readily discernible and communicative.

Dodge (1972) described a saturation campaign of personal pleas, posters, bumper stickers, pamphlets, and newspaper anti-litter notes. Data monitored in an Alaskan National Forest campsite showed that compared to pre-campaign conditions less litter was left at campsites, fewer campers littered the sites, and more campers actually cleaned their sites.

Finnie (1973) investigated the effects of a clean or littered environment, attractive trash cans, and extra trash cans on littering behavior. In one study, using a 2 X 2 design, extra litter cans or no litter cans were available in environments judged to be clean or dirty. The dependent measure was the proportion of persons who purchased hot dogs and littered the wrapper compared to the number of persons purchasing hot dogs. Not surprising, the least littering occurred in the clean environment with extra cans, and the most littering was observed in the dirty environment with no cans. Regardless of the

---

.[1]The authors are indebted to E. Scott Geller for bringing these studies to our attention.

number of cans, less littering occurred in the clean environment. It was also demonstrated that persons under 18 years of age littered more than older persons.

In another study, Finnie found that attractive cans which displayed the names of companies sponsoring a "Clean City Squares" project reduced the amount of litter on city blocks relative to blocks with regular cans or with no cans. The efficacy of these conditions, however, was not substantial, averaging only 3% litter reduction for the regular cans and 15% for the clean city cans.

In a third study, Finnie tried to reduce littering by placing trash cans along a highway with warning signs located one-quarter mile before the cans. This procedure was compared to a condition where cans were placed along the highway without signs, and a control condition with neither signs nor cans. Three highways were used in this 3-month study, with conditions rotated on each highway every month. The dependent measure consisted of monthly counts of litter in specified areas on the highway. It was found that litter cans with or without the signs reduced the amount of collected litter by approximately 29%.

A final study, performed on two 16-block sidewalk sections, involved the placement of trash cans on every block or every fourth block. There was also a no-trash-can control condition. A small reduction in littering was found with trash cans placed on every fourth block; a 17% reduction was observed for the "one can per block" condition. Apparently, if trash receptacles are readily available, at least some people will use them thereby producing a cleaner environment.

Geller (1973), working in six different settings (a college classroom, a college snack bar, the lobby of an academic building, a grocery store, and two movie theaters), varied written prompt conditions on soft drink cups, handbills, and flyers. "General" prompts usually told the person to dispose of litter properly, while "specific" prompts gave a particular location for litter disposal. Across the different settings, it was found that compared to no prompts, general prompts increased proper litter disposal; compared to specific prompts, the general condition resulted in less properly disposed litter. Tuso, Witmer, and Geller (1975) also discovered that a clean compared to a littered grocery store tended to decrease littering in the store, a finding consistent with Finnie (1973). (Additional work by Geller and his associates on the use of prompts for litter control is found in the section on recycling.)

In summary, increasing the number or attractiveness of trash cans, cleaning the environment, or prompting various disposal responses are antecedent manipulations which are moderately effective and practical in instigating litter reductions.

Positive Consequences

Studies that have reinforced litter removal are traceable to Burgess, Clark, and Hendee's (1974) classic report which sought to establish the use of positive incentives as an alternative litter control strategy to such apparently ineffective procedures as legal threats, attempts at attitude change, or discovery of a "litterbug personality." This study involved children who attended matinees at two theaters. Following the matinee, litter deposited in trash cans and litter dropped on the floor and deposited by usherettes into containers were weighed. The dependent measure was the percent of total litter in the theater that was deposited by the audience. The design involved introducing different experimental procedures for different matinee performances; baseline conditions were included also. Experimental conditions included doubling the number of trash cans in the theater, presenting an anti-litter film prior to the regular film, providing litter bags to each person entering the theater, providing litter bags plus instructions at intermission to put trash in the litter bags and place the bags in trash cans, giving litter bags plus instructions that returning a bag of litter to the lobby would result in a 10-cent prize, and providing each person with litter bags along with periodic announcements that a free ticket to a special movie would be given to each person returning a bag of litter.

The data indicated that during baseline conditions about 21% of the litter was returned by the audience; with extra trash cans, 16% of the litter was returned; the litter film resulted in 21% returned; litter bags alone produced a return of 31%; litter bags plus instructions yielded 57%; and litter bags plus 10 cents and litter bags plus a movie ticket resulted in 94% and 95% of the litter being returned by the audience. Clearly, the procedures providing immediate incentives and prompts for pro-environmental behaviors were much more effective than procedures which varied antecedents (e.g., films, extra trash cans, litter bags). Another indication of the magnitude of effect associated with incentive conditions was that the ratio of trash in the cans to that on the floor was 1:5 during baseline conditions, while the ratio was 19:1 during incentive conditions.

Clark, Burgess, and Hendee (1972) extended this work to a national forest campground that covered about 100 acres and attracted about 1,000 visitors at a time. In addition to its relevance for litter control, this study also provided a demonstration that behavioral procedures can work in open as opposed to circumscribed settings. The dependent variable was the number of pieces of planted litter found in the campground. Planted litter included deposit and nondeposit bottles, paper bags, and beverage cans. Before each of two mid-summer weekends, 169 pieces of litter were planted, thus creating a constant amount of litter. The location of each piece of planted litter was marked on a map which allowed later identification by observers. Thus, it was possible to see how much and what kind of litter was picked up at any given time. The intervention procedure is described below:

At 10:00 a.m. Saturday morning of the second weekend, one member of the research staff in a Forest Service uniform contacted seven families. The parents were informed that there was a litter problem in the campground, and they were asked if their children would be willing to help. The children were told that if they could help they could choose one of the following items: a Smokey Bear shoulder patch, a Junior Forest Ranger badge, a Smokey Bear comic book, a wooden ruler, a Keep Washington Green pin, or a small box of Chiclets gum. Each child was then given a large 30-gallon plastic bag and told in which general areas to look for litter . . . No specific amount of litter was required. They were informed that they had all day for the project and that the Rangers would be back at 7:00 p.m. to pick up their bags and to give them their reward. This was the only contact made with the participants until that evening. Their efforts were not monitored nor were they encouraged at any time to do a better job or to look in any specific area. (Clark et al., 1972, p. 3)*

The results of the study showed that for the first weekend (no treatment), the litter count was 160 on Thursday, 143 on Friday, 87 on Saturday, 63 on Sunday, and 56 on Monday. For weekend two, the Thursday litter count was 160, Friday 145, Saturday (when the procedure was put into effect) 24, and during the next two days 18 of the remaining 24 pieces were picked up. All four types of planted litter were picked up in about equal amounts during the incentive period, although bags and cans were unlikely to be picked up during baseline or incentive conditions. In addition, nonplanted, natural litter appeared to increase during both weekends, except for a temporary decline on the Saturday the incentive procedure was in effect. In all, about 150 to 200 pounds of litter were collected by the children in exchange for 21 Smokey Bear patches, four Junior Forest Ranger badges, and one Smokey Bear Fight Forest Fires pin. The incentives cost $3.00 and two hours were needed to set up the incentive procedures. If campground personnel would have had to pick up the litter, the cost would have been $50 to $60 for 16 to 20 hours of work.

It should be noted here in response to criticisms that such incentive procedures are "contrived," "unnatural," or "dehumanizing," that deposit bottles with a natural incentive value were picked up regardless of experimental conditions. Deposits could be placed on a variety of containers and bottles to promote their return, reduce littering, and aid the recycling of materials.

This procedure has become law in Oregon where nonreturnable beverage containers are no longer in use. Attempts to institute similar procedures in other states have been met by considerable opposition from the container industry and unions who argue that such laws would result in the loss of thousands of jobs. Environmentalists, however, counter this position by suggesting that losses in manufacturing jobs would be offset by new jobs created to transport and handle

---

*Clark, R. N. Burgess, R. V., and Hendee, J. C. The development of antilitter behavior in a forest campground. *Journal of Applied Behavior Analysis*, 1972, *5*, 1-5.

returnable containers, a position which is supported by data from a study by the Oregon State University School of Business and Technology (*The Courier-Journal*, 1975b). The deposit law in Oregon resulted in the loss of 350 production jobs, and the creation of 140 truck driving and 575 warehouse and handling jobs, or a net gain of 365 jobs. In addition, such legislation on recycling would undoubtedly save energy since the recycling process would require less energy than producing more throwaways. However, recycling bills have been defeated in many state legislatures. This state of affairs is an important reminder that demonstrating that a procedure works in one setting is merely a first step in having the procedure widely implemented (Fairweather et al., 1974; Winett, 1976a).

Kohlenberg and Phillips (1973) extended the technology developed in the previous two studies by examining the effects of a variable-ratio reinforcement schedule on litter disposal and the aesthetic appearance of an experimental area over one 8-week summer period (for 8 hours each day, 12:00 p.m. to 8:00 p.m.). The study was conducted at the Woodland Park Zoo in Seattle, a free admission zoo that attracts people of widely differing ages and socioeconomic backgrounds. A single trash receptacle located in the central portion of the zoo, an area having a good deal of ground litter, was selected as the experimental site. Litter deposits into the trash receptacle were recorded individually but were counted as a litter deposit only if a person deposited all the litter he or she was carrying. In addition, a person could not take litter out of other receptacles to deposit it in the designated one. Two sets of photographs of the experimental area were taken during the last 4 weeks of the study.

Four experimental conditions, each 2 weeks in duration, were included: (1) a baseline period, (2) a reinforcement period in which a progressively "thinned" (first VR 10, 7; later VR 20) variable ratio system was implemented and accompanied by a sign which announced the reinforcement contingengies (those receiving a coupon for litter disposal could redeem it for a Pepsi), (3) a modified baseline in which the sign was still present but no contingencies were in effect, and (4) a final reinforcement period using a VR 10 schedule.

The data showed that 4,577 and 6,032 litter deposits were made during the first and second reinforcement periods, with 723 and 2,403 litter deposits made during the first and second baselines. Two sets of slides depicting the experimental area were judged by five volunteers who indicated that for one set of the slides less litter was visible under reinforcement than baseline conditions, while for the other set of slides equal amounts of litter were perceived under reinforcement and baseline conditions. Additional analyses showed that when the litter deposit data were adjusted for sky conditions, temperature, and an estimate of total attendance, the original relationships still held. An analysis of the approximate age of the depositers indicated that from the second baseline to the second reinforcement condition the percentage of persons over 20 years old sharply decreased (34% to 7%), while the percentage for persons ages 10 to 20 years increased (16% to 44%). For both conditions, children under 10 years of age constituted about 50% of the depositers. Thus, either the Pepsi reinforcer or this particular approach to litter control might be effective only with children. The rate of litter depositing also sharply declined during the last hour to hour and one-half, indicating that the benefits of the program could have been maintained, but its costs reduced, if it were curtailed earlier in the day. In addition, while the design of the study did not provide a complete answer to the question of the relative effectiveness of VR 10 or 20 schedules, the data do suggest that if cost is a major concern a VR 20 schedule might result in litter being frequently deposited at less cost than a richer schedule.

Powers, Osborne, and Anderson (1973) also sought to establish litter control that would be effective in a large, natural setting, over a long period of time, yet would not require personal (and expensive) contact between the public and sanitation personnel. This study was conducted during a 21-week period (July to November; April to May) in Green Canyon, an undeveloped recreational area with little supervisory surveillance. The apparatus used for the study was three litter stations each containing two large deposit cans. The stations also contained large bags with attached data card that requested the person's name, address, telephone number, age, sex, and whether the person wanted 25 cents or a chance to win $20 (see below). A person was to fill the litter bag to a designated line, place the bag in the litter bin, and put the completed data card in an attached card container.

Baseline conditions were in effect for 2-week periods alternated with 3-week experimental conditions. In the latter case, a person filling a litter bag and completing the data card could choose between immediately being sent 25 cents or taking a chance in a weekly $20 lottery.

Of the 88 people submitting data cards, 56 were completed during the experimental conditions. Most of the respondents were male students between the ages of 11 and 25. Of the 187 bags (1,658 pounds) of litter picked up during the 21 weeks, 129 (74%) were picked up under the experimental conditions. Experimental conditions were particularly effective when first introduced (August) and when reintroduced (April and May). Ground surveys of paper and metal litter conducted during the last 6 weeks of the study showed litter reductions correlated with the experimental conditions. Seventy-three percent (101 bags) of the respondents turned in a data card for a chance in the lottery; 10 lottery checks (total of $200 were awarded during the experimental conditions; 24% (34 bags) were turned in for the 25 cents, and 3% (four bags) of the respondents indicated that they did not want any payment.

This study demonstrated that incentive procedures can promote litter removal by adults in an unsupervised area over extended time periods. It also showed that most adults would opt for a chance in a lottery, a procedure which was fairly simple to administer, required contact with only the winners, and offered a prize capable of motivating litter removal. However, on the average over 1,000 people visited the canyon, indicating that only a very small proportion (.004) of these visitors picked up litter. Further studies are needed to evaluate procedures that induce more people to pick up litter in relatively unsupervised areas.

Chapman and Risley (1974) compared the effectiveness of using incentives for picking up litter versus incentives for maintenance of a clean environment. The participants in this study were 132 children who resided in the Juniper Gardens Housing Project in Kansas City; all children were black, with an age range of 4 to 13 years. The project contained about 390 low-income and welfare families; about 1,000 children lived in the project. Target settings included residential yards, public yards, streets, and sidewalks. For purposes of this research, a piece of litter was defined as plastic, rubber, fabric, leather, paper, wood, glass, metal, food, or food by-products measuring two or more inches in diameter. The amount of litter in the study sites was observed and recorded daily. Additional daily measures included the number of children participating in litter collection and the weight of the litter collected. The study was conducted over a 5-month period with five separate conditions using a replication design.

In the *verbal-appeal condition*, a large litter basket was placed at the corner of a sidewalk near the project's community center. After a bell rang indicating the end of school for that day, an experimenter would approach the children and ask them if they wanted to help clean up litter in the area. This condition lasted for 30 minutes per day for 14 days. Observers also recorded the number of children receiving litter baskets and the number of children depositing litter in the baskets.

In the *payment-for-volume condition* (15 days), an experimenter approached the children and indicated that they would be paid 10 cents for returning a filled litter bag to a designated area. Unfilled bags or bags containing improper material were not counted, but the child was instructed to refill the bag.

The *no-payment condition* was in effect for 30 days followed by the payment-for-volume condition for 7 days, a no-payment condition for 11 days, and a return to a full-day payment-for-volume condition for 14 days. For the next 24 days, a *payment-for-clean-yards condition* was instituted. In this condition the experimenter assigned each child one or two yards in the project area. Yards to be cleaned were delegated so that previously cleaned yards were not assigned on a particular day. This procedure was in effect from 10:00 a.m. to 3:00 p.m. A child who cleaned a yard needed to have the experimenter check the yard for cleanliness and return the litter bag to the litter station. Payment was contingent on yard cleanliness. A 10-day no-payment condition followed this procedure.

The results indicated that there was less litter in the yards under the payment-for-volume or payment-for-cleanliness conditions. The verbal appeal and the no-payment conditions were associated with higher levels of litter in the yards. The overall weight of the litter collected was highest in the payment-for-volume condition (an average of 94 pounds per day compared to 28 pounds in the payment-for-cleanliness condition). About 10 children per day participated in litter collection under the verbal-appeal condition, while there were 25 per day in the payment-for-volume condition and 15 per day in the clean–yards condition. In this last condition, new children were frequently involved in litter collection on any given day.

However, in the verbal-appeal and the payment-for-volume conditions, the number of children participating and the amount of litter collected tended to decrease after the procedures had been in effect for a few days. More consistent litter collection and clean yards were observed when the children were paid to clean particular yards. This level of litter approached the level observed in a sample of middle-income yards. The successive assignment of yards also constituted a replication of the payment-for-clean-yards condition. The data indicated that each of the 10 yards showed a decrease in litter with the advent of the procedure.

Although more children participated and more litter (by weight) was collected in the payment-for-volume condition, children in this condition either collected bulkier litter leaving behind smaller pieces or collected garbage from trash containers. When the children were not paid for these inappropriately filled bags, they often dumped the bags' contents in the yards. While the payment-for-clean-yards condition circumvented these problems, it had to be continuously in effect because its ability to promote clean yards was not maintained after its withdrawal. Chapman and Risley (1974) estimated that a half-time maintenance worker recruiting the children and paying them $50 per week would be required to keep all the yards clean in the 15 square-block project. The cost of such an intervention would be less than $1 per housing unit per month.

Hayes, Johnson, and Cone (in press) have described a major weakness in many littering studies: the more trash that is produced or distributed the greater the density of reinforcement delivered. Thus, it is possible that over time the "trash buying" approach can produce an increase in both littering and anti-littering behaviors. Hayes et al. evaluated a procedure to circumvent this problem. In a study conducted at the Robert F. Kennedy Youth Center, a site with a large littering problem, specific litter items were marked surreptitiously by the experimenters. Center residents could earn special privileges or 25 cents for turning in a bag of trash that contained one of the specially marked items. Thus, the collection of marked litter (rather than quantity of litter) was reinforced.

Data from a multiple baseline design showed that the technique yielded litter reduction of about 70% in three specified areas. About one-quarter of the residents participated in the project, and about 70% of the marked items were returned. Residents apparently never were aware of the marked item code. The results indicated that if people curtail littering, the use of this technique will increase their chances for picking up a marked item. However, with the trash-buying procedures, once littering is decreased, the possibility of being reinforced also is decreased. A further advantages of the marked item technique is that small, unsightly pieces of litter will be deposited because even a small piece potentially could be a marked one. Tuso and Geller (1976) have noted, however, that this technique will generally influence those people who do not litter while leaving unaffected those who do. Therefore, it offers only a temporary solution to the litter problem.

Some interesting data on these issues were presented recently by LaHart and Bailey (1974). Working with groups of children in a natural setting, they found that an incentive similar to that of Clark et al. (1972) effectively influenced children to pick up marked litter while instructions, lectures, educational materials and statements about the problems of littering were not effective. However, the statement, lecture, and educational material were effective in reducing littering by the children while incentives had no effect on the amount of litter dropped in this setting. Since only the marked litter had incentive value, there was no consequence for leaving one's own litter. Not depositing litter and cleaning up others' litter may be two quite distinct behaviors with different procedures and explicit contingencies differentially effective with each one (Tuso & Geller, 1976).

The marked item technique might be used eventually on a community basis if surveillance substances and scanning devices (flourescent paint and a black light, isotopes and a gieger counter, etc.) could be used for mass screening of litter. Conceivably, a person disposing of litter in automatic bins could be reinforced immediately with mechanically delivered reinforcers. Problems such as notifying authorities about abandoned cars, pollution violations, or the presence of post-election posters might also use variants of this procedure. In addition, the marked item technique has the advantages of allowing a program administrator to control the upper limit of funding for litter removal projects and to allocate the number of marked items in a particular area in proportion to the importance of litter removal from that area compared to other sites. Unfortunately, the LaHart and Bailey study suggested that persons who are actually littering or violating environmental laws will be effected minimally by this procedure.

Recycling

The ecological imbalance due to the accumulation of nondegradable waste products in the environment is steadily increasing. For example, it was estimated that the average American disposed of a ton of solid waste in 1970, and that this amount per individual should almost double by 1980 . . . However, a large portion of household waste could be reused and thus become a resource rather than a pollutant. Such recycling requires appropriate relocation of particular trash items and therefore makes the consumer the first rather than the last link in the distribution channel. (Geller, Farris, & Post, 1973, p. 367)

Recycling can be conceptualized as a specific, very important aspect of the proper disposal of litter. For example, rather than throwing away soft drink bottles, consumers can be motivated to return them to a recycling plant. Clark et al. (1972) have demonstrated that returnable bottles with their built-in value are returned without any additional incentives. In areas of the country where nonreturnable, nondeposit bottles are still in use, a pro-environmental objective is a determination of how to induce consumers to purchase beverages in returnable bottles.

The seminal work on behavioral control of recycling is attributed to the research of E. Scott Geller and his colleagues at Virginia Polytechnic Institute and State University. Geller, Wylie, and Farris (1971) demonstrated that providing grocery store customers with a circular which urged them to buy drinks in returnable containers followed by social approval contingent on the appropriate purchases resulted in a greater proportion of customers purchasing their drinks in returnable bottles.

Geller et al. (1973) investigated different kinds of prompting procedures in a small grocery store in Blacksburg, Virginia, a community where about half of the residents are students or faculty. Any individual who entered the store and purchased soft drinks was a study participant. A "returnable container" customer was defined as a person who purchased more than half of his/her drinks in returnable containers, while a "nonreturnable" customer purchased more than half in nonreturnable containers. Purchases were observed at the check-out counter.

Using a Latin Square design to control for day and time of day, five prompting procedures were investigated over a 4-week period in which conditions were varied every 2 hours. In the *handbill* condition, patrons received a small poster that urged them to buy soft drinks in returnable bottles because beverages purchased this way were cheaper, fewer taxes would be required to clean up bottles, and recycled containers would help fight pollution. Finally, the handbill contained the statement, "Show concern: help us fight pollution" and indicated that such efforts would be reported in the local newspapers and at the American Psychological Association. Customers who indicated that they had already seen the handbill were not given another one.

In the *pollution chart* condition, handbills were distributed in the same way. However, the circular contained the additional statement that the customer's purchase would be recorded publicly. This was accomplished by using a large chart at the entrance that provided an updated tally of the number of "returnable" or "throwaway" customers. The pollution chart condition was also varied by occasionally surrounding the chart with five observers in an attempt to make the chart more salient and to place additional pressure on customers to buy drinks in recyclable containers. The effect of sex of the prompter or scorekeepers on the purchases of male and female customers was examined.

In this study all prompting conditions resulted in essentially equivalent increases in the proportion of returnable container customers. Approximately 60% purchased returnable containers under nonprompt conditions, while about 75-80% did so under prompt conditions. The addition of the chart and social pressure had no discernible effect over the handbill alone. There were no differential effects associated with the sex of the prompters or customers.

A weakness of this and other studies that do not record the same individual's behavior under varying conditions (i.e., the site becomes the organism) was that it was unclear if a person whose purchases were influenced by prompts tended to maintain this behavior under nonprompt conditions. In this study, because of their frequent visits to the store, many customers experienced several conditions. If generalization did occur, differences between conditions (particularly prompt and nonprompt conditions) might have been underestimated. However, the fact that differences between prompt and nonprompt conditions still did exist suggested that prompting effects might be relatively transient and require continual use to influence behavior. Future experimental analysis of such questions is essential to a more adequate understanding of issues concerning maintenance of behavior change and is of great practical significance in environmental work.

More recent research on prompts and instructions in inducing proper litter disposal and recycling has been conducted by Geller, Witmer, and Orebaugh (in press). In a study performed over a 40-day period from 5:00 to 7:00 p.m. at two large grocery stores, a Latin Square design was used to assess the impact of different instructions on handbill advertisements distributed to customers. Besides a baseline condition, instructions that were investigated included a *general* anti-litter prompt (*Please* don't litter. *Please* dispose of properly), a *specific* anti-litter prompt (*Please* don't litter. *Please* dispose in *green* trash can located at rear of store), a *demand* anti-litter prompt (*You must* not litter, *you must* dispose in *green* trash can located at rear of store), and a *recycle* prompt (*Please* help us *recycle*. Please dispose for *recycling* in *green* trash can located at rear of store).

The effects of the prompts were studied Monday through Friday. On Saturday and Sunday, two prompts were investigated that were designed to have customers avoid depositing handbills in shopping carts. One prompt designated a *specific alternative response* (*Please don't* dispose of in carts. Please dispose in *green* trash can located at rear of store) while the other designated a *general alternative* (*Please* don't dispose of in carts. *Please* dispose of properly.). Also, during the seventh week of the project, the effects of a pro-litter prompt (*Please* litter. Dispose of on *floor*) were studied.

For both stores, the "demand," "specific," and "recycle" prompts led to about four to five times the number of properly disposed handbills associated with the general prompt or baseline conditions. The effects of even the most potent prompts were rather limited; only 15-30% of the distributed handbills were disposed of correctly. An almost equal proportion of handbills was still left in the carts under demand, specific, and recycle prompt conditions. In general a large proportion of handbills was taken from the store regardless of prompt condition. A specific prompt for not disposing of the handbill in the cart was more effective than other prompt conditions in reducing the proportion of handbills left in the carts. In addition, the general prompt was as effective as the other prompts in decreasing the proportion of handbills left on shelves, counters, and tables in one of the stores. The pro-litter prompts generally influenced people to litter more than during other conditions.

The results of this study and a systematic replication (Geller, 1975) suggested that people tended to follow the specific instructions on the handbill even when told to litter. Geller et al. (in press) concluded that this "acquiescence phenomenon" could be used on a large scale to develop specific antipollution instructions that may set the occasion for littering. However, a remaining problem is the fact that the proportion of customers responding to such prompts was quite low (about 20%). In addition, since many customers experienced several prompt conditions but generalization was not readily apparent, the effects of prompts were probably quite transient. Prompts do appear to be simple, inexpensive interventions that can be implemented on a wide basis and result in at least minimum behavior change.

Geller, Chaffee, and Ingram (1975) and Witmer and Geller (1976) have investigated prompting and reinforcement conditions that promote recycling behaviors by motivating consumers to bring reusable waste to a recycling center. The study was conducted on the campus of Virginia Polytechnic Institute and State University and the participants were the residents of six campus dormitories. Three pairs of dorms, matched for sex of residents, designated a room as a paper collection center where students were to bring paper. Returned paper was collected by an ecologically concerned student group that sold the paper to industry for $15 a ton. For 4 months preceding the study and during the 6 weeks that the study was conducted, large posters on dormitory bulletin boards made a general appeal to recycle paper and specified the location of the dorm's recycling room.

Three different experimental conditions each lasting 2 weeks were used in each dorm following a Latin Square design. These conditions were: (1) a baseline identical to pre-study conditions except for the presence of data recorders in the recycling center; (2) a contest between men's and women's dorms with the dorm handing in the most paper receiving $15 (contest rules were announced on posters located next to the regular recycling posters); (3) a raffle in which each student bringing at least one 8½ x 11 sheet of paper or cardboard to the room received a ticket making him/her eligible for one of four prizes donated by local merchants; the raffle was also advertised with extra posters. The dependent variables were the number of visits to the recycling center and the size of the material brought to the room.

More paper was delivered to the recycling center at the monitored times under the contest and raffle conditions than during the baseline conditions. The total pounds delivered during the 6 weeks of the project was 845 for baseline, 1,420 for the contest, and 1,515 during the raffle condition. Generally more paper was brought to the room during the second week of the raffle or contest conditions; also more paper was delivered when more expensive raffle prizes were available. As might be expected, less paper by weight per visit was brought to the recycling room during the raffle condition because this condition resulted in more repeat visits by the same individual handing in a minimum amount of paper. A specific weight requirement for a raffle was introduced at a later time.

Unfortunately, only a small proportion of the dorm residents participated in this project under any of the experimental conditions. Geller et al. (1975), noting that participation increased during the second week of the raffle and contest conditions, attributed the low participation level to the limited awareness of the project rather than the ineffectiveness of the procedures. Whether more prompting coupled with similar reinforcement techniques could increase participation and hence amount of recycled paper was assessed in a subsequent study.

A systematic replication of this research was provided by Witmer and Geller (1976). Major changes from the initial study included a more thorough prompt condition in which flyers detailing experimental conditions were placed under the door of every room in experimental dorms and a revised raffle condition involving more prizes and the stipulation that one pound of paper needed to be returned to receive one raffle ticket. While the prompt condition led to only small increases in returned paper, the contest contingency and particularly the revised raffle condition were effective in promoting more paper recycling. The revised raffle condition lessened the number of repeat visits and led to greater volume of recycled paper than that observed in the earlier Geller et al. study (1975).

However, participation was still limited to fewer than 15% of the dorm residents. The prompt condition used in this study nullifies the previous hypotheses concerning lack of awareness of the contingencies and suggests the ineffectiveness of the present contingencies for most of the dorm residents. However, Geller's other work suggested that prompts may influence effectively more convenient behaviors such as buying drinks in recyclable rather than throwaway containers. This observation is consistent with the discovery that close proximity of a resident's room to the recycling center was associated with higher paper delivery levels (Witmer & Geller, 1976). Perhaps more recycling centers could be used that reinforce automatically the return of specified amounts of paper thereby enhancing the convenience of such ecological behaviors.

Some excellent studies in this area have been provided by Bailey and his associates (Luyben & Bailey, 1975; Reid, Luyben, Rawers, & Bailey, 1976). Working in apartment complexes, Reid et al. demonstrated that personal prompts (delivered as part of door-to-door interviews) and the placement of two additional containers resulted in the placement of 50-100% more newspapers in designated containers than a baseline condition in which only one container was available. Luyben and Bailey (1975), in a study conducted in mobile home parks, compared a simple *reward* procedure to a *proximity* condition. In both conditions, flyers announcing the conditions were placed at each residence. In the reward system, children who turned in newspapers at a designated time and location could choose a toy whose value varied on the amount of newspaper returned. In the proximity condition, seven containers in which newspapers could be recycled were placed in the park.

Each procedure had its advantages and disadvantages. The reward system was more effective than the proximity condition only when the mobile park had a large number of older children who could solicit customers and carry more newspapers. The reward procedure cost more to operate, but the initial expense was limited to the cost of one container. In addition, only one stop was required by persons picking up the newspapers. The proximity program was cheaper but required seven stops, and the seven containers reduced the aesthetic quality of the environment. Luyben and Bailey suggested that the proximity procedure might work in a retirement community while the reward system might be ideal for neighborhoods with many children in the 7-12 year range.

The work by Bailey's group is significant in several other respects. Luyben and Bailey (1975) recorded costs, person-hours, and miles traveled to implement the procedures. The researchers acknowledged that the eventual adaptability of their procedures is very dependent on these factors as well as the market value of recycled newspaper which in turn is dependent on the overall economic and political climate. Their work is also a good illustration of behavioral techniques and methodology applied to the actual change of neighborhood environments and resident behaviors.

The continued work of Geller's and Bailey's groups suggests that a personal or more dense system of prompts, prompts combined with other procedures, close proximity of recycling areas, and simple reward systems are effective methods to promote recycling. These studies also demonstrated that such programs could be implemented in communities with a minimum of personnel. Finances for such programs can come from the sale of recycled material to industry or local merchants' economic support of environmental projects in return for "good will" or the association of their names with a worthwhile program. Lottery procedures (Powers et al., 1973) or a differentiated raffle procedure based on amount of material delivered might also be instituted to attract more participants.

Geller et al. (1975) predicted that:

community merchants would willingly donate raffle prizes, and the local newspapers would not only print free advertisements of the program contingencies but also publish the names and pictures of both donators and winners of raffle prizes. Thus, with the availability of community support (following tactful solicitation) and model techniques for modifying ecology-related behaviors on large scales . . . , the most challenging feature of the urgent task to implement community programs for increasing the frequency of ecology-improving behaviors becomes one of prompting and reinforcing the necessary personnel to develop, maintain, evaluate and refine such programs. (p. 55)

The research on littering and recycling has focused on procedures that are simple, inexpensive, and can be applied on neighborhood and community levels. Their successful dissemination, as suggested by Geller et al. (1975) and Luyben and Bailey (1975) will depend on both economic considerations and the skillful use of the media to promote such programs. The next step likely will involve the development of more powerful reinforcers and the demonstration that a large-scale environmental protection program can be implemented and supported by communities.

Energy

Because the problems of energy conservation have received extensive media coverage in recent years, an elaborate review of this particular sociopolitical history seems unnecessary. There are, however, several issues that are extremely important to the present discussion.

While the causes of the energy crisis at the "macro-level" include the international economic situation, changes in the balance of trade and power, and the depletion of our energy sources, energy conservation policies such as differential prices (*The Courier Journal*, 1975b), peak pricing (Associated Press, 1975), special meters (*The Courier Journal*, 1975c), and rebates or low prices for "good" customers and high prices for "bad" customers (*The Courier Journal*, 1975c) ultimately must have the predicted effect on human behavior (the "micro level") if such approaches are to be successful. Both the design and evaluation of such proposals are clearly within the province of psychologists in collaboration with economists, planners, and government officials. Behavioral approaches to energy conservation also illustrate the desirability of specifying target behaviors and contingencies as an alternative to less precise conceptualizations and methodologies. In this regard, a coupling of the precision of behavior analysis and the perspective of community psychology can be found in efforts to disseminate findings from demonstration energy studies.

Presently there are five behavioral studies that have tried to change either the magnitude or pattern of energy use. Pattern, or peaking, refers to the variation in energy use during the day with greatest use usually occurring between 8:00 and 11:00 a.m. and between 5:00 and 9:00 p.m. A major part of the actual generating capacity that is needed for peak periods remains unused during times of lower demand. A reshaping of consumer demands to a more level pattern could lead to the construction of smaller power plants which could reduce the environmental impact of power production.

Amount of Use

Winett and Nietzel (1975), using a combined within- and between-subject design, matched two groups of volunteer residents on prior natural gas and electricity use. Following meetings with the participants and a 2-week baseline period, one group (n=15) received an information packet and forms to record their energy use; the packet was an 8-page manual which detailed energy conserving procedures. The other group (n=16) recieved the same information and recording sheets and in addition were placed on an incentive plan that paid $2 per week for a 5-10% reduction (average gas and electricity use) from baseline levels of use, $3 per week for an 11-19% reduction, and $5 per week for reduction greater than 20%. The participants averaging the greatest amount of reduction during the 4 weeks of this condition received a $25 bonus; "second place" was worth $15. Persons in the incentive condition received feedback every week on energy used, percent energy reduction from baseline, and amount of incentive earned. Total earnings were paid at the end of 4 weeks. The study included a 2-week and a 2-month follow-up. The data consisted of actual gas and electricity meter readings by meter readers unaware of the experimental assignment of the household. These readings were taken on the same day and time each week. Participants also were trained in meter reading and were encouraged to monitor their own levels of energy use.

The results indicated a highly significant effect of the monetary incentive on electricity use. The incentive group averaged about 15% more reduction than the information group, which averaged about an 8% reduction from baseline. Differences between the groups were also consistent across temperatures that ranged from a weekly average of 35 to 57 degrees. There was a trend for these differences to be maintained at the follow-up points. An examination of individual household data showed that while 9 of the 16 incentive households averaged more than a 20% reduction over the 4-week incentive condition and 2-week follow-up, only one of 15 participants in the information group displayed a reduction of this magnitude.

However, the data on natural gas use did not show any differences between the groups. The primary determinant of gas use was temperature. For example, compared to the baseline weeks when the temperature averaged 38 degrees, both groups used about 5% more gas when the weekly temperature averaged 35 degrees, but about 60% less when the weekly temperature averaged 57 degrees.

Post-hoc interviews with the six households making the largest reductions indicated that these participants not only made minor changes (turning off the lights, lowering the thermostat) but also installed insulation, repaired appliances, and curtailed or eliminated use of heating in certain rooms. In conjunction with the data on electricity, these results suggest that: (1) for most people, incentives can reduce unnecessary electricity use for lighting and minor appliances; (2) for most people, the type and magnitude of incentive used in this study will not reduce energy use directed at home heating; (3) heating reduction will require some major lifestyle and structural changes in the home probably not supportable by the kinds of incentives researched in this study.

Hayes and Cone (in press,a) extended this work by using a more precise within-subject design, separating the confounded effects of monetary payments from utility bill savings for reduced energy use, more thoroughly examining the effects of feedback alone which in Winett and Nietzel (1975) was a part of the incentive condition, and using participants who had not overtly volunteered for a study. Participants were four married couples who lived in identical West Virginia housing units. They were approached casually by the experimenters and and asked if they wanted to participate in a study about energy conservation.

Since space and water heating in these units were provided by gas, electricity consumption (the target behavior in this study) was not altered markedly by temperature changes. Billing for utilities was part of a monthly rental fee. While the apartments did not have individual meters, watt-hour meters were connected to each unit's electricity writing in a basement area inaccessible to the residents.

Treatment conditions included: (1) baseline recordings; (2) feedback on the amount of electricity consumed the previous day, the amount used so far during that week, the predicted amount for the full week, the percent above or below baseline for the predicted use rate, and the cost of the amount used the previous day; (3) information that included descriptions of ways to reduce energy use and listings of the amounts of energy used in kilowatt hours and cost by common household devices; (4) monetary payments at the end of each week based on reduction from baseline. A 100% payment schedule provided $3 for a 10-19% reduction, $6 for a 20-29% reduction, $9 for a 30-39% reduction, $12 for a 40-49%, and $15 for reductions over 50%. Conditions involving 50%, 25%, and 10% of the original payment schedule were also evaluated.

By designing the study so that the order of treatments varied across the units, the results clearly showed that information by itself or with a payment scheme had little effect, feedback had only minor temporary effects, and the 100% payment scheme produced immediate and stable reductions averaging about 33%. The average reduction was 32% for the 50% scheme, 27% for the 25% plan, and 23% for the 10% plan. Although smaller reductions were associated with smaller payments, the slope of this declining function was not steep with even small payments producing substantial savings. If replicated, this latter finding may be extremely important. Economically, the payments used by Winett and Nietzel (1975) and Hayes and Cone (in press,a) were essentially utility price changes. Given that the cost per kilowatt hour was 2.6 cents, the price reductions in these two studies were in the 100-500% range. These are probably not feasible price changes, although the Hayes and Cone 10% plan represented a more reasonable incentive level. Until smaller price reductions are shown to reduce residential energy use substantially, the combined results of these two studies indicate that only very large and probably impractical incentives can reduce electricity use that is associated largely with minor appliances and lighting.

Two recent studies have provided refinements of the early conservation research. A study conducted primarily by two economists (Kagel, Battalio, Winkler, & Winett, 1976) was concerned with energy use during the summer months in Texas. It was an expanded, systematic replication of the Winett and Nietzel (1975) study. Climate, time of year, and major means of consuming electricity (air conditioning) were different from Winett and Nietzel, a study run in Kentucky during the winter. As Sidman (1960) has noted, the possible payoffs from systematic rather than direct replications are numerous. Despite mostly nonsignificant results, the present study illustrates such advantages.

Participants in the Texas study were volunteers responding to a letter and a telephone call requesting their participation. After introductory meetings, training in meter readings, and baseline recording, participants (in groups of 18 to 29 persons) were assigned to either a high-price "rebate" group (a payment of 30 cents for each one percent reduction in weekly electricity use compared to the previous summer's average), a low-price "rebate" group (a 1.3 cent payment for each KWH reduction in weekly electricity use compared to the previous summer's average; this represented a 50% increase in savings since one KWH=2.6 cents), a feedback-only group, an information group (which received two conservation booklets also given to the previous groups), and a control group. Following a 2-week baseline, all groups were run for 4 weeks. At that point, the control group received energy conservation information. Two weeks later, the first information-only group was placed on a high-price reduction scheme, and after another 2 weeks the high and low price reductions were withdrawn from the first two groups.

Using either the 2-week baseline or the participants' level of energy use the previous year as a comparison, it generally was found that only the high-price condition resulted in reduced use compared to the other groups. This reduction was quite small (5-8%).

The primary means of consuming energy during the summer in the Southwest was air conditioning. One important conclusion of this study was that even large price reductions will not induce residents to curtail their air conditioning use in very hot, humid weather. Electricity consumption under these weather and price conditions is basically "inelastic." In other words, during the summer, in that part of the country with air conditioning as the specific behavior to be modified, a price reduction scheme effective with minor electricity use (Winett & Nietzel, 1975) does not appear to be an effective intervention for air conditioning use.

It may well be that it is necessary to become even more specific than "air conditioning use." For example, many residents may set their air conditioning systems or units to operate at the hottest, most humid conditions, unaware that at lower levels of humidity some minimum amount of air conditioning in associate with a dehumidifier might be a sufficient cooling strategy (Battalio, 1975). Some sort of feedback device might be installed on air conditioning units that could cue these sorts of behaviors. In addition, it might be possible to shape lesser levels of air conditioning use by providing either large incentives for initial curtailment of air conditioning followed by a fading of the incentives (Hayes & Cone, in press,a) or some continual, minimal incentive for gradually reducing air conditioning use. While each strategy seems consistent with behavioral principles, their actual implementation awaits future experimental assessment.

Kagel et al.'s (1976) phrasing of the incentive or rebate schemes in economic terms may have quelled some of the participants' excitement created by the "demand characteristics" of the more typical "reinforcement" or "incentive" program. In addition, data collected prior to the study indicated that over 90% of the participants were unaware of how many KWH they used per month, suggesting that price schemes or feedback tied to KWH use may have little salience to consumers. For example, consumers may have little idea of the savings in KWH associated with specific conservation behaviors. These points suggest the necessity for interventionists to study carefully the meaning that their change techniques have for others, the context in which techniques are implemented, and the procedures for allowing greater specification of ecological behaviors and outcomes.

Seaver and Patterson (1975), in a study conducted in the Northwest during the winter, noted that the manner in which fuel oil (for heating) is purchased and used (large and infrequent deliveries, variable weather conditions, automatic oil burners, and variations in the use of the home) makes it difficult for the resident to be aware of how much fuel has been used and saved. In addition, monthly billings which are based often on fluctuating prices make the amount of the bill a highly variable index of actual use and conservation. Taking these problems into account, Seaver and Patterson investigated the effects of feedback and feedback plus commendation on the fuel use of 122 households drawn randomly from a list of the customers of a local fuel oil distributor. Differential feedback was given to households following their first oil delivery. Specially prepared slips which accompanied the delivery ticket explained the following use indices: consumption rate, rate of use during the delivery period and the previous winter, percentage increase or decrease in consumption rate, and a figure indicating the customers' savings or loss compared to what they could expect to pay if their use level continued at the previous year's rate. This slip represented the information and feedback condition (n=35).

In the feedback and commendation condition (n=45), households received the same feedback plus a decal which said: "we are saving oil." Receiving the decal was contingent on reducing the rate of fuel consumption from the previous winter. No-feedback control participants (n=42) received only the usual delivery ticket.

The dependent measure consisted of fuel consumption recorded at the second delivery of the winter. In the feedback and decal condition, 75% of the households had reduced their use from the previous winter. Also, households in the feedback and decal condition had significantly reduced their fuel use compared to the control and information-with-feedback conditions, which did not differ significantly from each other. Households originally were assigned to groups using a matched blocks (fuel-use level) design. No significant differences were found for blocks by conditions suggesting that the feedback and commendation technique was not differentially effective with different use levels.

It is surprising that such a simple, low-cost procedure was effective particularly given the ineffectiveness of monetary incentives in the previously reviewed research. While this was a short-term demonstration and the social climate of the period (the winter of 1974) contributed to the meaning of the decal, it was a simple decal given only once. There were also some methodological problems in the study (unequal baseline levels, reduction from baseline not used as a dependent measure) which make definitive conclusions difficult. Nonetheless, this procedure would appear to warrant further empirical attention.

Perhaps there is much more that people can or are willing to do in colder weather to make themselves warmer, but "when you're hot, you're hot." What is required in the area of energy conservation research is a much greater specification of potentially effective conservation behaviors (Nietzel & Winett, in press). It is also important to discover what methods are used by successful energy conservers so that such behaviors and strategies can be incorporated into future conservation programs.

Peaking

While peak pricing has received some attention in the press (Associated Press, 1975), only one behavioral study on this topic has been performed. Kohlenberg, Phillips, and Proctor (1973) monitored the patterns of electricity use of three volunteer families for 14 days. Following this baseline, information was supplied to each family on the relationship of peaking and environmental degradation and the wattage ratings of different home appliances. Following this information, feedback was introduced in the form of in-home devices which turned on a light when a specified level of current was exceeded. After another baseline, a feedback-plus-payment condition was introduced which included (1) exhortations to the families to reduce peaking, (2) feedback about the effects of the previous experimental conditions, (3) training in reading their in-home recording device to allow monitoring of kilowatt hours used, and (4) a large payment (a 100% reduction in peaking was worth twice the value of the utility bill). The results revealed that information had little effect on peaking, feedback alone had some minimal effects, while payments plus feedback produced the greatest reduction in peaking.

Continued work in this area is important in terms of the previously described environmental issues and because unlike a "simple" reduction in energy use, which if successful would cost the utility companies greatly (Winett, 1976a), peak reduction through differential prices could still result in the same income for utility companies (Papamarcos, 1975). Unless social-political contingencies change drastically (e.g., socialization of utilities), procedures which reduce energy use through dramatic alterations in rate structures thereby contributing to profit losses are not likely to be adopted in this country (Winett, 1976a). It should be clear that effective peak shaping will probably require such additional and supportive lifestyle changes as staggered work hours perhaps with differential, high pay for working less desirable hours. Similar work schedules have been introduced previously for the alleviation of peaking in the use of public transportation and highways (Nietzel & Winnett, in press).

The Kohlenberg et al. study also is important because of its introduction of in-home meters. Feedback in the previous energy studies has had only weak effects, a fact attributable perhaps to the fact that such feedback was not delivered by clearly visible, easily monitored meters. Such meters might have two recorders for on and off peak use, indicate past consumption, predict future consumption, and record differential prices, current expenditures, and savings. In addition, a light or sound might cue overuse. A series of within-subject designs could indicate the most effective display and pricing systems. It is important that this work be done soon since there are indications (Neikirk, 1975) that such programs might be introduced with sufficient research verification.

Future vital developments of energy conservation research include the following components: (1) increased communication between researchers so as to maximize the possibility that a few well-integrated studies can evaluate the effectiveness of alternative conservation strategies and in turn focus the direction of future research; (2) input from policy makers and utility companies so that procedures to be investigated are both influential and cost-effective. (On the other hand, program innovators should resist the temptation to limit energy conservation strategies to those that are currently acceptable to utility companies. For example, when from the winter of 1973 through the summer of 1974 Winett and Nietzel [1975] first approached power companies on the idea of using incentives or differential pricing schemes, these possibilities were poorly received. By the winter of 1974 and spring of 1975—the time of rebate sales—the same plans became suddenly acceptable if not "fashionable"; see Winett

[1976a]); (3) public input on what energy conservation behaviors people are willing to try and for what types of supports.

Public surveys conducted in Lexington, Kentucky during the last 2 years (Nietzel & Winett, in press) have revealed a pattern indicating that respondents have engaged in few conservation behaviors themselves but are looking to the federal government for guidelines and policies on energy use; respondents also indicated that they probably would be willing to reduce their energy use in return for direct payments. Finally, as suggested in other sections of this chapter, behavior analysis of energy problems should be supplemented by prior and concomitant data sources, other research methodologies, and varied means of information gathering.

Transportation

From the behaviorist's perspective, it is easy to speculate that transportation problems will not be solved on the basis of physical technology (e.g., a new subway system). Physical technical advances must be accompanied by behavioral technology to deal effectively with issues that are, to a large degree, clearly behavioral (e.g., few individuals riding buses, too many individuals driving private automobiles). One might assume that use of mass transportation facilities, such as a bus system, is low in this country because it is met with aversive consequences (e.g., paying cash out of one's pocket, a reduction in schedule and route options relative to private car use, and/or the derogatory connotations of being a "bus rider") and that ridership would increase if any of these consequences were eliminated and/or potentially reinforcing events were scheduled to follow bus riding responses. (Everett, Hayward, & Meyers, 1974, p. 1)*

The main purpose of the Everett et al.'s (1974) study was to devise a token reinforcement system that was low cost, workable in an "open field" setting, yet attractive enough to induce residents, students, faculty, and staff of a university community to ride the bus. Unlike other token economy systems that have been implemented for relatively circumscribed populations and settings, in this study any of the community's members (about 56,000) were potential participants.

Two buses traversing the 2.5 mile campus route were used in the study. Advertisements in the university newspaper advised persons of the contingencies to be in effect on a bus during a given day. The advertisement presented a map of the bus route and stated that all persons boarding the "Red Star Bus" during specified days would receive a token redeemable for services and goods at local

---

*Everett, P. B. Hayward, S. C., and Meyers, A. W. The effects of a token reinforcement procedure on bus ridership. *Journal of Applied Behavior Analysis*, 1974, *1*, 1-9.

businesses that had contracted to participate in the study. Only previously specified items (food, movies, a free bus ride, publication of "eco-heroes" names in the paper) could be obtained for tokens at participating stores; the stores were reimbursed by the project for the token purchases.

Following the establishment of a stable, 16-day baseline level of bus ridership, each passenger boarding the "Red Star Bus" received a token from one of the experimenters. Persons boarding a control bus did not receive any tokens. These conditions were in effect for 8 days. After a clear trend had been demonstrated for ridership, the token condition was terminated with a return to the baseline condition, which was in effect for 12 days.

The results of the study showed that during the first baseline, the experimental bus averaged 280 riders per day while the control bus averaged 255 riders. During the token condition, the average number of riders on the experimental bus was 420 or 150% of baseline, while the control bus' ridership remained relatively constant (270). With the introduction of the second baseline, ridership on both buses was about the same as during the first baseline.

The token system for this study operated smoothly; about half the tokens were used for additional bus rides with the other tokens dispersed for the other back-up reinforcers. Bus ridership was not affected by weather, nor was the length of the ride affected by experimental conditions. Questionnaire data indicated that walkers, undergraduates, and persons making academically relevant trips were the individuals primarily attracted to bus ridership during the token condition; there was not a ridership increase from car drivers during this condition.

Several features of this study are particularly important. The token system worked very well and enabled individuals to redeem their tokens at reliable establishments at diverse times and at many different locations. The cooperation of local businesses that could profit from the publicity and additional sales generated by persons redeeming tokens suggests that such community token programs might be effective for other social problems such as the return of recyclable materials. It is also possible that these potential advantages to businesses could allow such a system to become self-supporting.

The use of accessory data (questionnaires, weather conditions, length of ride) allowed for a more thorough evaluation of the program's impact on different strata of the population under varying conditions and on nontargeted but related behaviors. These supplementary data are an essential adjunct to operant field studies which depart from single-subject methodology (Sidman, 1960). In the present case, the entire community was treated as a single organism with each bus ride considered a distinct response. While the additional data sources were inexpensive, they were able to suggest several directions for future research. This attention to a multiplicity of measures is indicative of Willems's (1974) concept of "ecological" research.

Deslauriers and Everett (1975) systematically replicated the previous study by comparing the effects of continuous and intermittent reinforcement schedules on bus ridership. The same bus route was used with ridership counts being made from 8:00 to 11:00 a.m., 11:00 to 2:00 p.m. and 2:00 to 5:00 p.m. on an experimental and control bus. After a 6-week baseline, a variable ratio -3 reinforcement system was instituted for 15 days on the experimental bus. At this time, large red stars were attached to the experimental bus. Tokens redeemable in the same manner as Everett et al. (1974) were given to approximately every third person boarding the bus. A sign mounted on the bus indicated the probability for that day of receiving a token. This information was also provided in newspaper advertisements. A 10-day continuous token reinforcement system was followed by a return to the variable ratio -3 schedule for 8 days. These contingency changes were announced on the bus and in the newspaper. Finally, a second baseline was instituted for 10 days.

The data revealed that the experimental bus' ridership increased during both the continuous and variable ratio reinforcement schedules. The control bus showed a decrease in riders during the 11:00 a.m. to 2:00 p.m. time period, while ridership on the experimental bus remained about the same during nonreinforcement time periods. There was no appreciable differences in ridership between the variable and continuous reinforcement schedules. The second baseline figures approximated the ridership counts for the first baseline. Questionnaire data indicated no significant changes in the type of passenger or trip length when baseline one was compared to the continuous reinforcement system. Evidently, car drivers still were not attracted to the bus. Seventy-one percent of the tokens were spent to procure a free bus ride.

The fact that the variable ratio schedule was as effective as continuous reinforcement suggests one way to economize reinforcement systems for transportation problems. In addition, Deslauriers and Everett reported that only a few passengers were upset when they did not receive a token during the variable ratio portion of the study. They also suggested investigating the effects on transportation behaviors of tokens with different values or lottery schemes similar to Powers et al. (1973).

At this stage of this research, it is extremely important to be able to specify which interventions will affect which types of potential users of which modes of transportation. For example, token procedures might induce walkers to ride the bus, but other procedures might be necessary to persuade people to abandon their cars. Mini-buses with convenient, specific routes might be necessary to persuade car drivers to use alternative means of transportation. Therefore, more specificity in procedures, modalities, and target groups is required in behavioral transportation research.

Two recent reports suggest that such investigations do have the potential to be used on a wide scale. In Seattle, free bus service directly to the center of the city apparently has decreased traffic congestion by inducing former car drivers to take the bus (C. Smith, 1975). The area served by the free bus service is the entire 111 square-block downtown business district. Buses make about 5,400 daily trips in and out of the free ride area. Riders pay the normal fare if they enter or leave the bus outside of the area. From the start of the 16-month experiment, the number of riders taking the bus downtown has tripled to 12,000 daily riders. The convenience of the service also has bolstered some businesses because workers will often take buses to different parts of the downtown area for lunch and shopping. This suggests that some tax on these businesses could halp defray part of the yearly $115,000 cost for operating this free service. In addition, free service might be used on a special part-time basis to encourage sampling of carless transportation. Some tentative evidence (Blumenthal, 1975) indicates that at least some people who curtailed use of their cars for public transportation during the height of the energy crisis have continued to use this mode of transportation.

MacCalden and Davis (1975) described an experiment on the San Francisco-Oakland Bay Bridge. Commuters who drove to San Francisco in car pools (three or more people in a car) were given cheaper monthly bridge fares and were allowed to use a faster moving priority lane. Though the results of this study did not show dramatic changes, there were some increases in use of car pools and municipal transportation attributable to the reduced rates and priority lane.

However, there were three shortcomings of this experiment. First, the priority lane was located in the center of the bridge, thereby virtually precluding the apprehension of noncarpool users who during the course of the study sabotaged or ignored the operative contingencies. Proper physical planning in terms of either new forms of transportation (e.g., mini-buses, electric cars) or alterations of transportation structures should accompany applications of behavioral technology in order to maximize its impact.

Second, the reinforcement system was a nondifferentiated one. Some of the procedures discussed in Deslauriers and Everett (1975) could be extended to this situation. Perhaps financial contingencies could be related to criteria such as make of car.

Finally, perusal of the newspaper before and during this project indicated that the community was unprepared for this experiment, creating somewhat of a public backlash against it. This suggests that efforts to inform the public and tap their opinions about such programs should precede attempts at actual implementation. However, unlike many programs, this project was identified as an experiment, not a panacea, an advisable policy for social reform efforts (Campbell, 1969). Another successful ingredient of this project was the computerization of car pools by bringing together the names of people who had similar departing points, routes, or final destinations. Such information efforts also were used by Deslauriers and Everett (1975) and Everett et al. (1974) and should be a routine component of future programs.

There are several other proposals which have been suggested for the alteration of our transportation habits and the problems related to the continued use of large, internal combustion engine automobiles. In almost all cases, the proposals are quite specific in terms of techniques and target behaviors and present the opportunity for behavior analysts to validate experimentally these proposals before their system-wide adoption. For example, will very high taxes on low-mileage cars or rebates on small cars lead to a decrease in large-car sales or a decrease in small-car sales? Which persons are most affected by such incentive schemes? Would building safe bicycle routes be associated with greater use of bicycles and a decline in the use of cars, or must other procedures accompany the construction of this transportation alternative? What is the relative cost of alternative porposals and how do they affect fuel consumption and air pollution levels? Both the urgency and the clarity of these questions suggest a fertile, socially significant area of research for behavior analysts.

Environmental research must also be understood as originating from and often paralleling social-political beliefs endemic to the environmental issues themselves (Maloney & Ward, 1973) and broader economic policies. For example, price changes may produce home energy conservation and reduce the use of the automobile. But the governmental policies most often discussed by recent administrations have involved across-the-board price increases for re-sources. Such increases are more likely to affect middle or lower class families than wealthier families, exposing them to the extremes of weather or inadequate and at times nonexistent public transportation facilities. Lest we who advocate price reductions or incentives for the "good consumer" blush in liberal pride, it should be clear that such incentives might promote conservation only among the poorer people in the country. At this time, systems based on large penalties for wealthy people and small penalties for poor people seem unworkable, while large incentives for the wealthy and small incentives for the poor are also not desirable. The point of this departure is to underscore both the political context of these questions and emphasize again that the behavior analyst does not work in a social vacuum.

As noted in the previous discussion of legislative bans on throwaway containers, the development of a technique for environmental protection is only the first step in instituting wider scale changes. A brief report on a transportation experiment in San Jose, California (Lindsey, 1975) illustrates this point. A mini-bus "dial-a-ride" mass transit system was in operation for about 6 months; this type of system has been considered crucial for cities that are more horizontal than vertical (e.g., Los Angeles). The history of this project reveals that the particular system failed because if anything it was too successful.

For 25 cents, the county provided door-to-door transportation between almost any two locations in an area covering about 200 square miles (with a one to two million population). A potential rider could call the bus company, and a computer would identify which of the buses was cruising closest to the person's home. The bus could then transport the person to his/her destination or to a conventional bus stop. A transfer could be arranged from the conventional bus to one of the mini-buses.

The services attracted many more consumers than expected, causing delays in the reception of calls and actual pickups; mechanical problems with the new equipment added to these problems. A labor settlement increased drivers' wages, escalating the cost of the system to community residents. A court decision ordered the transit district to buy all eight of the county's taxi companies since dial-a-ride buses were taking away their business. This decision was never enacted since the bus service was largely discontinued.

While the dial-a-ride buses carried up to 6,500 passengers per day, many of these people were "transit dependents"—young people, the elderly, and the poor. It was unclear whether the middle-class person who normally would drive a private car to work used the mini-buses. This is probably the key segment of the population that needs to be attracted to such a service to relieve traffic congestion and air pollution and provide the necessary political and fiscal support.

In response to these problems, Everett (1975) has described a number of urban (simulated) games for pre-testing and gaining preliminary information about large-scale interventions. He has developed one game that examines the effects of reinforcement contingencies on specific ridership behaviors. Everett's summary evaluation of these techniques is important in light of the introductory comments of this chapter in which it was noted that the restriction of the chapter to behavior analytic work should not be construed as meaning that such principles or procedures were complete solutions to environmental problems.

As operant psychology expands its scope of interest to broader more complex social settings, the radical behaviorist will have to forsake his rigidness and develop tools for gaining insight about potential behavior changes. It is often impossible (by economic, time, manpower, complexity, logistical criteria) to test an actual reinforcement-response relationship in the real settings of interest. Tools for gaining hunches, preliminary analyses, ideas, and parameters are needed. Existing models of large scale program implementation all demonstrate pretesting tools. People in marketing initiate market surveys, and then pilot sales programs. Engineers in the aircraft industry simulate a new model on a computer and then build an experimental model. Gaming techniques are simply one category of pretesting mechanisms. (Everett, 1975, p. 12)*

---

*Everett, P. B. A gaming simulation for pretesting large-scale operant manipulations: An urban transportation example. Unpublished manuscript. The Pennsylvania State University, 1975.

Architecture

One difficulty of behavior analysis of architectural design is the problem of manipulating aspects of a physical environment. However, the Twardosz et al. (1974) study which analyzed open and partitioned environments (described in Chapter 2) indicates that if the physical environment is built flexibly, systematic experimentation on the best behavior/environment fit becomes an ultimately feasible enterprise.

A recent study by Hayes and Cone (in press,b) also examplifies the rich possibilities of experimentation in this area. The problem behavior was destructive lawn walking in a university park comprised of grass islands and rock pathways. The park was traversed hourly by hundreds of people who walked across the grass islands, wearing dirt paths through them. As a result, the area was never used as a park. Of course, such destructive behavior is not unique to this setting; national forests, parks, zoos, and other natural environments often are used inappropriately.

Most behavioral methods developed for environmental problems generally require the active participation of someone to observe and reinforce behavior. In terms of influencing the behavior of masses of people for long periods of time, such strategies are inappropriate. What is needed are "passive interventions" (e.g., signs, aspects of the physical design) that can be built into a setting. Interventions that are adopted also should have some general applicability and be permanent, inexpensive, and supportive of the use of an area (e.g., putting insurmountable fences around park areas would not support park behaviors).

Three principles used by Hayes and Cone (in press,b) in developing their interventions were response consequences, chaining, and prompting. A prime determinant of destructive lawn walking may be the inconvenience of alternative responses. For example, if the distance required to traverse a park in an environmentally sound manner was increased, destructive lawn walking should increase. If it became more difficult to cross the park using the lawns, then the frequency of environmentally sound routes should increase. The authors also hypothesized that a person entering the park on a rock pathway would be more likely to follow the rock pathway as opposed to walking on the lawn (an example of chaining). General and specific prompts also might influence this type of behavior.

The experimental park was a large rectangle surrounded on three sides by sidewalks and on the other side by a building. Six islands of grass rimmed the perimeter of the park; three smaller islands were on the inside of the park. The areas between the islands were rock covered.

Interventions included: placing benches on the rock pathways so as to increase the distance required to walk in an environmentally sound manner; increasing the distance of nondestructive routes by placing chairs around the benches; locating benches on the dirt pathways so as to make walking on these routes more difficult; placing a chain fence at the northwest corner of the park by the lawn so as to steer walkers toward the rock pathway ("chaining"); marking the park area by placing six benches on the park's perimeter; prompting pro-environmental walking by placing two signs at the northwest corner of the park which said, "University Mini-Park—Please Don't Trample the Grass."

Treatment conditions were investigated using an A-B-A design. Each condition lasted 1 hour, and data were collected on 6 separate days with one treatment studied per day. The experiment was conducted over a 3-week period with observations taken only when the ground was firm and the temperature was between 50 and 70 degrees. Observers recorded the number of grass islands touched by a person walking through the park; a person could receive a score from 0 to 7. The walking behavior of 1,885 people was recorded.

The data indicated that placement of the benches on the dirt pathways in the lawns sharply reduced the incidence of lawn walking, the fence eliminated lawn walking on the grass island by which it was placed, and the specific sign prompt also decreased lawn walking. The two interventions designed to *increase* lawn walking revealed very limited effects. Interestingly, it was found that only during the conditions when the benches were on the grass islands was the park used as a park (sitting or lying down, leaning against a tree). In other conditions it was used simply as a thoroughfare. These data substantiate previous findings that the characteristics of environmental settings can exert substantial control over behavior (Moos & Insel, 1974; Proshansky et al., 1970) and that environment-behavior relationships can be studied within a behavior analytic framework. They further point toward the construction of flexible environments (Sommer, 1974) that can be manipulated experimentally to determine (1) the optimal behavior-environment fit, (2) the effects of discriminative stimuli and the social contingency functions of specific prompts, (3) other antecedent conditions of environmentally important behaviors, and (4) automatic or passive methods for reinforcing pro-environmental behavior.

The brevity of this section reflects the limited amount of experimental work concerning the manner in which physical environments influence behavior. Therefore, some conceptual and empirical input from Robert Sommer's (1974) book *Tight Spaces: Hard Architecture and How to Humanize It* is included because it provides a framework which is very consistent with an experimental orientation to environmental design. Sommer's major thesis is that our society's overemphasis on security and control has led to the use of "hard" architecture, originally used in the design of prisons and other institutions but increasingly finding its place in universities and schools, office buildings, apartments, airports, and shopping centers.

The physical characteristics of such architecture include: a lack of permeability (minimum contact between the inside and outside of structures), expensive construction with little possibility for change and expansion, clear differentiation of status levels, and uniformity of design and layout with the selection of materials and furnishings based on ease of purchase and maintenance. The behavioral manifestations of such environments are passive behaviors, limited interactions and range of activities, reduced experimentation with the environment, and reliance on external agencies or machines for security. In other words, the behaviors associated with these environments are the ones traditionally linked with prisons and mental hospitals (Goffman, 1961). Ironically, while there has been some recognition and modification of the pathology supporting aspects of institutional environments, this same architecture is becoming more common in noninstitutional settings.

Part of the solution to this situation rests in experimenting with different designs to assess their effect on behavior. In the design of physical settings, such as buildings, this step has occurred rarely. Usually "evaluation" is based on pictures, the opinions of experts, etc.; there is no actual observing of behavior *in vivo*. Sommer presented data, primarily based on a comparative research strategy, which attempted to examine behavior-setting relations. Studies were conducted on the effects of putting decorations in college classrooms and the relationship of student interaction patterns to classrooms of different designs. Classrooms designed as laboratories or workshops were associated with more participation and interaction. The decorations were found to increase students' ratings of the pleasantness, cheerfulness, comfort, and relaxing qualities of the classroom without disrupting concentration. Additional comparative data indicated that the typical structure of university buildings tended to limit a person's interactions with people of similar rank and status.

In brief, Sommer advocated "soft," flexible architecture that encourages people to experiment with and change ("humanize") their environments. Excellent examples of the potential of this area are found in the discussion in Chapter 2 of Risley's Living Environments Group which has initiated experimental investigations of the effects of open-setting child-care centers and various managerial procedures on diverse child and staff behaviors (Twardosz et al., 1974).

Population Change

Although empirical behavior research on population change is very limited, Zifferblatt and Hendricks (1974) have developed a framework for behavioral population change methods. Their behavioral approach is outlined as an adjunct to other technological advances and an alternative to the more traditional psychological approach to focusing on the modification of attitudes. For example:

A number of effective sanitation, birth control, nutrition and antipollution devices and products now exist yet their employment is somewhat unsystematic and thus ineffective. Quite often these problems relate to the behavior of people employing the technology. Scientific tools are used to create a physical technology. Similar scientific tools must be used in delivering, implementing and maintaining the use of this technology. Developing an effective birth control device is one thing, but designing an environment ensuring its proper use is quite another.

A common thread weaving its way through psychological research in population change and family planning is the search for underlying and common causal variables that transcend individual differences within a culture and account for the problem phenomena . . . Once these variables are identified through correlation and factorial research then hypotheses may be established and experimental research conducted. Finally, these hypotheses will hopefully lead to useful treatment strategies that eventuate in behavioral change. When behavior change or control over behaviors related to problem areas are used as criteria, these attempts have not borne fruit. (Zifferblatt & Hendricks, 1974, pp. 750-751)*

After reviewing several studies that have attempted to implement family planning programs, Zifferblatt and Hendricks concluded that such programs suffered from lack of specific behavioral goals, methods, and incentives for the monitoring and attainment of the target behaviors. Applications of the behavior analytic process could partially alleviate some of these deficits. Advantages of this process include the following elements: the clear specification of target behaviors (taking one contraceptive pill each morning, a functional analysis of potential antecedents and consequences which would support population control behaviors (placing the bottle of pills on the breakfast table, receiving prompts and approval from the spouse), the provision of naturalistic data collection to enable monitoring of the intervention's effectiveness, and development and implementation of intervention strategies based on the principles of behavioral control.

An especially significant contribution of this article was its emphasis on the cultural context of the behavior to be modified.

Systematic and knowledgeable guidance is required to isolate critical behaviors and events in the culturally unique environment of each individual. Different cultures, for instance, provide differential male sex roles and incentives (e.g., money versus status), religious practices, and social behaviors which may lead the scientist to observe and select

---

*Zifferblatt, S. M. and Hendricks, C. G. Applied behavioral analysis of societal problems: Population change, a case in point. *American Psychologist*, 1974, Vol. 29, 750-761.

different contingency arrangements in developing an intervention strategy for population change. (Zifferblatt & Hendricks, 1974, p. 755)

Given the idiosyncratic nature of family planning, population change, and specific milieu, the authors suggested the use of intensive n=1 designs to evaluate the effectiveness of interventions. The generality of the methods' effectiveness could be assessed by systematic replications. They also described the skills (e.g., observation, functional analysis, setting of objectives) needed by family planning workers and consumers to implement such programs and a behavioral taxonomy that would identify all potential behaviors and contingencies in a specific culture that might be salient to family planning programs. Decisions about which strategies to use in a specific case would depend on analyses of available and required behaviors for a family to use a given birth control procedure effectively. Following identification of the crucial behavioral requirements, intervention packages could be developed for application by the field staff. While this conceptualization offered a comprehensive framework and technology for family planning the prescribed interventions will require empirical validation in natural settings.

Conclusion

It is expected that the next few years will experience a much greater development of behavioral approaches to environmental protection. The current research, though limited in quantity, is of sufficient quality to engender optimism for the future of the field. In virtually all of the reviewed literature there was the clear intention of not only demonstrating functional relationships but building into initial studies the mechanisms which subsequently would allow wider scale applications. While some methodological limitations of the research were observed, (e.g., treating the site as the organism), much of the research also indicated that behavior modifiers are willing to incorporate other sources of data into their work, and that such a multimethod approach likely will have a beneficial impact on the planning, development, and analysis of current projects and perhaps extend behavioral work to new environmental problems.

Behaviorists' experimental approach to environmental problems also should make a unique contribution to environmental psychology which heretofore has relied on more "passive" methods. Most environmental research rests on a descriptive or comparative methodology (Ittelson et al., 1974). In contrast, the behavioral analytic approach manipulates antecedent or consequent events to decrease environmentally destructive behaviors or increase environmentally enhancing behaviors. Thus, a potential solution to a given environmental problem is field tested experimentally; the process of demonstrating behavioral control in turn yields new knowledge concerning the relationship of human behavior to a sound ecology.

Many of the alternative policies concerning environmental protection that are currently being debated can be analyzed and evaluated using the methods reviewed in this chapter. The ultimate aims of this research (e.g., wide-scale implementation) coupled with the growing acknowledgment of the political relevance and ramifications of environmental protection (Hayes & Cone, in press,a; Winett, 1976a) should enable behavioral researchers to influence substantially the environmental policies of the future.

Chapter 12
THE BEHAVIORAL PARADIGM AND COMMUNITY CHANGE

The progressively strengthened coalition between behaviorists and community psychologists has been described and welcomed in such terms as prescriptions for "positive deviance" (Ullmann & Krasner, 1975), operationalization of community psychology's interests and commitments (Winett, 1974), reconceptualizations of social problems in terms of collective human behavior (Maloney & Ward, 1973), and the advancement of community mental health by a behavioral-preventive approach to the development of self-controlling communities (Meyers, Craighead, & Myers, 1974). The foundations for such a collaboration are numerous and include such commonalities as a resolution to be relevant, a continuing commitment to applied research, and conceptual similarities regarding the etiology of psychosocial problems in living (see Chapter 1).

The preceding chapters have surveyed the extension of social learning procedures to several community problems which historically have not been the primary targets of psychologists. In many ways the extensions have been gratifying ones. Conditions which have been notoriously exasperating because of their resistance to change have responded to some extent to behavioral interventions. The facility with which social change can be reconceptualized in behavioral terms has rekindled the enthusiasm of many behavioral scientists who heretofore avoided issues for which they felt inadequately equipped. Finally, it should be obvious that applications of behaviorally based techniques to community modification have proliferated dramatically in recent years. In all areas reviewed in this book, the majority of programmatic interventions have appeared within the past 5 years.

Concurrent with the recognition and appreciation of behavioral contributions to the remediation of community problems, one must confront the fact that behavioral strategies for effecting generalized, sustained social change are more a future promise than a present reality. In this final chapter, we would like to identify the deficits of the current behavioral paradigm which contribute to the discrepancy between actuality and potential, and hopefully in the process, suggest some ways in which behavioral scientists can reconsider both their theoretical explanations of human problems and preferred means by which such problems can be eliminated, controlled, or prevented.

Domains in Need of Further Attention

Prevention

A cardinal feature of the social psychiatry-community psychology-community mental health movement, particularly in its early years, has been its insistence on interventions that seek to prevent rather than ameliorate "deviant," "unhealthy," or "improper" human behavior (Cowen, 1973; Kessler & Albee, 1975). Caplan (1964) has distinguished three types of prevention: primary, secondary, and tertiary.

Primary prevention involves the reduction and ultimate elimination of disorders by either modifying the pathogenic components of an environment or bolstering interpersonal-individual resources to the point where disorder does not occur. Primary preventive activities usually have involved either social action in which changes in community systems or institutions are planned so that the resources incompatible with problem development are available, or interpersonal action in which the targets of change are important policy makers whose position or status results in a "radiation" of the changes they might experience (Kessler & Albee, 1975; Zax & Specter, 1974). Examples of primary prevention through social action include compensatory education and school programs (Cowen, 1969; Griffin & Reinhorz, 1969), job-training programs (O'Connor & Rappaport, 1970), urban renewal, and varieties of social welfare (Kessler & Albee, 1969). Primary prevention via interpersonal action is exemplified by programs such as family intervention and parent education (e.g., Bolman, 1968), consultation to "essential service" agencies—e.g., police (Bard, 1969), and training of "community care givers" (Dorsey, Matsunaga, & Bauman, 1964; Hommen, 1972).

Secondary prevention aims at a reduction of the prevalence of disability through the coordinated efforts of early detection and rapid, effective intervention. Essential to secondary prevention is the development of instruments which allow reliable and valid diagnosis as early in the course of the problem as possible. Secondary prevention programs often have been directed at elementary school students because of the demonstrated relationship between early school maladaptation and later adjustment problems (Zax & Cowen, 1969) and the belief that the schools should be a primary vehicle for optimizing both educational and personal growth. An example of this approach is the Primary Mental Health Project (PMHP) of Cowen and his colleagues at the University of Rochester (Cowen, Dorr, Izzo, Madonia, & Trost, 1971). The PMHP uses quick-screening techniques for the identification of primary schoolers who are experiencing educational or behavioral problems (Cowen, Dorr, Clarfield, Kreling, Pokracki, Pratti, Terrell, & Wilson, 1973). At-risk children then are seen by trained, nonprofessional child aides who attempt to assist children in coping with their difficulties and building their adaptive skills (Cowen, Dorr, Trost, & Izzo, 1972). Outcome data on the PMHP suggest behavioral and educational improvements for program participants (Cowen & Schochet, 1973). The majority of preventive interventions in psychology continue to be at a secondary level reflecting the fact that at this time secondary prevention is more specific and feasible than programs aimed at primary prevention.

The history of the mental health fields could be chronicled as the persistent pursuit of *tertiary prevention*. The aims of tertiary prevention are to minimize the severity of dysfunction, reduce long- or short-term sequelae of the disorder, and contain the effects of the disturbance so that maximal personal effectiveness is retained. Zax and Cowen (1972) have argued that "tertiary prevention is prevention in name only" and is justified not because of its capacity to eliminate or forestall dysfunction but because of its compatibility with the "democratic-humanitarian goal of reducing human discomfort and providing maximal opportunity for all men to live effectively" (p. 453). Although almost any form of psychological and psychiatric intervention including hospitalization, psychotherapy, and pharmacotherapy could claim to embody tertiary levels of prevention, the uniqueness and utility of the term "prevention" is preserved only if we restrict its use to primary and early secondary interventions.

Behavior modifiers have yet to display an affinity for interventions aimed at more ambitious forms of prevention. Too often they have appeared content to discourage individuals from continuing their littering, drinking, stealing, or bizarre behavior. As a result, behavioral interventions have been tertiary and sporadic, with neither the etiological understanding nor breadth of focus necessary for primary prevention. It is encouraging that psychologists have established themselves as credible agents of action in schools (see Chapter 2), because early education systems provide one logical arena in which planned innovations can have preventive outcomes. While establishment of such power bases is an essential element in preventive programs, it does not obviate the need for understanding how to foster the learning histories and social-psychological environments most likely to promote maximally effective forms of behavior. At this point, we do not have the behavioral theories which would guide decisions about what types of learning histories would have a preventive or constructive impact. A concurrent constraint is behaviorists' tendency to focus on single-subject behavior change and research. This ideological mistrust of group data and interventions remains an obstacle to epidemiological investigations as well as appreciation of the preventionist credo that "no human disease is ever brought under control by the treatment of afflicted individuals" (Kessler & Albee, 1975, p. 567).

Consultation

Another identifying feature of community interventions has been the utilization of professionals in consultation capacities (Mannino & Shore, 1975; Woody, 1975). The consultation concept is an increasingly expansive one involving at least three discernible types of activity:

1)   Interprofessional consultation in which one professional shares his or her expertise with a second professional. The consultant may provide advice or assistance with the management of a particular professional case (client-centered consultation), the administration of social service programs (program-centered consultation), or the modification of the consultee's handling of individual cases or planning of mental health programs (consultee-centered case or administrative consultation) (Caplan, 1963).

2)   Preparation of volunteers, paraprofessionals, and nonprofessionals for behavior change functions typically reserved for the professional. The passage of several pieces of anti-poverty legislation within the past decade has created thousands of nonprofessional positions in community service agencies (Riessman, 1967). In turn the nonprofessional movement has been associated with a number of social advantages and ideological justifications including the creation of viable careers for poor people, the endorsement of the belief that troubled people can be helped by personnel with whom they share demographic characteristics, cultural heritage, or strong political commitments, and the recognition that new sources of mental health workers are necessary for adequate delivery of mental health services (Albee, 1959). Para- and nonprofessionals have been used most often as adjunct personnel in classrooms (Alden, Rappaport, & Seidman, 1975), counselors for drug addict populations (Dwarshuis et al., 1973), correctional agents in the criminal justice system (Twain, McGee, & Bennett, 1973), volunteer therapeutic aides for chronic mental patients (Holzberg, Knapp, & Turner, 1967; Rioch, Elkes, Flint, Usdansky, Newman, & Silber, 1963), participants in community mental health centers (Bartels & Tyler, 1975) and in juvenile justice system programs (Davidson et al., 1975).

3)   Training relatives (Guerney, 1969), peers (Harris & Sherman, 1973a), teachers (Meyers, 1975), and friends (Sulzer, 1965) to initiate behavior change conditions or to maintain contingencies and conditions that had been introduced during a professional intervention. This planned involvement of auxiliary personnel as treatment mediators has been a relatively popular addition to social learning interventions (Tharp & Wetzel, 1969; Wiltz & Patterson, 1974).

Most behavioral programs have not evidenced an interest in interprofessional or paraprofessional consultation. Despite their popular portrayal as a collection of principles and procedures which can be transmitted quickly and learned easily, behavior modification programs continue to be implemented, directed, staffed, and supervised mostly by psychologists and their graduate students. In fact there would appear to be little data inconsistent with the conclusion that most behavioral intervention programs terminate on dates which correspond closely to the appearance of a publication describing the project's "initial" results. The literature we have reviewed consists too often of "demonstration projects" whose resources and intentions are seldom sufficiently ambitious to allow serious efforts at professional dissemination or continuation of the program by subprofessional personnel. Fortunately, there are growing indications that behaviorists are prompting and training *in vivo* agents to continue therapeutic contingencies in an attempt to make intervention gains more durable and extensive. Nonetheless, traditionally trained behavior modifiers have been slow to extend or amplify their impact through the deliberate use of formalized consultation or the systematic instruction of nonprofessionals.

Activism

The social action dimensions of community psychology have been considered alternatively as an essential contribution and an unnecessary evil. Advocates of social action tactics claim that the professional's willingness to provoke, confront, agitate, and pressure is the *sine qua non* of effective community psychology. Opponents of professional social action argue that such activity is incompatible either with the spirit of professionalism or with the pursuit of truth through objective observation and the development of empirically based generalizations for which behavioral science should be responsible.

Behavior modification's position on the social action continuum seems relatively well defined. Either by deliberate choice or default, behavior modifiers have not exhibited a strong commitment to principled, provocative activisim as a style of social intervention. Only if one is willing to equate applied research with social action would it seem possible to attribute an activist contribution to behavior modification as historically practiced.

The advantages of such a position are neither surprising nor unimportant. It reduces the probability that "objectivity" will be jeopardized by political or self-interests. It limits professionals' attention to issues for which they have had extensive academic training. Finally, it is responsive to the reality that academic respectability is reserved for professionals who maintain a separation between their politics and their science.

These advantages aside, it would appear that a behavioral paradigm which is wedded to a commitment to some forms of social activism would be more influential and decisive than the same paradigm not augmented by such a commitment. Behavioral conceptions have provided political activists with a set of principles by which their political energies can be translated into effective social change tactics. The ideal fusion is the emergence of a social technology as creative and vigorous in changing social conditions as it is in understanding them. While we have yet to accomplish fully either of these objectives, it may be that the dual roles of "conceptualizer" and "participant changer" will require interdisciplinary involvement incorporating more than one type of professional. Regardless of the determinants of behaviorists' reluctance to be true activists, it would be shortsighted to obscure their potential conceptual-methodological importance to an effective community psychology because of their hesitancy in matters of activism.

Whether activism and conceptual rigor can be maintained best through a single or multiple type(s) of professionals, the goal remains to develop a social activism grounded on and contributing to empirically derived principles of behavior change. Sarason (1974) has commented on the potential use of social action as experimental intervention:

> The social action role as I have described it is not everybody's cup of tea. It is, however, a brew without which the social sciences will remain insipid and trivial. In their quest for scientific respectability the social sciences have erected "experimentation" and the "experimental attitude" as a supreme value. An essential feature of this attitude, so obvious that it rarely receives elaboration, is that if you want to understand how things work you have to *intervene*, you have to introduce something new into the accustomed order of things. The additional feature of manipulating variables, contrasting control and experimental conditions, is a consequence of the basic assumption that you must *intervene and change* things in some way. Social action is a form of intervention no less than changing the feeding schedules of rats is an intervention. Where it is possible to introduce controls one should do so, of course. But the fact that such controls may not be possible, or that they may fall short of the ideal mark, is an argument for caution in interpretation, and not an argument against intervention. One does the best one can and relies on the efforts and criticisms of others to do better the next time. *But that is also true for the most rigorous experimentalist.* In the final analysis the best control is in what others say and do in response to what one claims to have learned. Rigor is no guarantee of significance and importance. Calling something social action or fieldwork is no excuse for sloppiness. What we ask of everyone is that they do justice to themselves and to the problem, uninfluenced by fashion, unconstrained by narrow tradition, and unfearful of the new. (pp. 266-267)*

Psychological Sense of Community

The tendency for behavior modification to be a tertiary, professionally centered enterprise focusing in large measure on the individual has limited its potential to advance a comprehensive community psychology and instill what Sarason (1974) has termed the "psychological sense of community."

> I have never met anyone—young or old, rich or poor, black or white, male or female, educated or not—to whom I have had any great difficulty explaining what I meant by the psychological sense of community. My

---

*Sarason, S. B. *The psychological sense of community: Prospects for a community psychology.* San Francisco: Jossey-Bass, 1974.

explanation or language varied, of course, depending on whom I was talking with, but it never took long for them to comprehend that what I was getting at was the sense that one was part of a readily available, mutually supportive network of relationships upon which one could depend and as a result of which one did not experience sustained feelings of loneliness that impel one to actions or to adopting a style of living masking anxiety and setting the stage for later and more destructive anguish. It is not merely a matter of how many people one knows, or how many close friends one has, or even the number of loved ones—if they are scattered all over the country or world, if they are not part of the structure of one's everyday living, and if they are not available to one in a 'give and get' way, they can have little affect on one's immediate or daily sense of community. Indeed, for many people these treasured but only occasionally available relationships accentuate the lack of a feeling of community. At a social gathering a colleague of mine once remarked: 'If in the community you live you have more than two close friends, you have one more than par.' Nobody disagreed. Immersed as we all are in a sea of human interaction it is the rare person who does not feel adrift, without a secure compass, and perceiving the signs of impending storm. Alienation, anomie, isolation, and words of similar meaning have flooded our language and literature. And paralleling this flood has been an outpouring of social group techniques to give people at least a transient experience of "authenticity" and "togetherness." The group dynamics and encounter movements (a bewildering array of ideas and techniques), communes, the different youth countercultures, the increasing frequency of formation of new fundamentalist religious groups which give meaning and direction to every hour of a member's day—these are only some of the indications of how earnestly people strive to be and feel part of a network of intimate relationships that gives one the sense of willing identification with some overarching values.

The community in which we live is a geo-political entity with which we feel little kinship. We may work in the community, pay taxes, and vote, but in no other respect feel a part of it. In fact, we may feel repelled by it because of the violence, crime, and conflict within it. We wish things were otherwise, but we feel impotent to do anything. We are aware that much money is being spent to repair our community, socially and physically, but the feeling persists that the seams of the community are not being tightened. We do not feel *needed* in our community and we rarely if ever seriously think about how we can contribute to the solution of its problems. We are busy during the day, tired at night, and seek recreation and entertainment on the weekends. And if we are parents, there are children who need our attention everyday. Where is there time to engage in a community activity? What community activity? What do I have to contribute? Where am I *needed*? Our lives are circumscribed spatially and psychologically, and it all seems so natural except for those poignant moments, quite frequent for many people, when we yearn to be part of a larger network of relationships that would give greater expression to our needs for intimacy, diversity, usefulness, and belongingness. The concept of the psychological sense of community is like that of hunger: neither is easy to define, but there is no mistaking it when an individual experiences the lack of a psychological sense of community, just as there is no mistaking what we think an individual experiences as a result of starvation. (pp. 1-3)*

A community's shared perception of its own strengths, competencies, control, and interdependence will be enhanced by professionals and programs that aim not at treating the problems of its individual members, but rather at amplifying a community's internal resources for modification or replacement of harmful social systems and institutions (Rappaport et al., 1975). Unfortunately, the role of the community or its subgroups vis-à-vis the typical behavior modification program is usually one of target recipient rather than collaborative participant. Behaviorists have demonstrated little appreciation for the fact that the process of maximally involving the community in its own change may be more important than the immediate outcomes of such change efforts. In fact, the ultimate contribution which a community psychologist might make is not the solution of social problems but the strengthening of a community by the planning of its own change.

Behaviorists' contributions to building a psychological sense of community would be heightened by a redirection of the goals of behavior modification programs as well as the style of program initiation and delivery. First psychologists might wish to concentrate on enhancing the strength of a community rather than eliminating or remedying its deficits. An example of this strategy is provided by Rappaport et al.'s (1975) establishment of an infant day-care center for single parents which allowed the parents to pursue their otherwise precluded educational and employment interests. Second, behavior modifiers should consider replacing their usual role as professional with one in which they function as consulting partners with community residents whose decision-making powers are fully independent of professional "good will." Finally, behavior modification programs with a goal of improving a community's social competence could seek to increase or reinforce the "constructive diversity" which a community manifests. The ways in which a community achieves its education, promotes its physical and mental health, insures its safety, protects its environment, and enhances the sense of vitality in its citizens typically represent only a small portion of the available means to the desired ends. A behavioral psychology that enables a community to "expand its repertoire" or create effective alternatives to existing social institutions will

---

*Sarason, S. B. *The psychological sense of community: Prospects for a community psychology*. San Francisco: Jossey-Bass, 1974.

require that cultural differences and individual variability be treated as desirable assets rather than undesirable liabilities.

Dissemination Research

One potential vehicle for the expression of more comprehensive social policy and programming could take the form of research aimed at the diffusion of successful intervention programs. This approach constitutes a professsionally responsible avenue for the stimulation of social change. The demand is that the social researcher not only focus attention on the development of empirically validated social change procedures but also engage in systematic efforts to initiate the adoption of successful procedures in other communities. Coupled with this charge is the responsibility to monitor the quality of the implanted program, assess the replicability of the original research, and assist in needed modifications.

One promising development in this direction has been the dissemination work carried out by the Achievement Place Project at the University of Kansas. Although the final outcome data are not yet available, it can be said with considerable certainty that the Achievement Place Project has demonstrated a highly successful methodology for providing a positive alternative for youthful offenders. Recognizing their responsibility for the diffusion of this project, a training program for potential teaching parents from several communities around the nation was initiated. The first phase of the diffusion effort was primarily concerned with providing potential teaching parents with the information and principles necessary for operating a teaching-family model program. Training sessions consisted of didactic instruction in the procedures of the Achievement Place Program, drawing heavily on a handbook that had been developed for that purpose (Phillips, Phillips, Fixsen, & Wolf, 1972). The training program evolved to include increasing focus on direct training of interpersonal skills for handling particular situations with the target resident groups and community agencies. The program was also extended to include on-site consultation by the training staff once the trained teaching parents assumed the operation of their own group home. Finally, procedures were implemented for evaluating the progress of each set of teaching parents in meeting the criteria of a site visit team comprised of representatives from the training program, the youth involved in their program, and community members involved in the initiation of the various replication sites (Braukman et al., 1975).

The successful extension process of diffusing the Achievement Place program involved a number of complex behavioral repertoires. Only by systematically monitoring the *in vivo* progress of each program, instituting retraining sessions for programs which were having difficulty, and continuing expansion of the initial training component to include practical as well as academic performances were consistently positive replications of the original Achievement Place Model attained. This program, as well as the pioneering work of Fairweather et al.

(1974), discussed earlier, provide the models for a needed direction in the behavioral movement.

Conceptual Needs

Conceptually, the behavioral paradigm has been victimized by its own provincialism. While behaviorists tend to view their theoretical background as one which emanates from general psychological principles, the theoretical model of most behavioral therapist-researchers remains one whose predominant roots are traceable to operant or respondent learning theories and not major psychological traditions such as social psychology, individual differences, organizational and physiological bases of behavior, cognition, and perception. To the extent that these traditions have been included, they have received their attention only recently and have served all too often only as positions against which behaviorists have reacted or have translated into the more "objective" semantics of behaviorism.

Apart from its selectiveness within the field of psychology, the behavior modification movement has allowed itself little interdisciplinary nourishment. Discussions of "reinforcement contingencies" and "behavior deficits" typically proceed without the encumbrance of considering economic, political, sociological, or bureaucratic-organizational contributions to human problems. Behavioral scientists have rarely been able to articulate theoretical rationales that were broad enough to support the social programs and policies that they might favor (Goodwin & Tu, 1975). At the same time, the conceptual narrowness of many behaviorists has prevented them from considering the functional relationships between the social systems in which they participate and the official designation of certain populations as problems, deviants, or victims. The ultimate danger of such theoretical sterility is that the behavioral paradigm will become as entrenched in institutionalized forms of service delivery and person-blaming as the ideologies it sought to replace (Rappaport et al., 1975).

The deficiencies of the behavioral paradigm in relation to the requirements of community psychology can be corrected by appropriate paradigmatic innovation. Following are three recommended paradigm expansions the pursuit of which could strengthen substantially the impact of behavioral interventions for community change.

1. Community psychology requires a paradigm whose involvement and abilities in active interventions are equal to its capacities for developing an empirically based science of social change. There is a need for professionals who are committed to being both advocates for the populations they serve and pursuers of data from which to create maximum impact programs for the creation of resourceful and resilient schools, environments, primary care services, and communities.

2. Another paradigm requirement is the theoretical flexibility to consider both the psychological factors that are excluded from the relatively prosaic

notions of learning histories, conditioning, and operant reinforcement as well as the extra-psychological influences (i.e., political, economic, and bureaucratic) that either mitigate or agitate social problems.

3.   A final innovation requires a paradigm whose view of community service is increasingly expansive such that the professional is viewed less often as a direct interventionist and more often as a program planner, consultant, trainer, and supervisor.

Training Models

One likely source of paradigm change is the development of new training models and programs for behavioral scientists. Most community psychologists, behavioral or not, have received their formal professional preparation in programs whose viability and existence have depended on their continuing alliance with clinical training programs in academic psychology departments. The product of this historically endorsed training has been what Sarason (1973) has termed the community clinical psychologist, a person whose efforts have been directed at (1) bringing clinical services to poor, disenfranchised groups, (2) inventing new clinical programs to meet the specific needs of those consumers, and (3) assessing the parameters of psychological and social disturbance in the community. The importance of these "person-centered" innovations (Cowen, 1973) to increased community mental health and the evolution of community psychology is substantial. However, the full achievement of a community psychology which aims at social system intervention for the purpose of disability prevention, constructive social change, and community growth will require the evolution of training programs which provide behavioral scientists with an interdisciplinary conception of behavior, an ability to function as system or program developers and consultants as well as direct interventionists, and an ideological and personal willingness for responsible activism coupled with careful empiricism.

Innovations in behaviorally based community psychology programs have occurred. At the University of Illinois, Seidman and Rappaport (1974) have developed an *educational pyramid* which uses professional, experienced psychologists as consultants and teachers of a larger number of graduate students who in turn train and supervise a larger number of undergraduates and other nonprofessionals as direct interventionists in various social systems such as the elementary schools, the juvenile justice system, psychiatric hospitals, and nursing facilities for the aged (see Fig. 12-1). Krasner (1975) has developed a similar program at the State University of New York at Stony Brook.

The educational pyramid is directed at four crucial needs of community psychology: "First, it includes a conceptual-methodological schema for understanding and evaluating the impact of community interventions at multiple levels of society. Second, it offers a model for training future professionals and nonprofessionals in their specific career goals. Third, the paradigm calls for

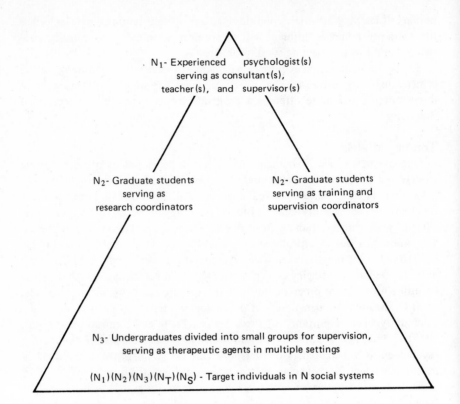

Fig. 12-1. The Educational Pyramid Applied to a University Setting. Note: The pyramid diagrammed represents one social system where N_1 refers to number of experienced psychologists; N_2 refers to the number of graduate student pairs supervised by each psychologist; N_3 refers to number of undergraduate therapeutic agents supervised by each graduate student pair; N_T refers to number of target individuals per therapeutic agent. In this particular case it is assumed that the above terms are constant across N_S, where N_S refers to number of social systems. Thus, $(N_1) (N_2) (N_3) (N_T) (N_S)$ equals the total number of people served by N_1 experienced psychologists. In the more general case when the above terms are not constant across N_S, the appropriate formula calls for an addition across

$$N_S \text{ or } \sum_{i=1}^{N_S} (N_1 \cdot N_2 \cdot N_3 \cdot N_T).$$

(From Seidman, E. and Rappaport, J. The educational pyramid: A paradigm for training, research and manpower utilization. *American Journal of Community Psychology*, 1974, *2*, 79-130.)

rigorous and systematic evaluation of human service programs. Fourth, and most obviously, the paradigm allows for efficient deployment of mental health manpower" (Seidman & Rappaport, 1974, p. 120). In addition, by formalizing two professional degree programs, the model has responded to the requirement that community psychologists be activist and empirical as well as the recognition that one type of professional might not choose to emphasize both dimensions equally. Graduate students in the Doctor of Psychology program are trained as intervention planners and coordinators with the expectation that they will assume career roles as directors and supervisors of social change programs. PhD students, on the other hand, receive predominantly research-oriented training in anticipation of their role as evaluators of program effectiveness and conceptualizers of novel programs.

Others have advocated a departure from the scientist-professional training model which has dominated both clinical and community psychology. For example, Libo (1974) has called for a two-track training program in which students specialize in either community psychology service or community psychology research. Both tracks would be preceded by a core curriculum in general and community psychology.

Programs whose faculty size or university resources prohibit a two-track system could consider developing training components that maximize the relevance of research to service functions. Leitenberg (1974) has described such a training model for the University of Vermont clinical program, which seeks to integrate service and research activities. The sequence involves the following components: (1) the student must generate a full-scale dissertation proposal relevant to a community problem encountered in each facility in which she or he is placed; the prevailing expectation is that the research will be of an applied nature; (2) each proposal must be presented to and approved by the student's faculty committee as well as the administrators of the placement facility; (3) one of these proposals is conducted as the student's dissertation research; (4) in most cases it is expected that some type of funding will be necessary for such research. Students will be responsible (with faculty consultation) for the preparation of grant proposals as a means of obtaining either intramural (university sources) or extramural (often the placement agency) research support; (5) in addition to the full dissertation report, the student must prepare the research for dissemination to both professional and public audiences.

A recurring theme of many new community psychology training models is the necessity of interdisciplinary preparation (Libo, 1974; Newbrough, 1973; Sarason, 1973). At the most basic level, students should be exposed to the nonpsychological factors which shape social systems and policies in which community psychologists are most likely to intervene. Sarason (1973) has identified several such areas including demography, labor relations, economy, politics, government, law, and public administration. Interdepartmental collaboration is essential to the adequate inclusion of these disciplines into community training programs.

At a more intense level, students could supplement this broadened perspective with a specific competence in some specialized area (e.g., criminal justice system, child care, environmental protection, educational innovation). In addition to didactic instruction in the specialty area, students would participate in supervised practica and/or "modularized internships" in the nontraditional settings associated with the area (Newbrough, 1973). Community placements could occur in any of a number of social service systems including (1) law enforcement or judicial agencies, (2) special rehabilitation programs (halfway houses, drug programs), (3) governmental settings (city councils, offices of urban planning, boards of education, human relations councils), (4) interdisciplinary research centers, and (5) academic programs with strong emphasis on specific social changes or populations (e.g., black studies, urban affairs, women's studies). In this same regard, Sarason (1973) has argued that "one of the greatest educational challenges confronting community psychology is the need for its students to have exposure to the full panoply of problems that impinge on communities large and small" (p. 96).

The most ambitious level of training innovation is represented by the suggestion that community psychology programs not be confined to traditional departments of psychology. Libo has expressed doubt that "any department of psychology, or any other single department for that matter, can, by itself, launch a functional training program [that] can do justice to what community psychology purports to cover" (Libo, 1974, p. 177). Alternatives to departmentally based training include multidisciplinary programs (e.g., environmental or behavioral sciences), college-wide divisions (e.g., allied health professions), and target-area programs which seek to train specialist professionals in areas such as the criminal justice system and city planning.

The second decade of applied behavior analysis has witnessed the extension of the paradigm from the chronic populations and closed institutions in which it was introduced to areas involving educational development, juvenile and adult crime, unemployment, environmental protection, alcoholism and drug abuse, community mental health, and aging. Behavior modifiers have applied their technology to these social problems with considerable amounts of energy and ingenuity. Our view of behavior modification's prospects for creating decisive and durable social change is cautiously optimistic. Although the behavioral paradigm has yet to outgrow the narrowness of its theoretical preferences and single-subject orientation, it represents an orientation which is potentially translatable into broader conceptualizations of behavior change and is sympathetic to the spirit of intervention research. The recent history of behavior modification as a source of educational innovations (Chapter 2) portends its ability to conceptualize and promote institutional change as opposed to the "psychoadaptation" of target populations (Renner, 1974).

Our survey of behavioral approaches to community problems has emphasized the current limitations that prevent behavior modification from attaining full status as a science and strategy of social change. This emphasis has been inspired by both a desire to portray realistically the empirically evaluated accomplishments of behavioral interventions and to guard against underestimating the gap between the present state of applied behavioral procedures and the requirements of an effective community psychology. At the same time, we are confident that we have not overestimated the resourcefulness and vitality of the behavioral paradigm to respond to the need for the applied and conceptual innovations that we have identified.

Our chosen emphasis on the current limitations of the behavioral paradigm is intended neither to dampen nor deter those involved in its application and extension to community problems. On the contrary, we would hope that this survey stimulates the innovations that would enable current practices to be replaced by more productive ones. A future of energetic innovation will insure that the initial achievements of behavioral community psychology are continued.

REFERENCES

Abel, G., Blanchard, E.B., Barlow, D.H., & Flanagan, B.A. A controlled behavioral treatment of a sadistic rapist. Paper presented at the ninth annual convention of the Association for the Advancement of Behavior Therapy, San Francisco, 1975.

Abelson, H., Cohen, R., Schrayer, D., & Rappeport, M. Drug experiences, attitudes and related behavior among adolescents and adults. In *Drug use in America: Problem in perspective*. Washington, D.C.: Government Printing Office, 1973.

Abraham, K. The psychological relations between sexuality and alcoholism. *International Journal of Psychoanalysis*, 1926, **7**, 2-10.

Adam, E.E. An analysis of changes in performance quality with operant conditioning procedures. *Journal of Applied Psychology*, 1972, **56**, 480-486.

Adams, G.M. & deVries, H.A. Physiological effects of an exercise training regimen upon women aged 52 to 79. *Journal of Gerontology*, 1973, **28**, 50-55.

Adams, K.A. The child who murders: A review of theory and research. *Criminal Justice and Behavior*, 1974, **1**, 51-61.

Adams, S. Evaluative research in corrections: An abbreviated tour guide. *Federal Probation*, 1974, March, **38**, 14-20.

Adams v. Carlson, 488 f 2nd 619 (7th Cir. 1973).

Adler, A. The individual psychology of the alcoholic patient. *Journal of Criminal Psychopathology*, 1941, **3**, 74-77.

Albee, G.W. *Mental health manpower trends*. New York: Basic Books, 1959.

Albee, G.W. The relation of conceptual models to manpower needs. In E.L. Cowen, E.A. Gardner, & M. Zax (Eds.), *Emergent approaches to mental health problems*. New York: Appleton-Century Crofts, 1967.

Albee, G.W. Conceptual models and manpower requirements in psychology. *American Psychologist*, 1968, **23**, 317-320.

Alden, L., Rappaport, J., & Seidman, E. College students as interventionists for primary-grade children: A comparison of structured academic and companionship programs for children from low-income families. *American Journal of Community Psychology*, 1975, **3**, 261-272.

Alexander, J.F. Defensive and supportive communications in normal and deviant families. *Journal of Consulting and Clinical Psychology*, 1973, **40**, 223.

Alexander, J.F., & Parsons, B.V. Short-term behavioral intervention with delinquent families: Impact on family process and recidivism. *Journal of Abnormal Psychology*, 1973, **81**, 219-225.

Altman, J. An operant analysis of heroin self-administration in man. Paper presented at the 82nd convention of the American Psychological Association, New Orleans, 1974.

Alvord, J.R. The home token economy: A motivational system for the home. *Corrective Psychiatry and Journal of Social Therapy*, 1971, **17**, 6-13.

American Enterprise Institute for Public Policy Research. *Manpower Training and Employment Proposals: Legislative Analysis*. Washington, D.C.: American Enterprise Institute, 1970.

Amir, M., & Berman, Y. Chromosomal deviation and crime. *Federal Probation*, 1970, **34**, 55-62.

Anant, S.S. A note on the treatment of alcholics by a verbal aversion technique. *Canadian Psychologist*, 1967, **8**, 19-22.

Anant, S.S. Former alcoholics and social drinking: An unexpected finding. *The Canadian Psychologist*, 1968a, **9**, 35.

Anant, S.S. Treatment of alcoholics and drug addicts by verbal conditioning techniques. *International Journal of the Addictions*, 1968b, **3**, 381-388.

Anderson, L.T., & Alpert, M. Operant analysis of hallucination frequency in a hospitalized schizophrenic. *Journal of Behavior Therapy and Experimental Psychiatry*, 1974, **5**, 13-18.

Anderson, L.T., Lubetkin, B., Logan, D., & Alpert, M. Comparison of relaxation methods for alcoholics: Differential relaxation vs. sensory awareness. *Proceedings of the 81st convention of the American Psychological Association*. Washington, D.C.: APA, 1973.

Ankus, M., & Quarrington, B. Operant behavior in the memory-disordered. *Journal of Gerontology*, 1972, **27**, 500-510.

Arehart, J.L. The search for a heroin "cure." *Science News*, 1972, **101**, 250-251.

Argyle, M. *The social psychology of work*. New York: Taplinger, 1972.

Arie, T. Day care in geriatric psychiatry. *Gerontologia Clinica*, 1975, **17**, 31-39.

Arkowitz, H. College dating inhibitions: Assessment and treatment. Paper presented at the annual meeting of the American Psychological Association, Montreal, 1973.

Arnon, D., Kleinman, M., & Kissin, B. Psychological differentiation in heroin addicts. *The International Journal of the Addictions*, 1974, **9**, 151-160.

Aron, W., & Daily, D. Short- and long-term therapeutic communities: A follow-up and cost effectiveness comparison. *The International Journal of the Addictions*, 1974, **9**, 619-636.

Arthur, G.L., Donnan, H.H., & Lair, C.V. Companionship therapy with nursing home aged. *Gerontologist*, 1973, **13**, 167-170.

Arvey, R.D., & Mussio, S.J. Job expectation and valences of job rewards for culturally disadvantaged and advantaged clerical employees. *Journal of Applied Psychology*, 1974, **59**, 230-232.

Ashem, B., & Donner, L. Covert sensitization with alcoholics: A controlled replication. *Behavior Research and Therapy*, 1968, **6**, 7-12.

Associated Press. Zarb backs new utility rate schedules. In *The Louisville Courier-Journal*, June 12, 1975.

Atthowe, J.M. Behavior innovation and persistence. *American Psychologist*, 1973a, **28**, 34-41.

Atthowe, J.M. Token economics come of age. *Behavior Therapy*, 1973b, **4**, 646-654.

Atthowe, J.M. Behavioral rehabilitation of hospitalized patients. In R.A. Winett (chair), *Behavior modification in the community: Progress and problems.* Symposium presented at the 83rd convention of the American Psychological Association, Chicago, 1975.

Atthowe, J.M., & Krasner, L. Preliminary report on the application of contingency response procedures (token economy) on a "chronic" psychiatric ward. *Journal of Abnormal Psychology*, 1968, **73**, 37-43.

Ayllon, T., & Azrin, N.H. *The token economy: A motivational system for therapy and rehabilitation.* New York: Appleton-Century-Crofts, 1968.

Ayllon, T., & Kelly, K. Effects of reinforcement on standardized test performance. *Journal of Applied Behavior Analysis*, 1972, **5**, 477-484.

Ayllon, T., Layman, D., & Burke, S. Disruptive behavior and reinforcement of academic performance. *The Psychological Record*, 1972, **22**, 315-323.

Ayllon, T., Layman, D., & Kandel, H.J. A behavioral-educational alternative to drug control of hyperactive children. *Journal of Applied Behavior Analysis*, 1975, **8**, 137-147.

Ayllon, T., & Roberts, M. Eliminating discipline problems by strengthening academic performance. *Journal of Applied Behavior Analysis*, 1974, **7**, 71-76.

Azrin, N.H., Flores, T., & Kaplan, S.J. Job-finding club: A group-assisted program for obtaining employment. *Behaviour Research and Therapy*, 1975, **13**, 17-27.

Azrin, N.H., & Holz, W.C. Punishment. In W.K. Honig (Ed.), *Operant behavior: Areas of research and application.* New York: Appleton, 1966.

Bahn, A.K. An outline for community mental health research. *Community Mental Health Journal*, 1965, **1**, 23-28.

Bailey, J. *Correctional outcome: An evaluation of 100 reports.* School of Social Welfare, University of California at Los Angeles, 1961.

Bailey, J.S., Timbers, G.D., Phillips, E.L., & Wolf, M.M. Modification of articulation errors of pre-delinquents by their peers. *Journal of Applied Behavior Analysis*, 1971, **4**, 265-281.

Bailey, J.S., Wolf, M.M., & Phillips, E.L. Home-based reinforcement and the modification of pre-delinquents' classroom behavior. *Journal of Applied Behavior Analysis*, 1970, **3**, 223-233.

Ballard, K.D., & Glynn, T. Behavioral self-management in story writing with elementary school children. *Journal of Applied Behavior Analysis*, 1975, **8**, 387-398.

Bander, K.W., Steinke, G.V., Allen, G.J., & Mosher, D.L. Evaluation of three dating-specific treatment approaches for heterosexual dating anxiety. *Journal of Consulting and Clinical Psychology*, 1975, **43**, 259-265.

Bandura, A. *Principles of behavior modification*. New York: Holt, Rinehart & Winston, 1969.

Bandura, A. *Aggression: A social learning analysis*. Englewood Cliffs, N.J.: Prentice-Hall, 1973.

Bandura, A. Behavior theory and the models of man. *American Psychologist*, 1974, **29**, 859-869.

Bandura, A., & Walters, R. *Social learning and personality development*. New York: Holt, Rinehart & Winston, 1964.

Barbee, J.R., & Keil, E.C. Experimental techniques of job interview training for the disadvantaged: Videotape feedback, behavior modification, and microcounseling. *Journal of Applied Psychology*, 1973, **58**, 209-213.

Bard, M. Family intervention teams as a community mental health resource. *Journal of Criminal Law, Criminology and Police Science*, 1969, **60**, 247-250.

Barnes, J.A. Effects of reality orientation classroom on memory loss, confusion, and disorientation in geriatric patients. *Gerontologist*, 1974, **14**, 138-142.

Barrish, H.H., Saunders, M., & Wolf, M.M. Good behavior game effects of individual contingencies for group consequences on disruptive behavior in a classroom. *Journal of Applied Behavior Analysis*, 1969, **2**, 119-124.

Barrow, G.M. Physicians' attitudes toward aging and the aging process. *Dissertation Abstracts International*, 1971, **32**, (4-A), 2205.

Bartels, B.D., & Tyler, J.D. Paraprofessionals in the community mental health center. *Professional Psychology*, 1975, **6**, 442-452.

Bass, B.M., & Alexander, R.A. Climate, economy, and the differential migration of white and nonwhite workers. *Journal of Applied Psychology*, 1972, **56**, 518-521.

Bass, H., & Brown, B. Methadone maintenance and methadone detoxification: A comparison of retention rates and client characteristics. *The International Journal of the Addictions*, 1973, **8**, 889-896.

Bassett, J., Blanchard, E.B., Harrison, H., & Wood, R. Applied behavior analysis on a county penal farm: A method of increasing attendance at a remedial education center. *Proceedings of the 81st Annual Convention of the American Psychological Association*. Washington, D.C.: APA, 1973.

Battalio, R. Personal communication. Summer 1975.

Beasley, R.W., & Antunes, G. The etiology of urban crime: An ecological analysis. *Criminology*, 1974, **11**, 439-461.

Beatty, R.W. Supervisory behavior related to job success of hard-core unemployed over a two-year period. *Journal of Applied Psychology*, 1974, **59**, 38-42.

Beaubrun, M Treatment of alcoholism in Trinidad and Tobago, 1956-1965. *British Journal of Psychiatry*, 1967, **113**, 643-658.

Becker, H. *Outsiders: Studies in the sociology of deviance.* Glencoe, Ill.: The Free Press, 1963.

Becker, J.M., Haber, W., & Levitan, S.A. *Programs to aid the unemployed in the 1960's.* Kalamazoo: Upjohn Institute for Employment Research, 1965.

Becker, W.C. *Parents are teachers: A child management program.* Champaign, Ill.: Research Press, 1969.

Bednar, R.L., Zelhart, P.F., Greathouse, L., & Weinberg, S. Operant conditioning principles in the treatment of learning and behavior problems with delinquent boys. *Journal of Counseling Psychology*, 1970, **17**, 492-497.

Bell, B.D. Mobile medical care to the elderly: An evaluation. *Gerontologist*, 1975, **15**, 100-103.

Bell, W.G., & Olsen, W.T. An overview of public transportation and the elderly: New directions for social policy. *Gerontologist*, 1974, **14**, 324-330.

Bellack, L. (Ed.) *Handbook of community psychiatry and community mental health.* New York: Grune & Stratton, 1964.

Bellack, L. Overview and introduction: Community mental health – ten years later. In L. Bellack (Ed.) *A concise handbook of community psychiatry and community mental health.* New York: Grune & Stratton, 1974.

Bender, L. Psychopathic behavior disorders in children. In R. Linder & R. Seliger (Eds.), *Handbook of correctional psychology.* New York: Philosophical Press, 1947.

Bennett, C.C., Anderson, L.S., Hassol, L., Klein, D., & Rosenblum, G. (Eds.) *Community psychology: A report of the Boston conference on the education of psychologists for community mental health.* Boston: Boston University & South Shore Mental Health Center, 1966.

Bennis, W.G., Benne, K.D., & Chin, R. *The planning of change* (2nd ed.). New York: Holt, Rinehart & Winston, 1969.

Bereiter, C., & Englemann, S. *Teaching disadvantaged children in the preschool.* Englewood Cliffs, N.J.: Prentice-Hall, 1966.

Berg, W.E., Atlas, L., & Zeiger, J. Integrated homemaking services for the aged in urban neighborhoods. *Gerontologist*, 1974, **14**, 338-393.

Bergler, E. Personality traits of alcohol addicts. *Quarterly Journal of Studies on Alcohol*, 1946, **1**, 356-361.

Bernstein, D. Modification of smoking: An evaulative review. *Psychological Bulletin*, 1969, **71**, 418-440.

Berwick, P., & Morris, U. Token economies: Are they doomed? *Professional Psychology*, 1974, **5**, 434-439.

Berzins, J.I., Therapist-patient matching. In A.S. Gurman & A.M. Razin (Eds.), *Effective Psychotherapy.* Elmsford, N.Y.: Pergamon Press, in press.

Berzins, J.I., Bednar, R.L., & Severy, L. The problem of intersource consensus in measuring therapeutic outcomes: New data and multivariate perspectives. *Journal of Abnormal Psychology*, 1975, **84**, 10-19.

Berzins, J.I., & Ross, W. Experimental assessment of the responsiveness of addict patients to the "influence" of professionals versus other addicts. *Journal of Abnormal Psychology*, 1972, **80**, 141-148.

Biase, D. A comparative study of addicted community and penitentiary volunteers NACC (967-968) for treatment at Phoenix House. Unpublished manuscript, 1970.

Bigelow, G.E., Cohen, M., Liebson, I., & Faillace, L. Abstinence and moderation: Choice by alcoholics. *Behaviour Research and Therapy*, 1972, **10**, 209-214.

Bigelow, G.E., Lawrence, C., Harris, A., & D'Lugoff, B. Contingency management and behavior therapy in a methadone maintenance program. Paper presented at the 82nd convention of the American Psychological Association, New Orleans, 1974.

Bigelow, G.E., Liebson, I., & Griffiths, R. Experimental analysis of alcoholic drinking. In C.M. Franks (chair), *Can alcoholics learn to control their drinking?* Symposium at the meeting of the American Psychological Association, Montreal, 1973.

Bigelow, G.E., Liebson, I., & Griffiths, R. Alcoholic drinking: Suppression by a behavioral time-out procedure. *Behaviour Research and Therapy*, 1974, **12**, 107-115.

Birkett, D.P., & Boltuch, B. Remotivation therapy. *Journal of the American Geriatric Society*, 1973, **21**, 368-371.

Birnbaum, B. The right to treatment. *American Bar Association Journal*, 1960, **46**, 499.

Blachly, P.H. An "electric needle" for aversive conditioning of the needle ritual. *The International Journal of the Addictions*, 1971, **6**, 327-328.

Blachly, P.H. Naloxone for diagnosis in methadone programs. *Journal of the American Medical Association*, 1973, **224**, 334.

Blackford, L. *Student drug use surveys: San Mateo County, California.* San Mateo: County Department of Health and Welfare, 1974.

Blake, B.G. The application of behavior therapy to the treatment of alcoholism. *Behaviour Research and Therapy*, 1965, **3**, 75-85.

Blake, B.G. A follow-up of alcoholics treated by behavior therapy. *Behaviour Research and Therapy*, 1967, **5**, 89-94.

Blonsky, L.E. Problems in development of a community action program for the elderly. *Gerontologist*, 1974, **14**, 394-401.

Bloom, B.L. *Community mental health: A historical and critical analysis.* Morristown, N.J.: General Learning Press, 1973.

Bloom, R., & Barry, J.R. Determinants of work attitudes among Negroes. *Journal of Applied Psychology*, 1967, **51**, 291-294.

Bloomfield, H.H. Assertive training in an outpatient group of chronic schizo-phrenics: A preliminary report. *Behavior Therapy*, 1973, **4**, 227-281.

Blum, E. Psychoanalytic views of alcoholism. *Quarterly Journal of Studies on Alcohol*, 1966, **27**, 259-299.

Blum, R.H., & Braunstein, L. Mind-altering drugs and dangerous behavior: Alcohol. In U.S. President's Commission, *Task Force Report: Drunkenness.* Washington, D.C.: Government Printing Office, 1967.

Blumenthal, R. Many transport systems retain crisis-won riders. *The New York Times*, June 2, 1975.

Boehm, V.R. Negro-white differences in validity of employment and training selection procedures: Summary of research evidence. *Journal of Applied Psychology*, 1972, **56**, 33-39.

Bolin, D.C., & Kivens, L. Evaluation in a community mental health center: Huntsville, Alabama. *Evaluation*, 1974, **2**, 26-35.

Bolman, W.M. An outline of preventive psychiatric programs for children. *Archives of General Psychiatry*, 1968, **17**, 5-8.

Bolstad, S.R., & Johnson, S.M. Self-regulation in the modification of disruptive classroom behavior. *Journal of Applied Behavior Analysis*, 1972, **5**, 443-454.

Boren, J., & Colman, A. Some experiments on reinforcement principles within a psychiatric ward for delinquent soldiers. *Journal of Applied Behavior Analysis*, 1970, **3**, 29-38.

Bornstein, P., Bugge, I., & Davol, G. Good principle, wrong target — An exten-sion of "Token economies come of age." *Behavior Therapy*, 1975, **6**, 63-67.

Bottrell, J. Behavior modification programs: Analogies from prisons to mental institutions. Paper presented at the 82nd annual convention of the American Psychological Association, New Orleans, 1974.

Boudin, H. Contingency contracting as a therapeutic tool in the deceleration of amphetamine use. *Behavior Therapy*, 1972, **3**, 604-608.

Boudin, H., Valentine, V., Ingraham, R., Brantley, J., Ruiz, M., Smith, G., Catlin, R., & Regan, E. Contingency contracting with drug addicts in the natural environment. Unpublished manuscript, University of Florida, 1974.

Bourne, P., Alford, J., & Bowcock, J. Treatment of skid-row alcoholics with Disulfiram. *Quarterly Journal of Studies on Alcohol*, 1966, **27**, 42-48.

Bowles, P.E., & Nelson, R.O. The efficacy of an inservice workshop and the bug-in-the-ear technique in training teachers as mediators. Unpublished manu-script, University of North Carolina at Greensboro, 1974.

Boyd, R., & Oakes, C. (Eds.) *Foundations of practical gerontology.* Columbia: University of South Carolina Press, 1969.

Brakel, S. Diversion from the criminal process: Informal discretion, motivation and formalization. *Denver Law Journal*, 1971, **48**, 211-227.

Braukmann, C.J., Fixsen, D.L., Kirigin, K.A., Phillips, E.A., Phillips, E.L., & Wolf, M.M. Dissemination of the teaching-family model. In R. Winett (chair), *Symposium on behavior modification in the community: Progress and prob-lems.* 83rd convention of the American Psychological Association, Chicago, 1975.

Braukmann, C.J., Maloney, D.M., Fixsen, D.L., Phillips, E.L., & Wolf, M.M. An analysis of the effects of training on interview skills. Presented at the convention of the American Psychological Association, Washington, D.C., September 1971.

Braun, S.H. Ethical issues in behavior modification. *Behavior Therapy*, 1975, **6**, 51-62.

Braverman, J. Report on state licensure regulations: Codes contribute to low standards of care. *Modern Nursing Home*, 1970, **24**, 5-9.

Brayfield, A.H. Community mental health center programs. *American Psychologist*, 1967, **22**, 670-673.

Brecher, E. *Licit and illicit drugs*. Boston: Little, Brown, 1972.

Brigham, T.A., Finfrock, S.R., Breunig, M.K., & Bushell, D., Jr. The use of programmed materials in the analysis of academic contingencies. *Journal of Applied Behavior Analysis*, 1972, **5**, 177-182.

Brigham, T.A., Graubard, P.S., & Stans, A. Analysis of the effects of sequential reinforcement contingencies on aspects of composition. *Journal of Applied Behavior Analysis*, 1972, **5**, 421-429.

Brill, L. Some comments on the paper "Social control in therapeutic communities" by Dan Waldorf. *The International Journal of the Addictions*, 1971, **6**, 45-50.

Briscoe, N., Hoffman, D., & Bailey, J. Behavioral community psychology: Training a community board to problem solve. *Journal of Applied Behavior Analysis*, 1975, **8**, 157-168.

Broden, M., Bruce, C., Mitchell, M.A., Carter, V., & Hall, R.V. Effects of teacher attention on attending behavior of two boys at adjacent desks. *Journal of Applied Behavior Analysis*, 1970, **3**, 199-203.

Brodsky, S.L. *Psychologists in the criminal justice system*. Urbana, Ill.: University of Illinois Press, 1973a.

Brodsky, S.L. Prometheus in the prison: Informed participation by convicted persons. Paper presented at the 81st annual convention of the American Psychological Association, Montreal, 1973b.

Brody, E.M., Kleban, M.H., Lawton, M.P., & Moss, M. A longitudinal look at excess disabilities in the mentally impaired aged. *Journal of Gerontology*, 1974, **29**, 79-84.

Bronfenbrenner, U. *Two worlds of childhood*. New York: Russel Sage, 1970.

Bronfenbrenner, U. Developmental research, public policy, and the ecology of childhood. *Child Development*, 1974, **45**, 1-5.

Brook, R., & Whitehead, P. Colloquialisms of the therapeutic community: Treatment of the adolescent drug abuser. *Federal Probation*, 1973, **37**, 46-49.

Brotman, H.B. *Who are the aged: A demographic view*. Occasional papers in gerontology number 1 of the Institute of Gerontology. Ann Arbor: University of Michigan, 1968.

Brown, A.S. Satisfying relationships for the elderly and their patterns of disengagement. *Gerontologist*, 1974, **14**, 258-262.

Brown, G.D., & Tyler, V.O. Time out from reinforcement: A technique for dethroning the "duke" of an institutionalized delinquent group. *Journal of Child Psychology and Psychiatry*, 1968, **9**, 203-211.

Brown, R.E., Copeland, R.E., & Hall, R.V. The school principal as a behavior modifier. *Journal of Educational Research*, 1972, **66**, 175-180.

Bruun, K. Significance of role and norms in the small group for individual behavioral changes while drinking. *Quarterly Journal of Studies on Alcohol*, 1959, **20**, 53-64.

Buehler, R.E., Patterson, G.R., & Furniss, J.M. The reinforcement of behavior in institutional settings. *Behaviour Research and Therapy*, 1966, **4**, 157-167.

Burchard, J.D. Systematic socialization: A programmed environment for the habilitation of antisocial retardates. *Psychological Record*, 1967, **17**, 461-476.

Burchard, J.D., & Barrera, F. An analysis of time out and response cost in a programmed environment. *Journal of Applied Behavior Analysis*, 1972, **5**, 271-282.

Burchard, J.D., & Tyler, V. The modification of delinquent behavior through operant conditioning. *Behaviour Research and Therapy*, 1965, **2**, 245-250.

Burgess, R.L., Clark, R.N., & Hendee, J.C. An experimental analysis of anti-litter procedures. *Journal of Applied Behavior Analysis*, 1971, **4**, 71-75.

Burrill, R.H., McCourt, J.F., & Cutter, H.S.G. Beer: A social facilitator for PMI patients. *Gerontologist*, 1974, **14**, 430-431.

Burvill, P.W. Physical illness in the elderly. *Gerontologia Clinica*, 1970, **12**, 288-296.

Butler, R.N. Summary statement on psychiatric perspective. *Interdisciplinary Topics in Gerontology*, 1969, **3**, 137-144.

Cahoon, D.D., & Crosby, C. A learning approach to chronic drug use: Sources of reinforcement. *Behavior Therapy*, 1972, **3**, 64-71.

Caird, F.I., Judge, T.G., & Macleod, C. Pointers to possible malnutrition in the elderly at home. *Gerontologia Clinica*, 1975, **17**, 47-54.

Callahan, E.J., & Leitenberg, H. Aversion therapy for sexual deviation: Contingent shock and covert sensitization. *Journal of Abnormal Psychology*, 1973, **81**, 60-73.

Callner, D. Behavioral treatment approaches to drug abuse: A critical review of the research. *Psychological Bulletin*, 1975, **82**, 143-164.

Callner, D.A., & Ross, S.M. The assessment and training of assertive skills with drug addicts: A preliminary study. Paper presented at the annual meeting of the American Psychological Association, Montreal, 1973.

Campbell, D.T. Reforms as experiments. *American Psychologist*, 1969, **24**, 409-429.

Campbell, D.T., & Fiske, D.W. Convergent and discriminant validation by the multi-trait multi-method matrix. *Psychological Bulletin*, 1959, **24**, 409-429.

Campbell, D.T., Sanderson, R.E., & Laverty, S.G. Characteristics of a conditioned response in human subjects during extinction trials following a single traumatic conditioning trial. *Journal of Abnormal and Social Psychology*, 1964, **68**, 627-639.

Campbell, D.T., & Stanley, J. *Experimental and quasi-experimental designs for research*. Chicago: Rand McNally, 1966.

Campbell, J.P., & Dunnette, M.D. Effectiveness of T-group experiences in managerial training and development. *Psychological Bulletin*, 1968, **70**, 73-104.

Cantrell, R.P., Cantrell, M.L., Huddleston, C.M., & Woolridge, R.L. Contingency contracting with school problems. *Journal of Applied Behavior Analysis*, 1969, **2**, 215-220.

Caplan, G. Types of mental health consultation. *American Journal of Orthopsychiatry*, 1963, **33**, 470-481.

Caplan, G. *Principles of preventive psychiatry*. New York: Basic Books, 1964.

Caplan, H., & Nelson, S. The nature and consequences of psychological research on social problems. *American Psychologist*, 1973, **28**, 199-211.

Cappell, H., & Herman, C.P. Alcohol and tension reduction: A review. *Quarterly Journal of Studies on Alcohol*, 1972, **33**, 33-64.

Cartwright, D., Kirtner, W., & Fiske, D. Method factors in changes associated with psychotherapy. *Journal of Abnormal and Social Psychology*, 1963, **66**, 164-175.

Casriel, D., & Amen, G. *Daytop*. New York: Hill & Wang, 1971.

Caudill, B., & Marlatt, G. Modeling influences in social drinking: An experimental analogue. *Journal of Consulting and Clinical Psychology*, 1975, **43**, 405-415.

Cautela, J.R. Behavior therapy and geriatrics. *Journal of Genetic Psychology*, 1966, **108**, 9-17.

Cautela, J.R. Covert sensitization. *Psychological Reports*, 1967, **20**, 459-468.

Cautela, J.R. The treatment of alcoholism by covert sensitization. *Psychotherapy: Theory, Research, and Practice*, 1970, **7**, 86-90.

Cautela, J.R., & Rosenstiel, A.K. Use of covert sensitization in treatment of drug abuse. *The International Journal of the Addictions*, 1975, **10**, 277-303.

Cayner, J.J., & Kiland, J.R. Use of brief time out with three schizophrenic patients. *Journal of Behavior Therapy and Experimental Psychiatry*, 1974, **5**, 141-145.

Chafetz, M.E. Addictions III: Alcoholism. In A.M. Freedman & H.I. Kaplan (Eds.), *Comprehensive textbook of psychiatry*. Baltimore: Williams & Wilkins, 1967.

Chafetz, M.E., & Demone, H.W. Jr. *Alcoholism and society*. New York: Oxford University Press, 1962.

Chapanis, A. Human engineering environments for the aging. *Gerontologist*, 1974, **14**, 228-235.

Chapman, C., & Risley, T.R. Anti-litter procedures in an urban high-density area. *Journal of Applied Behavior Analysis*, 1974, **7**, 377-383.

Chatfield, S. Pretrial disposition in the Twin Cities. *American Bar Association Journal*, 1974, **60**, 1089-1092.

Cheek, F., Tomarchio, T., Standen, J., & Albahary, R. Methadone plus – A behavior modification training program in self-control for addicts on methadone maintenance. *The International Journal of the Addictions* 1973, **8**, 969-996.

Chein, L., Gerard, D., Lee, R., & Rosenfeld, E. *The road to H*. New York: Basic Books, 1964.

Chinlund, S. Urgent questions about heroin maintenance programs. *Federal Probation*, 1973, **37**, 43-45.

Christensen, A., & Arkowitz, H. Preliminary report on practice dating and feedback as treatment for college dating problems. *Journal of Counseling Psychology*, 1974, **21**, 92-95.

Christensen, A., Arkowitz, H., & Anderson, J. Beaus for cupid's errors: Practice dating as treatment for college dating inhibitions. Unpublished manuscript, University of Oregon, 1975.

Cicchetti, D.V., Fletcher, C.R., Lerner, E., & Colemen, J.V. Effects of a social medicine course on the attitudes of medical students toward the elderly: A controlled study. *Journal of Gerontology*, 1973, **28**, 370-373.

Claeson, L.E., & Malm, U. Electro-aversion therapy of chronic alcoholism. *Behaviour Research and Therapy*, 1973, **11**, 663-66.

Clancy, J., VanderHoff, E., & Campbell, D. Evaluation of an aversive technique as a treatment for alcoholism: Controlled trial with succinylcholine-induced apnea. *Quarterly Journal of Studies on Alcohol*, 1967, **20**, 476-485.

Clark, H.B., & Boyd, S.B., & Macrae, J.W. A classroom program teaching disadvantaged youths to write biographic information. *Journal of Applied Behavior Analysis*, 1975, **8**, 67-75.

Clark, H.B., & Macrae, J.W. The use of imposed and self selected training packages to establish classroom teaching skills. *Journal of Applied Behavior Analysis*, 1976, **9**, 105.

Clark, H.B., & Risley, T.R. Experimentally specifying and effectively disseminating normal child rearing procedures. Paper at sixth Banff International conference on behavior modification, Canada, 1974.

Clark, J.V., & Arkowitz, H. The behavioral treatment of social inhibition: A case report. Unpublished manuscript, University of Oregon, 1974.

Clark, R. *Crime in America*. New York: Simon & Schuster, 1970.

Clark, R.N., Burgess, R.L., & Hendee, J.C. The development of anti-litter behavior in a forest campground. *Journal of Applied Behavior Analysis*, 1972, **5**, 1-5.

Clegg, R. *Probation and parole: Principles and practices*. Springfield, Ill.: Thomas, 1964.

Clemente, F., & Summers, G.F. Industrial development and the elderly: A longitudinal analysis. *Journal of Gerontology*, 1973, **28**, 479-483.

Clements, C., & McKee, J. Programmed instruction for institutionalized offenders: Contingency management and performance contracts. *Psychological Reports*, 1968, **22**, 957-964.

Clonce V. Richardson, 379 F Supp 338 (W.D. Mo, 1974).

Clore, G.L. *Interpersonal attraction – An overview*. Morristown, N.J.: General Learning Press, 1974.

Cloward, R.D. Studies in tutoring. *Journal of Experimental Education*, 1967, **36**, 14-25.

Cloward, R., & Ohlin, L. *Delinquency and opportunity: A theory of delinquent gangs*. New York: The Free Press, 1960.

Cobb, J.A. Relationship of discrete classroom behaviors to fourth-grade academic achievement. *Journal of Educational Psychology*, 1972, **63**, 74-80.

Coghlan, A., Dohrenwend, E., Gold, S., & Zimmerman, R. A psychobehavioral residential drug abuse program: A new adventure in adolescent psychiatry. *The International Journal of the Addictions*, 1973, **8**, 767-778.

Cohen, H.L. Educational therapy: The design of learning environments. *Research in Psychotherapy*, 1968, **3**, 21-58.

Cohen, H.L., & Filipczak, J. *A new learning environment*. San Francisco: Jossey-Bass, 1971.

Cohen, J. *Secondary motivation: Eyewitness series in psychology*. Chicago: Rand McNally, 1970.

Cohen, M., Liebson, I.A., & Faillace, L.A. Modification of drinking in chronic alcoholics. In N. Mello & J. Mendelson (Eds.), *Recent advances in studies of alcoholism*. Washington, D.C. Government Printing Office, 1971a.

Cohen, M., Liebson, I.A., & Faillace, L.A. The role of reinforcement contingencies in chronic alcoholism: An experimental analysis of one case. *Behaviour Research and Therapy*, 1971b, **9**, 375-379.

Cohen, M., Liebson, I.A., & Faillace, L.A. Controlled drinking by chronic alcoholics over extended periods of free access. *Psychological Reports*, 1973, **32**, 1107-1110.

Cohen, M., Liebson, I.A., Faillace, L.A., & Allen, R.P. Moderate drinking by chronic alcoholics. *Journal of Nervous and Mental Diseases*, 1971, **153**, 434-444.

Cohen, M., Liebson, I.A., Faillace, L.A., & Speers, W. Alcoholism: Controlled drinking and incentives for abstinence. *Psychological Reports*, 1971, **28**, 575-580.

Coleman, J. *Abnormal psychology and modern life*. (4th ed.) Glenview, Ill.: Scott, Foresman, 1972.

Coleman, R. Response generalization in two categories of classroom behavior. *Psychological Reports*, 1974, **34**, 1167-1173.

Collier, W., & Hijazi, Y. A follow-up of former residents of a therapeutic community. *The International Journal of the Addictions*, 1974, **9**, 805-826.

Collins, R.W., & Plaska, T. Mowrer's conditioning treatment for enuresis applied to geriatric residents of a nursing home. *Behavior Therapy*, 1975, **6**, 632-638.

Colman, A., & Baker, S. Utilization of an operant conditioning model for the treatment of character and behavior disorders in a military setting. *American Journal of Psychiatry*, 1969, **125**, 101-109.

Colman, A., & Boren, J. An information system for measuring patient behavior and its use by staff. *Journal of Applied Behavior Analysis*, 1969, **2**, 207-214.

Colthart, S.M. A mental health unit in a skilled nursing facility. *Journal of the American Geriatric Society*, 1974, **22**, 453-456.

Columbia Journal of Law and Social Problems, Nondelinquent children in New York: The need for alternatives to institutional treatment. 1972, **8**(3), 251-284.

Cone, J.D. Assessing the effectiveness of programmed generalization. *Journal of Applied Behavior Analysis*, 1973, **6**, 713-718.

Conger, J.J. Alcoholism: Theory, problem and challenge. II. Reinforcement theory and the dynamics of alcoholism. *Quarterly Journal of Studies on Alcohol*, 1956, **17**, 291-324.

Conrad, J. *Crime and its correction*. Berkeley: University of California Press, 1965.

Cooper, M.L., Thomson, C.L., & Baer, D.M. The experimental modification of teacher attending behavior. *Journal of Applied Behavior Analysis*, 1970, **3**, 153-157.

Copeland, R.E., Brown, R.E., Axelrod, S., & Hall, R.V. Effects of a school principal praising parents for school attendance. *Educational Technology*, 1972, **12**, 56-59.

Copeland, R.E., Brown, R.E., & Hall, R.V. The effects of principal-implemented techniques on the behavior of pupils. *Journal of Applied Behavior Analysis*, 1974, **7**, 77-86.

Corey, J.R., & Shamow, J. The effects of fading on the acquisition and retention of oral reading. *Journal of Applied Behavior Analysis*, 1972, **5**, 311-315.

Cossairt, A., Hall, R.V., & Hopkins, B.L. The effects of experimenter's instructions, feedback, and praise on teacher praise and student attending behavior. *Journal of Applied Behavior Analysis*, 1973, **6**, 89-104.

Costello, R.M. Alcoholism treatment and evaluation: In search of methods. *The International Journal of the Addictions*, 1975, **10**, 251-275.

The Courier-Journal. Both consumers and utilities need help (editorial). *The Courier Journal*. Louisville, Kentucky, March 31, 1975a.

The Courier-Journal. Deposit law can cut litter, save energy (editorial). *The Courier-Journal*, Louisville, Kentucky, August 5, 1975b.

The Courier-Journal. Utility rates should hit the biggest users the hardest (editorial). *The Courier-Journal*, Louisville, Kentucky, May 6, 1975c.

Cowen, E.L. Mothers in the classroom. *Psychology Today*, 1969, **2**, 36-39.

Cowen, E.L. Social and community interventions. *Annual Review of Psychology*, 1973, **24**, 423-472.

Cowen, E.L., Dorr, D., Clarfield, S.P., Kreling, B., Pokracki, F., Pratt, D.M., Terrell, D.L., & Wilson, A.B. The AML: A quick screening device for early detection of school maladaptation. *American Journal of Community Psychology*, 1973, **1**, 12-35.

Cowen, E.L., Dorr, D., Izzo, L.D., Madonia, A.J., & Trost, M.A. The primary mental health project: A new way of conceptualizing and delivering school mental health services. *Psychology in the Schools*, 1971, **5**, 216-225.

Cowen, E.L., Dorr, D., Trost, M.A., & Izzo, L.D. A follow-up study of maladapting school children seen by nonprofessionals. *Journal of Consulting and Clinical Psychology*, 1972, **36**, 235-238.

Cowen, E.L., Gardner, E.A., & Zax, M. (Eds.) *Emergent approaches to mental health problems*. New York: Meredith, 1967.

Cowen, E.L., & Schochet, B.V. Referral and outcome differences between terminating and nonterminating children seen by nonprofessionals in a school mental health project. *American Journal of Community Psychology*, 1973, **1**, 103-112.

Cox, T., & Longwell, B. Reliability of interview data concerning current heroin use from heroin addicts on methadone. *The International Journal of the Addictions*, 1974, **9**, 161-166.

Craig, M., & Furst, P.W. What happens after treatment. Report from New York City Youth Board, Research Department, 1965. *Social Service Review*, 1965, **39**, 165-171.

Craighead, W.E., Mercatoris, M., & Bellack, B. A brief report on mentally retarded residents as behavioral observers. *Journal of Applied Behavior Analysis*, 1974, **7**, 333-340.

Cressey, D. Achievement of an unstated organizational goal: An observation on prisons. In L. Hazelrigg (Ed.), *Prison within society*. Garden City, N.J.: Anchor Books, 1969.

Curran, J.P. Social skills training and systematic desensitization in reducing dating anxiety. *Behaviour Research and Therapy*, 1975, **13**, 65-68.

Cutler, S.J. The availability of personal transportation, residential location, and life satisfaction among the aged. *Journal of Gerontology*, 1972, **27**, 390-392.

Cutler, S.J. Transportation and changes in life satisfaction. *Gerontologist*, 1975, **15**, 155-159.

Cutter, H.S., Schwaab, E.L., & Nathan, P.E. Effects of alcohol on its utility for alcoholics and nonalcoholics. *Quarterly Journal of Studies on Alcohol*, 1970, **31**, 369-378.

Dale, R., & Dale, F. The use of methadone in a representative group of heroin addicts. *The International Journal of the Addictions*, 1973, **8**, 293-308.

Damich, E. The right against treatment: Behavior modification and the involuntarily committed. *Catholic University Law Review*, 1974, **23**, 774-787.

Davidson, L.M. The process of employing the disadvantaged. Unpublished doctoral dissertation, Massachusetts Institute of Technology, 1973.

Davidson, W.S. Studies of aversive conditioning for alcoholics: A critical review of theory and research methodology. *Psychological Bulletin*, 1974, **81**, 571-581.

Davidson, W.S. The diversion of juvenile delinquents: An examination of the processes and relative efficacy of behavioral contracting and child advocacy. Unpublished doctoral dissertation, University of Illinois, mimeo. 1975.

Davidson, W.S., Rappaport, J., Seidman, E., Berck, D., & Herring, J. The diversion of juvenile delinquents: An experimental examination. Unpublished manuscript, University of Illinois, Champaign, 1975.

Davidson, W.S., & Robinson, M.R. Community psychology and behavior modification: A community based program for the prevention of delinquency. *Corrective and Social Psychiatry and Journal of Behavior Technology Methods and Therapy*, 1975, **21**, 1-12.

Davidson, W.S., & Wolfred, T.R. A community based residential program for the prevention of delinquency: The success of failure. *Community Mental Health Journal*, in press.

Davies, D.L. Normal drinking in recovered alcohol addicts. *Quarterly Journal of Studies on Alcohol*, 1962, **23**, 94-104.

Davis, W.J. The Berkeley big brother project. In A. de Grazia (Ed.), *Grass roots private welfare*. New York: New York University Press, 1957. Pp. 41-44.

Davison, G.C. Appraisal of behavior modification techniques with adults in institutional settings. In C.M. Franks (Ed.), *Behavior therapy: Appraisal and status*. New York: McGraw-Hill, 1969.

Davison, G.C., & Neale, J.M. *Abnormal psychology: An experimental clinical approach*. New York: Wiley, 1974.

Davison, G.C., & Stuart, R.B. Behavior therapy and civil liberties. *American Psychologist*, 1975, **30**, 755-763.

DeAngelis, G. Testing for drugs – I: Techniques and issues. *The International Journal of the Addictions*, 1973, **8**, 997-1014.

DeCarlo, T.J. Recreation, participation patterns and successful aging. *Journal of Gerontology*, 1974, **29**, 416-422.

DeGrazia, F. Diversion from the criminal process: The "mental health" experiment. *Connecticut Law Review*, 1974, **6**, 432-528.

DeLong, J. The drugs and their effects. In P.Wald & P. Hutt (Eds.), *Dealing with drug abuse*. New York: Praeger, 1972a.

Delong, J. Treatment and rehabilitation. In P. Wald & P. Hutt (Eds.), *Dealing with drug abuse*. New York: Praeger, 1972b.

Deslauriers, B.C., & Everett, P.B. The effects of intermittent and continuous token reinforcement on bus ridership. Unpublished manuscript, The Pennsylvania State University, 1975.

Dineen, J.P., Clark, H.B., & Risley, T.R. Peer tutoring in elementary students: Educational benefits to the tutor. *Journal of Applied Behavior Analysis*, in press.

Dirks, S. Aversion therapy: Its limited potential for use in the correctional setting. *Stanford Law Review*, 1974, **26**, 1327-1341.

Doctor, R., & Polakow, R. A behavior modification program for adult probationers. *Proceedings of the 81st Annual Convention of the American Psychological Association*. Washington, D.C.: APA, 1973.

Dodge, M.C. *Modification of littering behavior: An exploratory study*. Unpublished master's thesis, Utah State University, 1972.

Doke, L.A., & Risley, T.R. The organization of day-care environments: Required versus optional activities. *Journal of Applied Behavior Analysis*, 1972, **5**, 405-420.

Dolch, E.W. *Basic Sight Vocabulary Cards*. Champaign, Ill: Garrard, 1949.

Dole, V. Research on methadone maintenance treatment. *The International Journal of the Addictions*, 1970, **5**, 359-369.

Dole, V. Methadone maintenance treatment for 25,000 heroin addicts. *Journal of the American Medical Association*, 1971, **215**, 1131-1134.

Dole, V., & Nyswander, M. A medical treatment for diacetylmorphine (heroin) addiction. *Journal of the American Medical Association*, 1965, **193**, 80.

Dole, V., Nyswander, M., & Warner, A. Successful treatment of 750 criminal addicts. *Journal of the American Medical Association*, 1968, **206**, 2708-2711.

Donaldson v. O'Connor, 493 F. 2d. 507 (5CA 1974).

Donaldson v. O'Connor, _____ U.S._____, 43 L. W. 4929 (1975).

Dorsey, J.R., Matsunaga, G., & Bauman, G. Training public health nurses in mental health. *Archives of General Psychiatry*, 1964, **11**, 214-222.

Drabman, R.S. Child-versus teacher-administered token programs in a psychiatric hospital. *Journal of Abnormal Child Psychology*, 1973, **1**, 68-87.

Drabman, R.S., & Spitalnik, R. Training a retarded child as a behavioral teaching assistant. *Journal of Behavior Therapy and Experimental Psychiatry*, 1973, **4**, 269-279.

Drabman, R.S., Spitalnik, R., & O'Leary, K.D. Teaching self control to disruptive children. *Journal of Abnormal Psychology*, 1973, **82**, 10-16.

Droppa, D. Behavioral treatment of drug addiction: A review and analysis. *The International Journal of the Addictions*, 1973, **8**, 143-162.

Dulany, D. Awareness, rules, and propositional control: A confrontation with S-R behavior theory. In T. Dixon & D. Horton (Eds.), *Verbal behaviour and general behaviour theory*. Englewood Cliffs, N.J.: Prentice-Hall, 1968.

Dunn, A., & Strang, C.D. Ward hostess experiment. *Gerontologia Clinica*, 1970, **12**, 267-274.

DuPont, R.L. The future of the federal drug abuse program. Paper presented at the 36th Annual Scientific Meeting of the Commission of Problems of Drug Dependence. Mexico City, 1974.

DuPont, R., & Katon, R. Development of a heroin-addiction treatment program: Effect on urban crime. *Journal of the American Medical Association*, 1971, **216**, 1320-1324.

Dwarshuis, L., Kolton, M., & Gorodezky, M. Role of volunteers in innovative drug treatment programs. *Proceedings of the 81st convention of the American Psychological Association*. Washington, D.C.: APA, 1973.

Edlund, C.V. The effect on the behavior of children, as reflected in the IQ scores, when reinforced after each correct response. *Journal of Applied Behavior Analysis*, 1972, **5**, 317-319.

Eisler, R.M., Hersen, M., & Miller, P.M. Effects of modeling on components of assertive behavior. *Journal of Behavior Therapy and Experimental Psychiatry*, 1973, **4**, 1-6.

Eisler, R.M., Hersen, M., & Miller, P.M. Shaping components of assertive behavior with instructions and feedback. *American Journal of Psychiatry*, 1974, **131**, 1344-1347.

Eisler, R.M., Miller, P.M., Hersen, M., & Alford, H. Effects of assertive training on marital interaction. *Archives of General Psychiatry*, 1974, **30**, 643-649.

Elkins, R. Aversion therapy for alcoholism: Chemical, electrical, or verbal imaginary. *The International Journal of the Addictions*, 1975, **10**, 157-209.

Elliot, D.S., & Voss, H.L. *Delinquency and dropout*. Lexington, Mass. Lexington Books, 1974.

Empey, L.T. *Alternatives to institutionalization*. Washington, D.C.: Government Printing Office, 1967.

Emrick, C.D. A review of psychologically oriented treatment of alcoholism II: The relative effectiveness of different treatment approaches and the effectiveness of treatment versus no treatment. *Quarterly Journal of Studies on Alcohol*, 1975, **36**, 88-108.

Epstein, L.H., & Peterson, C.L. Control of undesired behavior by self-imposed contingencies. *Behavior Therapy*, 1973, **4**, 91-95.

Epstein, N., & Guild, J. Further clinical experience with tetraethylthiuram disulfide in the treatment of alcoholism. *Quarterly Journal of Studies on Alcohol*, 1951, **17**, 366-380.

Epstein, N., & Shainline, A. Paraprofessional parent-aides and disadvantaged families. *Social Casework*, 1974, **55**, 230-236.

Erickson, M.L. Group violations, socioeconomic status, and official delinquency. *Social Forces*, 1973, **52**, 41-52.

Eriksson, J., Götestam, K., Melin, G., & Öst, L. A token economy treatment of drug addiction. *Behaviour Research and Therapy*, 1975, **13**, 113-126.

Erwin, W.S. Consumer participation in aging planning. *Gerontologist*, 1974, **14**, 245-248.

Esser, P.H. Evaluation of family therapy with alcoholics. *British Journal of Addictions*, 1971, **66**, 251-255.

Estes, C.L. Community planning for the elderly: A study of goal displacement. *Journal of Gerontology*, 1974, **29**, 684-691.

Estes, W.K. An experimental study of punishment. *Psychological Monographs*, 1944, **57**, (Whole No. 263).

Everett, P.B. A gaming simulation for pretesting large scale operant manipulations: An urban transportation example. Unpublished manucript, The Pennsylvania State University, 1975.

Everett, P.B., Hayward, S.C., & Meyers, A.W. The effects of a token reinforcement procedure on bus ridership. *Journal of Applied Behavior Analysis*, 1974, **1**, 1-9.

Eysenck, H.J. *Crime and personality*. Boston: Houghton Mifflin, 1964.

Fairweather, G.W. *Methods for experimental social innovation*. New York: Wiley, 1967.

Fairweather, G.W. *Social change: The challenge to survival*. Morristown, N.J.: General Learning Press, 1972.

Fairweather, G.W., Sanders, D.H., Maynard, H., & Cressler, D.L. *Community life for the mentally ill*. Chicago: Aldine, 1969.

Fairweather, G.W., Sanders, D.H., & Tornatzky, L.G. *Creating change in mental health organizations*. New York: Pergamon Press, 1974.

Farrar, C.H., Powell, B.J., & Martin, L.K. Punishment of alcohol consumption by apneic paralysis. *Behaviour Research and Therapy*, 1968, **6**, 13-16.

Faust, F.L. Delinquency labelling: Its consequences and implications. *Crime and Delinquency*, 1973, **19**, 41-48.

Federal Bureau of Investigation, *Federal Crime Reporting*. Washington, D.C.: Department of Justice, 1965-1975.

Federal Bureau of Investigation, *Uniform Crime Reports*. Washington, D.C.: Government Printing Office, 1973.

Feigenbaum, E.M. Geriatric psychopathology — Internal or external. *Journal of the American Geriatric Society*, 1974, **22**, 49-55.

Feldman, J.M. Race, economic class, and perceived outcomes of work and unemployment. *Journal of Applied Psychology*, 1973, **58**, 16-22.

Feldman, J.M. Race, economic class, and the intention to work: Some normative and attitudinal correlates. *Journal of Applied Psychology*, 1974, **59**, 179-186.

Feldman, R.A., Wodarski, J.S., Flax, N., & Goodman, M. Treating delinquents in traditional avenues. *Social Work*, 1972, **17**, 71-78.

Feldstein, M.S. *Lowering the permanent rate of unemployment: A study prepared for the use of the Joint Economic Committee of the Congress of the United States*. Washington, D.C.: Government Printing Office, Stock no. 5270-01991, 1973.

Fenichel, O. *The psychoanalytic theory of neurosis*. New York: Norton, 1945.

Fensterheim, H. Assertive methods and marital problems. Paper presented at the annual meeting of the Association for the Advancement of Behavior Therapy, New York, 1972.

Ferguson, R.H. *Unemployment: Its scope, measurement, and effect on poverty* (2nd ed.). Ithaca: New York State School of Industrial and Labor Relations, Cornell University, 1971.

Ferritor, D.C., Buckholdt, D., Hamblin, R.L., & Smith, L. The noneffects of contingent reinforcement for attending behavior on work accomplished. *Journal of Applied Behavior Analysis,* 1972, **5**, 7-18.

Field, M. *Depth and extent of the geriatric problem.* Springfield, Ill.: Thomas, 1970.

Fineman, K.R. An operant conditioning program in a juvenile detention facility. *Psychological Reports,* 1968, **22**, 1119-1120.

Finkestein, M., & Rosenberg, G. New lifestyle for the aged in a long-term hospital. *Journal of the American Geriatric Society,* 1974, **22**, 525-527.

Finnie, W.C. Field experiments in litter control. *Environment and Behavior,* 1973, **5**, 123-144.

Fixsen, D.L., Phillips, E.L., & Wolf, M.M. Achievement Place: The reliability of self-reporting and peer reporting and their effects on behavior. *Journal of Applied Behavior Analysis,* 1972, **5**, 19-30.

Fixsen, D.L., Phillips, E.L., & Wolf, M.M. Achievement Place: Experiments in self-government with pre-delinquents. *Journal of Applied Behavior Analysis,* 1973, **6**, 31-47.

Fodor, I.E. The use of behavior modification techniques with female delinquents. *Child Welfare,* 1972, **51**, 93-101.

Foote, C. The coming constitutional crisis in bail. *University of Pennsylvania Law Review,* 1965, **113**, 959-999.

Fowler, R.W., Fordyce, W.E., & Berni, R. Operant conditioning in chronic illness. *American Journal of Nursing,* 1969, **69**, 1226-1228.

Fox, V. Crime as a social problem. In J. Cull & R. Hardy (Eds.), *Fundamentals of criminal behavior and correctional systems.* Springfield: Thomas, 1973.

Foy, D.W., Eisler, R.M., & Pinkston, S. Modeled assertion in a case of explosive rages. *Journal of Behavior Therapy and Experimental Psychiatry,* 1975, **6**, 135-137.

Franks, C.M. Behavior therapy, the principles of conditioning and the treatment of the alcoholic. *Quarterly Journal of Studies on Alcohol,* 1963, **24**, 511-529.

Franks, C.M. Conditioning and conditioned aversion therapies in the treatment of the alcoholic. *International Journal of the Addictions,* 1966, **1**, 61-98.

Franks, C.M. (Ed.) *Behavior therapy: Appraisal and status,* New York: McGraw-Hill, 1969.

Franks, C.M. Alcoholism, In C.G. Costello (Ed.), *Symptoms of psychopathology,* New York: Wiley, 1970.

Freed, E.X. Alcohol and conflict: Role of drug dependent learning in the rat. *Quarterly Journal of Studies on Alcohol,* 1971, **32**, 13-28.

Frekany, G.A., & Leslie, D.K. Effects of an exercise program on selected flexibility measurements of senior citizens. *Gerontologist,* 1975, **15**, 182-183.

Freud, S. *Three contributions to the theory of sex.* (4th ed.). Washington, D.C.: Nervous and Mental Diseases Publishing Co., 1930.

Freud, S. *New introductory lectures on psychoanalysis.* New York: Norton, 1933.

Friedlander, F., & Greenberg, S. Effect of job attitudes, training, and organizational climate on the performance of the hard-core unemployed. *Journal of Applied Psychology,* 1971, **55,** 287-295.

Friedman, P.H. The effects of modeling and roleplaying on assertive behavior. Paper presented at the annual meeting of the Association for the Advancement of Behavior Therapy, Washington, 1969.

Fromm, E., & Maccoby, M. *Social character in a Mexican village: A sociopsychoanalytic study.* Englewood Cliffs, N.J.: Prentice-Hall, 1970.

Gaitz, C.M. & Scott, J. Analysis of letters to "Dear Abby" concerning old age. *Gerontologist,* 1975, **15,** 47-50.

Galassi, J.P., Galassi, M.D., & Litz, M.C. Assertive training in groups using video feedback. *Journal of Counseling Psychology,* 1974, **21,** 390-394.

Galassi, J.P., Kostka, M.P., & Galassi, M.D. Assertive training: A one-year follow-up. *Journal of Counseling Psychology, 1975,* **22,** 451-452.

Gambrill, E.D. A behavioral program for increasing social interaction. Paper presented at the annual meeting of the Association for the Advancement of Behavior Therapy, Chicago, 1973.

Gardner, J.M. Teaching behavior modification to nonprofessionals. *Journal of Applied Behavior Analysis,* 1972, **5,** 517-522.

Gardner, W. *Behavior modification in mental retardation.* New York: Aldine, 1971.

Garetz, F.K., & Garetz, D. Age as a factor in the referral and treatment of psychiatric patients by internists. *Journal of the American Geriatric Society,* 1973, **21,** 129-133.

Garfinkel, H. Conditions of successful degradation ceremonies. *American Journal of Sociology,* 1956, **61,** 421-422.

In re Gault, 387 U.S. 1 (1967).

Gay, G., Matzger, A., Bathurst, W., & Smith, D. Short-term heroin detoxification on an outpatient basis. *The International Journal of the Addictions,* 1971, **6,** 241-264.

Gazda, G.M., Parks, J., & Sisson, J. The use of a modified marathon in conjunction with group counseling in short-term treatment of alcoholics. *Rehabilitation Counseling Bulletin,* 1971, **15,** 97-105.

Gearing, F. Evaluation of a methadone maintenance treatment program. *The International Journal of the Addictions,* 1970, **5,** 517-543.

Geiger, O.G., & Johnson, L.A. Positive education for elderly persons: Correct eating through reinforcement. *Gerontologist,* 1974, **14,** 432-436.

Geller, E.S. Attempts to implement behavioral technology in Virginia corrections. Colloquium presentation at Florida State University, October 1974.

Geller, E.S. Prompting anti-litter behaviors. *Proceedings of the 81st Annual Convention of the American Psychological Association,* 1973, **8,** 901-902 (Summary).

Geller, E.S. Increasing desired waster disposals with instructions. *Man-Environment Systems*, 1975, **5**, 125-128.

Geller, E.S., Chaffee, J.L., & Ingram, R.E. Promoting paper recycling on a university campus. *Journal of Environmental Systems*, 1975, **5**, 39-57.

Geller, E.S., Farris, J.C., & Post, D.S. Prompting a consumer behavior for pollution control. *Journal of Applied Behavior Analysis*, 1973, **6**, 367-376.

Geller, E.S., & Johnson, D. Letter to the *APA Monitor*, November 1974, **5**.

Geller, E.S., Witmer, J.F., & Orebaugh, A.L. Instructions as a determinant of paper-disposal behaviors. *Environment and Behavior*, in press.

Geller, E.S., Wylie, R.G., & Farris, J.C. An attempt at applying prompting and reinforcement toward pollution control. *Proceedings of the 79th Annual Convention of the American Psychological Association*, 1971, **6**, 701-702 (Summary).

Gentile, J.R., Roden, A.H., & Klein, R.D. An analysis-of-variance model for the intrasubject replication design. *Journal of Applied Behavior Analysis*, 1972, **5**, 193-198.

Gerard, D.L., Saenger, G., & Wile, R. The abstinent alcoholic. *Archives of General Psychiatry*, 1962, **6**, 99-111.

Gilligan, J. Review of the literature. In M. Greenblatt, M.H. Soloman, A.S. Evans, & G.W. Brooks (Eds.), *Drug and social therapy in chronic schizophrenia*. Springfield, Ill.: Thomas, 1965.

Ginsburg, A.B., & Goldstein, S.G. Age bias in referral for psychological consultation. *Journal of Gerontology*, 1974, **29**, 410-415.

Glaser, D. *The effectiveness of a prison and parole system*. Indianapolis: Bobbs-Merrill, 1964.

Glass, E., Wilson, V., & Gottman, J. *The design and analysis of time series experiments*. Boulder, Col.: Laboratory of Educational Research Press, 1973.

Glickman, H., Plutchik, R., & Landau, H. Social and biological reinforcement in an open psychiatric ward. *Journal of Behavior Therapy and Experimental Psychiatry*, 1973, **4**, 121-124.

Glicksman, M., Ottomanelli, G., & Cutler, R. The earn-your-way credit system: Use of a token economy in narcotic rehabilitation. *The International Journal of the Addictions*, 1971, **6**, 525-531.

Glueck, S., & Glueck, E. *Unraveling juvenile delinquency*. Cambridge, Mass.: Harvard University Press, 1951.

Glueck, S., & Glueck, E. *Towards a typology of juvenile offenders*. New York: Grune & Stratton, 1970.

Glynn, E.L. Classroom applications of self-determined reinforcement. *Journal of Applied Behavior Analysis*, 1970, **3**, 123-132.

Glynn, E.L., & Thomas, J.D. Effects of cueing on self-control of classroom behavior. *Journal of Applied Behavior Analysis*, 1974, **7**, 299-306.

Glynn, E.L., Thomas, J.D., & Shee, S.M. Behavioral self-control of on-task behavior in an elementary classroom. *Journal of Applied Behavior Analysis*, 1973, **6**, 105-114.

Gobert, J. Psychosurgery, conditioning, and the prisoner's right to refuse "rehabilitation." *Virginia Law Review,* 1975, **61,** 155-196.

Goetz, E.M., & Baer, D.M. Social control of form diversity and the emergence of new forms in children's blockbuilding. *Journal of Applied Behavior Analysis,* 1973, **6,** 209-217.

Goffman, E. *Asylums.* Garden City, N.Y.: Doubleday Anchor, 1961.

Gold, J. Comparison of protective services projects. *Gerontologist,* 1972, **12,** 85 (abstract).

Gold, M., & Mann, D. Delinquency as defense. *American Journal of Orthopsychiatry,* 1972, **42,** 463-479.

Goldenberg, I. *Build me a mountain.* Cambridge, Mass.: M.I.T. Press, 1971.

Goldiamond, I. Toward a constructional approach to social problems. *Behaviorism,* 1974, **2,** 1-84.

Goldsmith, J.B., & McFall, R.M. Development and evaluation of an interpersonal skill-training program for psychiatric inpatients. *Journal of Abnormal Psychology,* 1975, **84,** 51-58.

Goldstein, A. Blind dosage comparisons and other studies in a large methadone program. *Journal of Psychedelic Drugs,* 1971, **4,** 177-181.

Goldstein, A.P., Heller, K., & Sechrest, L.B. *Psychotherapy and the psychology of behavior change.* New York: Wiley, 1966.

Goldstein, A.P., Martens, J., Hubben, J., vanBelle, H.A., Schaaf, W., Wiersma, H., & Goedhart, A. The use of modeling to increase independent behavior. *Behaviour Research and Therapy,* 1973, **11,** 31-42.

Goldstein, S. A critical appraisal of milieu therapy in a geriatric day hospital. *Journal of the American Geriatric Society,* 1971, **19,** 693-699.

Goodale, J.G. Effects of personal background and training on work values of the hard-core unemployed. *Journal of Applied Psychology,* 1973, **57,** 1-9.

Goodman, P.S., Salipant, P., & Paransky, H. Hiring, training, and retaining the hard-core unemployed: A selected review. *Journal of Applied Psychology,* 1973, **58,** 23-33.

Goodwin, D. Alcohol in suicide and homicide. *Quarterly Journal of Studies on Alcohol,* 1973, **34,** 144-156.

Goodwin, L., & Tu, J. The social psychological basis for public acceptance of the social security system: The role for social research in public policy formation. *American Psychologist,* 1975, **30,** 875-883.

Gordon, M.E., Arvey, R.D., Daffron, W.C., & Umberger, D.L. Racial differences in the impact of mathematics training at a manpower development program. *Journal of Applied Psychology,* 1974, **59,** 253-258.

Gordon, W.W. The treatment of alcohol (and tobacco) addiction by differential conditioning. *American Journal of Psychotherapy,* 1971, **25,** 394-417.

Gorham, D.C., Green, L.W., Caldwell, L.R., & Bartlett, E.R. Effect of operant conditioning techniques on chronic schizophrenia. *Psychological Reports,* 1970, **27,** 223-234.

Gormally, J., Hill, C.E., Otis, M., & Rainey, L. A microtraining approach to assertion training. *Journal of Counseling Psychology,* 1975, **22,** 299-303.

Götestam, K., & Melin, L. Covert extinction of amphetamine addiction. *Behavior Therapy,* 1974, **5,** 90-92.

Gottesman, L.E., & Bourestom, N.C. Why nursing homes do what they do. *Gerontologist,* 1974, **14,** 501-506.

Gottman, J.M. N-of-one and N-of-two research in psychotherapy. *Psychological Bulletin,* 1973, **80,** 93-105.

Graubard, P.S., Rosenburg, H., & Miller, M.B. Student applications of behavior modification to teachers and environments or ecological approaches to social deviancy. In E.A. Ramp & B.L. Hopkins (Eds.), *A new direction for education: Behavior analysis.* Lawrence, Kansas: Support and Development Center for Follow Through, 1971.

Grauer, H. Institutions for the aged — Therapeutic communities? *Journal of the American Geriatric Society,* 1971, **19,** 687-692.

Grauer, H., Betts, D., & Birnbom, F. Welfare emotions and family therapy in geriatrics. *Journal of the American Geriatric Society,* 1973, **21,** 21-24.

Gray, B.B., Baker, R.D., & Stancyk, S.E. Performance determined instruction for training in remedial reading. *Journal of Applied Behavior Analysis,* 1969, **2,** 255-264.

Greenwood, C.R., Hops, H., Delquadri, J., & Guild, J. Group contingencies for group consequences in classroom management: A further analysis. *Journal of Applied Behavior Analysis,* 1974, **7,** 413-426.

Greenwood, C.R., Hops, H., & Walker, H.M. The Program for Academic Survival Skills (Pass): Maintenance of changes in student behavior within the same school year. Report from Center at Oregon for Research in the Behavioral Education of the Handicapped, Center on Human Development, University of Oregon, 1975.

Greenwood, C.R., Sloane, H.N., Jr., & Baskin, A. Training elementary aged peer-behavior managers to control small group programmed mathematics. *Journal of Applied Behavior Analysis,* 1974, **7,** 103-114.

Grey, A.L., & Dermody, H.E. Reports of casework failure. *Social Casework,* 1972, **16,** 207-212.

Griffin, C.L., & Reinhorz, H.Z. Prevention of the "failure syndrome" in the primary grades: Implications for intervention. *American Journal of Public Health,* 1969, **59,** 2029-2034.

Griffiths, R.R., Bigelow, G.E., & Liebson, I.A. Alcohol self-administration and interaction in alcoholics. *Proceedings of the 81st Annual Convention of the American Psychological Association,* 1973, **8,** 1035-1036.

Griffiths, R., Bigelow, G.E., & Liebson, I. Suppression of ethanol self-administration in alcoholics by contingent time-out from social interactions. *Behaviour Research and Therapy,* 1974, **12,** 327-334.

Gripp, R.F., & Magaro, P.A. A token economy program evaluation with control ward comparisons. *Behaviour Research and Therapy,* 1971, **9**, 137-149.

Gripp, R.F., & Magaro, P.A. The token economy program in the psychiatric hospital: A review and analysis. *Behaviour Research and Therapy,* 1974, **12**, 205-228.

Gross, N., & Nerviano, V. The prediction of dropouts from an inpatient alcoholism program by objective personality inventory. *Quarterly Journal of Studies on Alcohol,* 1973, **34**, 514-515.

Grossman, H. Community treatment of adolescents. *Police,* 1972, **16**, 48-51.

Gruver, G.G. College students as therapeutic agents. *Psychological Bulletin,* 1971, **76**, 111-127.

Gubrium, J.F., & Ksander, M. On multiple realities and reality orientation. *Gerontologist,* 1975, **15**, 142-145.

Guerney, B.G., Jr. (Ed.) *Psychotherapeutic agents: New roles for nonprofessionals, parents, and teachers.* New York: Holt, Rinehart & Winston, 1969.

Gurel, L. Release and community stay in chronic schizophrenia. *American Journal of Psychiatry,* 1966, **122**, 892-899.

Gurian, B.S., & Scherl, D.J. A community-focused model of mental health services for the elderly. *Journal of Geriatric Psychiatry,* 1972, **5**, 77-86.

Gutride, M.E., Goldstein, A.P., & Hunter, G.F. The use of modeling and role playing to increase social interaction among asocial psychiatric patients. *Journal of Consulting and Clinical Psychology,* 1973, **40**, 408-415.

Haberman, P.W., & Baden, M.M. Alcoholism and violent death. *Quarterly Journal of Studies on Alcohol,* 1974, **35**, 221-231.

Hall, R.V., Cristler, C., Cranston, S.S., & Tucker, B. Teachers and parents as researchers using multiple baseline designs. *Journal of Applied Behavior Analysis,* 1970, **3**, 247-260.

Hall, R.V., Fox, R., Willard, D., Goldsmith, L., Emerson, M., Owen, M., Davis, F., & Porcia, E. The teacher as observer and experimenter in the modification of disputing and talking-out behaviors. *Journal of Applied Behavior Analysis,* 1971, **4**, 141-149.

Hall, R.V., Panyon, M., Rubon, D., & Broden, M. Instructing beginning teachers in reinforcement procedures which improve classroom control. *Journal of Applied Behavior Analysis,* 1968, **1**, 315-322.

Hallam, R., Rachman, S., & Falkowski, W. Subjective, attitudinal, and physiological effects of electrical aversion therapy. *Behaviour Research and Therapy,* 1972, **10**, 1-13.

Halleck, S.L. Legal and ethical aspects of behavior control. *American Journal of Psychiatry,* 1974, **131**, 381-385.

Hamburg, S. Behavior therapy in alcoholism: A critical review of broad-spectrum approaches. *Quarterly Journal of Studies on Alcohol,* 1975, **36**, 69-87.

Harris, R. *The fear of crime.* New York: Praeger, 1968.

Harris, R. Breaking the barriers to better health-care delivery for the aged. *Gerontologist,* 1975, **15**, 52-56.

Harris, V.W., & Sherman, J.A. Effects of peer tutoring and consequences on the math performance of elementary classroom students. *Journal of Applied Behavior Analysis,* 1973a, **6**, 587-598.

Harris, V.W., & Sherman, J.A. Use and analysis of the "good behavior game" to reduce classroom behavior. *Journal of Applied Behavior Analysis,* 1973(b), **6**, 405-417.

Harris, V.W., & Sherman, J.A. Homework assignments, consequences, and classroom performance in social studies and mathematics. *Journal of Applied Behavior Analysis,* 1974, **7**, 505-520.

Harry, J. Social class and delinquency. *Sociological Quarterly,* 1974, **15**, 294-301.

Harshberger, D., & Maley, (Eds.) *Behavior analysis and systems analysis: An integrative approach to mental health programs.* Kalamazoo, Mich.: Behaviordelia, 1974.

Hart, B.M., & Risley, T.R. Establishing use of descriptive adjectives in the spontaneous speech of disadvantaged preschool children. *Journal of Applied Behavior Analysis,* 1968, **1**, 109-120.

Hart, B.M., & Risley, T.R. Using preschool materials to modify the language of disadvantaged children. *Journal of Applied Behavior Analysis,* 1974, **7**, 243-257.

Hart, B.M., & Risley, T.R. Incidental teaching of language in the preschool. *Journal of Applied Behavior Analysis,* 1975, **8**, 411-420.

Hartman, C. Group relaxation training for control of impulsive behavior in alcoholics. *Behavior Therapy,* 1973, **4**, 173-174.

Haskett, G.J., & Lenfestey, W. Reading-related behavior in an open classroom: Effects of novelty and modeling on preschoolers. *Journal of Applied Behavior Analysis,* 1974, **7**, 233-242.

Hauserman, N., Walen, S.R., & Behling, M. Reinforced racial integration in the first grade: A study in generalization. *Journal of Applied Behavior Analysis,* 1973, **6**, 193-200.

Hayes, S.C., & Cone, J.D. Reducing residential electrical energy use: Payment, information, and feedback. *Journal of Applied Behavior Analysis,* in press (a).

Hayes, S.C., & Cone, J.D. Decelerating environmentally destructive lawnwalking behavior. *Environment and Behavior,* in press(b).

Hayes, S.C., Johnson, V.S., & Cone, J.D. The marked item technique: A practical procedure for litter control. *Journal of Applied Behavior Analysis,* in press.

Haynes, S.N., & Geddy, P. Suppression of psychotic hallucinations through timeout. *Behavior Therapy,* 1973, **4**, 123-127.

Hazell, K. *Social and medical problems of the elderly.* London: Hutchinson Medical Publications, 1960.

Heap, R.F., Boblitt, W.E., Moore, C.H., & Hord, J.E. Behavior milieu therapy with chronic neuropsychiatric patients. *Journal of Abnormal Psychology,* 1970, **76**, 349-354.

Hedberg, A.G., & Campbell, L. A comparison of four behavioral treatments of alcoholism. *Journal of Behavior Therapy and Experimental Psychiatry*, 1974, 5, 251-256.

Hedquist, F.J., & Weinhold, B.K. Behavioral group counseling with socially anxious and unassertive college students. *Journal of Counseling Psychology*, 1970, 17, 237-242.

Heldman, A. Social psychology vs. the first amendment freedoms, due process liberty and limited government. *Cumberland-Samford Law Review*, 1973, 4, 1-40.

Heldman, U. Behavior modification and other legal imbroglios of human experimentation. *Journal of Urban Law*, 1974, 52, 155-175.

Herbert, E.W., Pinkston, E.M., Hayden, M.L., Sajwaj, T.F., Pinkston, S., Cordua, G., & Jackson, C. Adverse effects of differential parental attention. *Journal of Applied Behavior Analysis*, 1973, 6, 15-30.

Herman, S.H., & Tramontana, J. Instructions and group versus individual reinforcement in modifying disruptive group behavior. *Journal of Applied Behavior Analysis*, 1971, 4, 113-119.

Hersch, C. From mental health to social action: Clinical psychology in historical perspective. *American Psychologist*, 1969, 24, 909-916.

Hersch, C. Social history, mental health, and community control. *American Psychologist*, 1972, 27, 749-754.

Hersen, M., & Eisler, R.M. Social skills training. In W.E. Craighead, A.E. Kazdin, & M.J. Mahoney (Eds.), *Behavior modification: Principles, issues, and applications*. Boston: Houghton Mifflin, 1976.

Hersen, M., Miller, P.M., & Eisler, R.M. Interactions between alcoholics and their wives: A descriptive analysis of verbal and nonverbal behavior. *Quarterly Journal of Studies on Alcohol*, 1973, 34, 516-520.

Hershenson, D.B. Stress-induced use of alcohol by problem drinkers as a function of their sense of identity. *Quarterly Journal of Studies on Alcohol*, 1965, 26, 213-222.

Hickey, T., & Spinetta, J.J. Bridging research and application. *Gerontologist*, 1974, 14, 526-530.

Higgins, R.L., & Marlatt, G.A. The effects of anxiety arousal upon the consumption of alcohol by alcoholics and social drinkers. *Journal of Consulting and Clinical Psychology*, 1973, 41, 426-433.

Hill, M.J., & Blane, H.T. Evaluation of psychotherapy with alcoholics: A critical review. *Quarterly Journal of Studies on Alcohol*, 1967, 28, 76-104.

Hilts, P. *Behavior mod.* New York: Harper's Magazine Press, 1974.

Himes, J. Work values of Negroes. In L.A. Ferman, J.L. Kornbluh, & J.A. Miller (Eds.), *Negroes and jobs.* Ann Arbor: University of Michigan Press, 1968.

Hindelang, M. A learning theory analysis of the correctional process. *Issues in Criminology*, 1970, 5, 43-58.

Hitz, D. Drunken sailors and others: Drinking problems in specific occupations.

Quarterly Journal of Studies on Alcohol, 1973, **34**, 496-505.

Holahan, C. Seating patterns and patient behavior in an experimental dayroom. *Journal of Abnormal Psychology,* 1972, **80**, 115-124.

Holland, J.G. Behavior modification for prisoners, patients, and other people as a prescription for the planned society. Paper presented at the meeting of the Eastern Psychological Association, 1974.

Hollingshead, A.B., & Redlich, F.C. *Social class and mental illness.* New York: Wiley, 1958.

Holt v. Sarver, 309 F. Supp. 362 (E.D. Ark. 1970).

Holzberg, J.D., Knapp, R.H., & Turner, J.L. College students as companions to the mentally ill. In E.L. Cowen, E.A. Gardner, & M. Zax (Eds.), *Emergent approaches to mental health problems.* New York: Appleton-Century-Crofts, 1967.

Holzinger, R., Mortimer, R., & Van Dusen, W. Aversion conditioning treatment of alcoholism. *American Journal of Psychiatry,* 1967, **124**, 246-247.

Hommen, D. An assessment of the effects of a community mental health center laboratory training-education-consultation program in bereavement ministry for parish clergymen. *Dissertation Abstracts International,* 1972, **33**, 1818A.

Hopkins, B.L., Schutte, R.C., & Garton, K.L. The effects of access to a play-room on the rate and quality of printing and writing of first- and second-grade students. *Journal of Applied Behavior Analysis,* 1971, **4**, 77-87.

Hops, H., & Cobb, J.A. Initial investigations into academic survival-skill training, direct instruction, and first-grade achievement. *Journal of Educational Psychology,* 1974, **66**, 548-553.

Horton, G.O. Generalization of teacher behavior as a function of subject matter specific discrimination training. *Journal of Applied Behavior Analysis,* 1975, **8**, 311-320.

Horton, L.E. Generalization of aggressive behavior in adolescent delinquent boys. *Journal of Applied Behavior Analysis,* 1970, **3**, 205-211.

Hospital and Community Psychiatry (Editorial). A rehabilitation center for the mentally handicapped. *Hospital and Community Psychiatry,* 1972, **23**, 311-314.

Hoyer, W.J., Kafer, R.A., Simpson, S.C., & Hoyer, F.W. Reinstatement of verbal behavior in elderly mental patients using operant procedures. *Gerontologist,* 1974, **14**, 149-152.

Hoyer, W.J., Mishara, B.L., & Reidel, R.G. Problem behaviors as operants: Applications with elderly individuals. *Gerontologist,* in press.

Hsu, J. Electroconditioning therapy of alcoholics: A preliminary report. *Quarterly Journal of Studies on Alcohol,* 1965, **26**, 449-459.

Huber, H., Karlin, R., & Nathan, P. Blood alcohol level discrimination by non-alcoholics: The role of internal and external cues. Unpublished manuscript, Rutgers University, 1975.

Hudson, J.H. Decision. *American Journal of Nursing,* 1970, **70**, 760-769.

Hulin, C.L. Effects of community characteristics on measures of job satisfaction. *Journal of Applied Psychology*, 1966, **50**, 185-192.

Hulin, C.L. Effects of changes in job satisfaction levels of employee turnover. *Journal of Applied Psychology*, 1968, **52**, 122-126.

Hunt, G.M., & Azrin, N.H. The community-reinforcement approach to alcoholism. *Behaviour Research and Therapy*, 1973, **11**, 91-104.

Hurvitz, N. Psychotherapy as a means of social control. *Journal of Consulting and Clinical Psychology*, 1973, **40**, 232-239.

Irvine, R.E. (Ed.) Symposium on day care. *Gerontologia Clinica*, 1974, **16**, 235-326.

Irwin, J. The trouble with rehabilitation. *Criminal Justice and Behavior*, 1974, **1**, 139-149.

Ittelson, W.H., Proshansky, H.M., Rivlin, L.G., & Winkel, G.H. *An introduction to environmental psychology,* New York: Holt, Rinehart & Winston, 1974.

Iwata, B.A., Bailey, J.S., Brown, K.M., Foshee, T.J., & Alpern, M. Modification of institutional staff behavior using a performance-based lottery. Unpublished manuscript, Sunland Center, Tallahassee, Florida, 1975.

Jackson, B.T. A case of voyeurism treated by counter-conditioning. *Behaviour Research and Therapy*, 1969, **7**, 133-134.

Jacobs, J. *The death and life of great American cities.* New York: Random House, 1961.

Jaffe, J.H. Further experience with methadone in the treatment of narcotics users. *The International Journal of the Addictions*, 1970, **5**, 375-389.

Jaffe, J.H., & Brill, L. Cyclazocine, a long-acting narcotic antagonist: Its voluntary acceptance as a treatment modality by narcotics abusers. *The International Journal of the Addictions*, 1966, **1**, 99-123.

James, H. *Children in trouble: A national scandal.* New York: Christian Science Monitor Publishers. 1969.

Jarvik, L., Klodin, V., & Matsuyama, S. Human aggression and the extra Y chromosome: Fact or fantasy? *American Psychologist*, 1973, **28**, 674-682.

Jeffrey, C. *Crime prevention through environmental design.* Beverly Hills, Calif.: Sage, 1971.

Jellinek, E.H. *The disease concept of alcoholism.* New Haven: College and University Press, 1960.

Jesness, C.F. Comparative effectiveness of behavior modification and transactional analysis programs for delinquents. California Youth Authority, mimeo., 1974.

Jesness, C.F., & DeRisi, W.J. Some variation in techniques of contingency management in a school for delinquents. In J. Stumphauser (Ed.), *Behavior therapy with delinquents.* Springfield, Ill.: Thomas, 1973.

Johnson, D., & Geller, E. *Operations manual. Contingency management program.* Blacksburg, Va.: Virginia Polytechnic Institute and State University, 1973.

Johnson, E.H. *Crime, correction, and society.* Homewood, Ill.: Dorsey Press, 1964.

Johnson, M., & Bailey, J.S. Cross-age tutoring: Fifth graders as arithmetic tutors for kindergarten children. *Journal of Applied Behavior Analysis,* 1974, 7, 223-232.

Johnson, S.M., Bolstad, O.D., & Lobitz, G.K. Generalization and contrast phenomena in behavior modification with children. Paper presented at the Sixth Annual International Conference on Behavior Modification, Banff, Canada, 1974.

Joint Commission on Correctional Manpower and Training. *A time to act.* Lebanon, Penn.: Sowers, 1970.

Joint Commission on Mental Health of Children. Report of Task Force VI. *Social change and the mental health of children.* New York: Harper & Row, 1973.

Jones, F.H., & Eimers, R.C. Role playing to train elementary teachers to use a classroom management "skill package." *Journal of Applied Behavior Analysis,* 1975, 8, 421-434.

Jones, R., & Kazdin, A.E., Programming response maintenance after withdrawing token reinforcement. *Behavior Therapy,* 1975, 6, 153-164.

Jordan, V.E. The system propagates crime. *Crime and Delinquency,* 1974, 20, 233-240.

Kagel, J.H., Battalio, R.C., Winkler, R.C., & Winett, R.A. Energy conservation strategies: An evaluation of the effectiveness of price changes and information on household-demand for electricity. Unpublished manuscript, Texas A. and M. University, 1976.

Kahn, R.L. The mental health system and the future aged. *Gerontologist,* 1975, 15, 24-31.

Kaimowitz and Doe v. Department of Mental Health for the State of Michigan, C. A. 73-19434-AW (Cir. Court for Wayne, Michigan, July 10, 1973).

Kale, R.J., Kaye, J.H., Wheelan, P.A., & Hopkins, B.L. The effects of reinforcement on the modification, maintenance, and generalization of social responses of mental patients. *Journal of Applied Behavior Analysis,* 1969, 1, 307-314.

Kalish, R.A. Social values and the elderly. *Mental Hygiene,* 1971, 55, 51-54.

Karen, A., & Bower, R. A behavioral analysis of a social control agency: Synanon. *Journal of Research in Crime and Delinquency,* 1968, 5, 18-34.

Karoly, P. Ethical considerations in the application of self-control techniques. *Journal of Abnormal Psychology,* 1975, 84, 175-177.

Kastenbaum, R. Persepctive on the development and modification of behavior in the aged: A developmental-field perspective. *Gerontologist,* 1968, 8, 280-283.

Katz, I., & Cohen, J. The effects of training Negroes upon cooperative problem solving in biracial teams. *Journal of Applied Psychology,* 1962, 63, 319-325.

Katz, I., Goldston, J., & Benjamin, L. Behavior and productivity in birarcial work groups. *Human Relations,* 1958, II, 123-141.

Kaufman, K.F., & O'Leary, K.D. Reward, cost, and self-evaluation procedures for disruptive adolescents in a psychiatric hospital school. *Journal of Applied Behavior Analysis*, 1972, **5**, 293-309.

Kazdin, A.E. Methodological and assessment considerations in evaluating reinforcement programs in applied settings. *Journal of Applied Behavior Analysis*, 1973a, **6**, 517-531.

Kazdin, A.E. The failure of some patients to respond to token programs. *Journal of Behavior Therapy and Experimental Psychiatry*, 1973b, **4**, 7-14.

Kazdin, A.E. Comparative effects of some variations of covert modeling. *Journal of Behavior Therapy and Experimental Psychiatry*, 1974a, **5**, 225-232.

Kazdin, A.E. Effects of covert modeling and model reinforcement on assertive behavior. *Journal of Abnormal Psychology*, 1974b, **83**, 240-252.

Kazdin, A.E. *Behavior modification in applied settings*. Homewood, Ill.: Dorsey Press, 1975a.

Kazdin, A.E. The impact of applied behavior analysis on diverse areas of research. *Journal of Applied Behavior Analysis*, 1975b, **8**, 213-229.

Kazdin, A.E., & Bootzin, R.R. The token economy: An evaluative review. *Journal of Applied Behavioral Analysis*, 1972, **5**, 343-372.

Kazdin, A.E., & Erickson, L.M. Developing responsiveness to instructions in severely and profoundly retarded residents. *Journal of Behavior Therapy and Experimental Psychiatry*, 1975, **6**, 17-21.

Keith, C. Specialized treatment for homosexuals in institutions. Paper presented at the 82nd annual convention of the American Psychological Association, New Orleans, 1974.

Kellam, A.M. Shoplifting treated by aversion to a film. *Behaviour Research and Therapy*, 1969, **7**, 125-127.

Kelly, D.H. Track position and delinquent involvement: A preliminary analysis. *Sociology and Social Research*, 1974, **58**, 380-386.

Kelly, J.C. Ecological constraints on mental health services. *American Psychologist*, 1966, **21**, 535-539.

Kelly, J.G. The quest for valid preventive interventions. In C.D. Spielberger (Ed.), *Current topics in clinical and community psychology*. New York: Academic Press, 1971.

Kepner, E. Application of learning theory to the etiology and treatment of alcoholism. *Quarterly Journal of Studies on Alcohol*, 1964, **25**, 279-291.

Kessler, M., & Albee, G.W. Primary prevention. *Annual Review of Psychology*, 1975, **26**, 557-592.

Keve, P. *Prison life and human worth*. Minneapolis: University of Minnesota Press, 1974.

Kiesler, D. Some myths of psychotherapy research and the search for a paradigm. *Psychological Bulletin*, 1966, **65**, 110-136.

Kifer, R.E., Ayala, H.E., Fixsen, D.L., Phillips, E.L., & Wolf, M.M. The teaching family model: An analysis of the self-government system. Unpublished manuscript, University of Kansas, 1975.

Kifer, R.E., Lewis, M.A., Green, D.R., & Phillips, E.L. Training predelinquent youth and their parents to negotiate conflict situations. *Journal of Applied Behavior Analysis*, 1974, 7, 357-364.

Killinger, G., & Cromwell, P. (Eds.) *Alternatives to imprisonment: Corrections in the community*. St. Paul, Minn.: West, 1974.

Killingsworth, C.C. The bottleneck in labor skills. In A.M. Okum (Ed.), *The battle against unemployment*. New York: Norton, 1965.

Kirby, F.D., & Shields, F. Modification of arithmetic response rate and attending behavior in a seventh-grade student. *Journal of Applied Behavior Analysis*, 1972, 5, 79-84.

Kirigin, K.A., Phillips, E.L., Fixsen, D.L., Atwater, J.A., Taubman, M.T., & Wolf, M.M. Overall evaluation of the Achievement Place Program. In Achievement Place Project Phase III Final Report. Lawrence, Kansas: Department of Human Development, University of Kansas, 1974.

Kirigin, K.A., Phillips, E.L., Fixsen, D.L., & Wolf, M.M. Modification of the homework behavior and academic performance of predelinquents with home-based reinforcement. Symposium on Behavior Analysis in Education, Lawrence, Kansas, 1971.

Kirkpatrick, J.J. Occupational aspirations, opportunities, and barriers. In K.S. Miller & R.M. Dreger (Eds.), *Comparative studies of blacks and whites in the United States*. New York: Seminar Press, 1973.

Kirschner, N. A group assertive training procedure: Its evaluation and an examination of therapist assertiveness effects. Paper presented at the annual meeting of the Midwestern Psychological Association, Chicago, May 1975.

Kittrie, N.N. *The right to be different*. Baltimore: The John Hopkins Press, 1971.

Klein, D.C. The community and mental health: An attempt at a conceptual framework. *Community Mental Health Journal*, 1965, 1, 301-308.

Klein, M.W. *Street gangs and street workers*. Englewood Cliffs, N.J.: Prentice-Hall, 1971.

Knapczyk, D.R., & Livingston, G. The effects of prompting question-asking upon on-task behavior and reading comprehension. *Journal of Applied Behavior Analysis*, 1974, 7, 115-121.

Knecht V. Gillman, 488 F. and 1136-1137 (8'th cir. 1973).

Knight, R.P. The psychodynamics of chronic alcoholism. *Journal of Nervous and Mental Diseases*, 1937, 86, 538-548.

Kohlenberg, R.J. Treatment of a homosexual pedophiliac using *in vivo* desensitization: A case study. *Journal of Abnormal Psychology*, 1974, 83, 192-195.

Kohlenberg, R.J., & Phillips, T. Reinforcement and rate of litter depositing. *Journal of Applied Behavior Analysis*, 1973, 6, 391-396.

Kohlenberg, R.J., Phillips, T., & Proctor, A. A behavioral analysis of peaking in residential electrical energy consumers. Paper presented at the American Psychological Association meeting, Montreal, 1973.

Kraft, T. Successful treatment of a case of Drinamyl addiction. *British Journal of Psychiatry*, 1968, 114, 1363-1364.

Kraft, T. Alcoholism treated by systematic desensitization: A follow-up of eight cases. *Journal of the Royal College of General Practice*, 1969a, **18**, 336-340.

Kraft, T. Successful treatment of a case of chronic barbiturate addiction. *British Journal of Addictions*, 1969b, **64**, 115-120.

Kraft, T. Treatment of Drinamyl addiction. *The International Journal of the Addictions*, 1969c, **4**, 59-64.

Kraft, T. Successful treatment of Drinamyl addicts and associated personality changes. *Canadian Psychiatric Association Journal*, 1970a, **15**, 223-227.

Kraft, T. Treatment of Drinamyl addiction. *Journal of Nervous and Mental Diseases*, 1970b, **150**, 138-144.

Kraft, T., & Al-Issa, I. Alcoholism treated by desensitization: A case report. *Behaviour Research and Therapy*, 1967, **5**, 69-70.

Krasnegor, L., & Boudin, H. Behavior modification and drug addiction: The state of the art. *Proceedings of the 81st convention of the American Psychological Association, Montreal*. Washington, D.C.: APA, 1973.

Krasner, L. The classroom as a planned environment. Invited address at the annual meeting of the American Educational Research Association, Washington, 1975.

Krasner, L., & Ullmann, L.P. *Behavior influence and personality*. New York: Holt, Rinehart & Winston, 1973.

Krueger, D.E. Operant group therapy with delinquent boys using therapist's versus peer's reinforcement. Unpublished doctoral dissertation, University of Miami, 1971.

Kurland, A., Hanlon, T., & McCabe, O. Naloxone and the narcotic abuser: A controlled study of partial blockade. *The International Journal of the Addictions*, 1974, **9**, 663-672.

Kushner, M. The reduction of a long-standing fetish by means of aversive conditioning. In L.P. Ullmann & L. Krasner (Eds.), *Case studies in behavior modification*. New York: Holt, Rinehart & Winston, 1965.

Kuypers, J.A., & Bengston, V.L. Social breakdown and competence: A model of normal aging. *Human Development*, 1973, **16**, 181-201.

LaHart, D.E., & Bailey, J.S. The analysis and reduction of children's littering on a nature trail. Unpublished manuscript, Florida State University, 1974.

Lahey, B.B. Modification of the frequency of descriptive adjectives in the speech of Head Start children through modelling without reinforcement. *Journal of Applied Behavior Analysis*, 1971, **4**, 19-22.

Lahey, B.B., & Drabman, R.S. Facilitation of the acquisition of sight-word vocabulary through token reinforcement. *Journal of Applied Behavior Analysis*, 1974, **7**, 307-312.

Lahey, B.B., McNees, M.P., & Brown, C.C. Modification of deficits in reading comprehension. *Journal of Applied Behavior Analysis*, 1973, **6**, 474-480.

Lana, R.E. Pretest sensitization. In R. Rosenthal & R.L. Rosnow (Eds.), *Artifact in behavioral research*. New York: Academic Press, 1969.

Langley, M.H., Graves, H.R., & Norris, B. The juvenile court and individualized treatment. *Crime and Delinquency*, 1972, **18**, 79-92.

LaRosa, J., Lipsius, S., & LaRosa, J. Experiences with a combination of group therapy and methadone maintenance in the treatment of heroin addiction. *The International Journal of the Addictions*, 1974, **9**, 605-617.

Laster, R. Criminal restitution: A survey of its past history and an analysis of its present usefulness. *University of Richmond Law Review*, 1970, **5**, 71-98.

Laverty, S.G. Aversion therapies in the treatment of alcoholism. *Psychosomatic Medicine*, 1966, **28**, 651-666.

Laws, D. The failure of a token economy. *Federal Probation*, September 1974, **38**, 33-37.

Lazarus, A.A. Towards the understanding and effective treatment of alcoholism. *South African Medical Journal*, 1965, **39**, 736-741.

Leeke, W., & Clements, H. Correctional systems and programs — An overview. In J. Cull & R. Hardy (Eds.), *Fundamentals of criminal behavior and correctional systems*. Springfield, Ill.: Thomas, 1973.

Lefcourt, H. The function of the illusions of control and freedom. *American Psychologist*, 1973, **28**, 417-425.

Lehr, U., & Dreher, G. Determinants of attitudes toward retirement. In R.J. Havighurst, J.M.A. Munnichs, B. Neugarten, & H. Thomae (Eds.), *Adjustment to retirement: A cross-national study*. Assen, The Netherlands: Royal Van Gorcum, 1969.

Lehrman, N.S. Follow-up of brief and prolonged psychiatric hospitalization. *Comprehensive Psychiatry*, 1961, **4**, 227-240.

Leitenberg, H. Training clinical researchers in psychology. *Professional Psychology*, 1974, **5**, 59-69.

LeLaurin, K., & Risley, T.R. The organization of day-care environments; "Zone" versus "man to man" staff assignments. *Journal of Applied Behavior Analysis*, 1972, **5**, 225-232.

Lemere, F. What happens to alcoholics. *American Journal of Psychiatry*, 1953, **109**, 674-676.

Lemere, F., & Voetglin, W.L. An evaluation of the aversion treatment of alcoholism. *Quarterly Journal of Studies on Alcohol*, 1950, **11**, 199-204.

Lemert, E.M. *Human deviance, social problems and social control*. Englewood Cliffs, N.J.: Prentice-Hall, 1967.

Lemert, E.M. Beyond Mead: The societal reaction to deviance. *Social Problems*, 1974, **21**, 457-461.

Lennard, H., & Allen, S. The treatment of drug addiction: Toward new models. *The International Journal of the Addictions*, 1973, **8**, 521-536.

Leonard, L.E., & Kelly, A.M. The development of a community-based program for evaluating the impaired older adult. *Gerontologist*, 1975, **15**, 114-118.

Leopold, R.L. Toward health maintenance organization. In L. Bellack (Ed.), *A concise handbook of community psychiatry and community mental health*. New York: Grune & Stratton, 1974.

Lesser, E. Behavior therapy with a narcotics user: A case report. *Behaviour Research and Therapy*, 1967, 5, 251-252.

Lester, D., & Greenberg, L.A. Nutrition and the etiology of alcoholism: The effect of sucrose-saccharin and fat on the self-selection of ethyl alcohol by rats. *Quarterly Journal of Studies on Alcohol*, 1952, 13, 553-560.

Levinson, P. Theory and practice of behavior modification in the Federal Bureau of Prisons. Paper presented at the 82nd convention of the American Psychological Association, New Orleans, 1974.

Levitt, E.L. Research on psychotherapy with children. In A. Bergin & S.L. Garfield (Eds.), *Handbook of psychotherapy and behavior change*. New York: Wiley, 1971.

Lewinsohn, P.M., & MacPhillamy, D.J. The relationship between age and engagement in pleasant activities. *Journal of Gerontology*, 1974, 29, 290-294.

Lewis, M.A., Kifer, R., Green, D.R., Roosa, J.B., & Phillips, E.L. The S.O.C.S. model: A technique for training communication skills to predelinquents. Paper presented at the annual meeting of the American Psychological Association, Montreal, 1973.

Lewis, S. A patient-determined approach to geriatric activity programming within a state hospital. *Gerontologist*, 1975, 15, 146-149.

Lewis, S., & Trickett, E. Correlates of differing patterns of drug use in a high school population. *American Journal of Community Psychology*, 1974, 2, 337-350.

Ley, R. Labor turnover as a function of worker differences, work environment, and authoritarianism of foremen. *Journal of Applied Psychology*, 1966, 50, 497-500.

Libb, J.W., & Clements, C.B. Token reinforcement in an exercise program for hospitalized geriatric patients. *Perceptual and Motor Skills*, 1969, 28, 957-958.

Liberman, R. Aversive conditioning of drug addicts: A pilot study. *Behaviour Research and Therapy*, 1968, 6, 229-231.

Libet, J.M., & Lewinsohn, P.M. Concept of social skill with special reference to the behavior of depressed persons. *Journal of Consulting and Clinical Psychology*, 1973, 40, 304-312.

Libo, L. A research vs. service model for training in community psychology. *American Journal of Community Psychology*, 1974, 2, 173-178.

Libow, L.S. Pseudo-senility: Acute and reversible organic brain syndromes. *Journal of the American Geriatric Society*, 1973, 21, 112-120.

Licensed Beverage Industries, Inc. *The alcohol beverage industry: Social and economic progress.* New York: Licensed Beverage Industries, 1973.

Lichtman, C.M., & Hunt, R.G. Personality and organization theory: A review of some conceptual literature. *Psychological Bulletin*, 1971, 76, 271-294.

Liebson, I., & Bigelow, G.E. A behavioral-pharmacological treatment of dually addicted patients. *Behaviour Research and Therapy*, 1972, 10, 403-405.

Likert, R., & Bowers, D.G. Organizational theory and human resource accounting. *American Psychologist*, 1969, **24**, 585-592.

Lindesmith, A. *The addict and the law*. Bloomington: Indiana University Press, 1965.

Lindsey, R. Dial-a-ride buses prove too successful to succeed. *The New York Times*, May 13, 1975.

Litow, L., & Pumroy, D.K. A brief review of classroom group-oriented contingencies. *Journal of Applied Behavior Analysis*, 1975, **8**, 341-347.

Lloyd, K.E., & Garlington, W.K. Weekly variations in performance on a token economy psychiatric ward. *Behaviour Research and Therapy*, 1968, **6**, 407-410.

Lombroso, C. *Crime, its causes and remedies*. Translated by H. Horton. Boston: Little, Brown, 1911.

Lomont, J.F., Gilner, F.H., Spector, N.J., & Skinner, K.K. Group assertion training and group insight therapies. *Psychological Reports*, 1969, **25**, 463-470.

London, P. The end of an ideology in behavior modification. *American Psychologist*, 1972, **27**, 913-1120.

Long, J.D., & Williams, R.L. The comparative effectiveness of group and individually contingent free time with inner-city junior high school students. *Journal of Applied Behavior Analysis*, 1973, **6**, 465-474.

Longin, H.E., & Rooney, W.M. Assertion training as a programmatic intervention for hospitalized mental patients. Paper presented at the annual meeting of the American Psychological Association, Montreal, 1973.

Lorenze, E.J., Hamill, C.M., & Oliver, R.C. The day hospital: An alternative to institutional care. *Journal of the American Geriatric Society*, 1974, **22**, 316-320.

Lorion, R.P. Patient and therapist variables in the treatment of low income patients. *Psychological Bulletin*, 1974, **81**, 344-354.

Lovaas, O.I., Koegel, R., Simmons, J.Q., & Long, J. Some generalization and follow-up measures on autistic children in behavior therapy. *Journal of Applied Behavior Analysis*, 1973, **6**, 131-166.

Lovibond, S.H., & Caddy, G. Discriminated aversive control in the moderation of alcoholics' drinking behavior. *Behavior Therapy*, 1970, **1**, 437-444.

Lovitt, T.C., & Curtiss, K.A. Academic response rate as a function of teacher- and self-imposed contingencies. *Journal of Applied Behavior Analysis*, 1969, **2**, 49-54.

Lowenthal, M.F. Psychosocial variations across the adult life course: Frontiers for research and policy. *Gerontologist*, 1975, **15**, 6-12.

Lubetkin, B., & Fishman, S. Electrical aversion therapy with a chronic heroin user. *Journal of Behavior Therapy and Experimental Psychiatry*, 1974, **6**, 193-195.

Luger, M. Tomorrow's training schools: Problems, progress and challenges. *Crime and Delinquency,* 1973, **19**, 545-550.

Luyben, P.D., & Bailey, J.S. *Newspaper recycling behavior: The effects of reinforcement versus proximity of containers.* Unpublished manuscript, Florida State University, 1975.

MacAndrew, C., & Edgerton, R.B. *Drunken comportment: A social explanation.* Chicago: Aldine, 1969.

MacCalden, M., & Davis, C. Report on priority lane experiment on the San Francisco-Oakland Bay Bridge. California: Department of Public Works, 1972.

MacCulloch, M.J., Feldman, M.D., Orford, J.E., & MacCulloch, M.L. Anticipatory avoidance learning in the treatment of alcoholism: A record of therapeutic failure. *Behaviour Research and Therapy,* 1966, 4, 187-196.

MacDonald, M.L. The forgotten Americans: A sociopsychological analysis of aging and nursing homes. *American Journal of Community Psychology,* 1973, **1**, 272-294.

MacDonald, M.L. A behavioral assessment methodology applied to the measurement of assertion. Unpublished doctoral dissertation, University of Illinois, 1974a.

MacDonald, M.L. Handling problems with female employees. Paper presented at the annual meeting of the Illinois Executives' Conference. Champaign, June 1974b.

MacDonald, M.L. Methods for the assessment of change in hospitalized psychiatric populations: A substantive review. *Catalog of Selected Documents in Psychology,* 1974c, ms. no. 780.

MacDonald, M.L. Teaching assertion: A paradigm for therapeutic intervention. *Psychotherapy: Theory, Research, and Practice,* 1975a.

MacDonald, M.L. Assessment strategies for describing social performance levels. Paper presented at the annual meeting of the Association for the Advancement of Behavior Therapy, San Francisco, 1975b.

MacDonald, M.L. Reversal of disengagement: Inducing social interaction in the institutionalized elderly. *Gerontologist,* in press.

MacDonald, M.L., & Butler, A.K. Reversal of helplessness: Producing walking behavior in nursing home wheelchair residents using behavior modification procedures. *Journal of Gerontology,* 1974, **29**, 97-101.

MacDonald, M.L., Lindquist, C.U., Kramer, J.A., McGrath, R.A., & Rhyne, L.D. Social skills training: Behavior rehearsal in groups and dating skills. *Journal of Counseling Psychology,* 1975, **22**, 224-230.

MacDonald, M.L., & Settin, J.M. Reality orientation versus remotivation therapy for the institutionalized aging. *Journal of Gerontology,* in press.

MacDonald, M.L., & Tobias, L.L. Withdrawal causes relapse? Our response. *Psychological Bulletin,* 1976, **83**, 448-451.

MacDonald, W.S., Gallimore, R., & MacDonald, G. Contingency counseling by school personnel: An economical model of intervention. *Journal of Applied Behavior Analysis,* 1970, **3**, 175-182.

Mackay v. Procunier, 477 F. 2nd 877 (9th cir. 1973).

Macleod, R.D.M. "Unrealistic" discharges. *Gerontologia Clinica,* 1970, **12**, 33-39.

Maddox, G.L. Activity and morale: A longitudinal study of selected elderly subjects. *Social Forces,* 1963, **42**, 195-204.

Maddox, G.L., & Douglass, E.B. Aging and individual differences: A longitudinal analysis of social, psychological, and physiological indicators. *Journal of Gerontology,* 1974, **29**, 555-563.

Madill, M.F., Campbell, D., Laverty, S.G., Sanderson, S.E., & VanderWater, S.L. Aversion treatment of alcoholics by succinylcholine-induced apneic paralysis. *Quarterly Journal of Studies on Alcohol,* 1966, **27**, 483-509.

Magnum, G.L., & Robson, R.T. *Metropolitan impact of manpower programs: A four-city comparison.* Salt Lake City: Olympus, 1973.

Maher, B. A theory of schizophrenic cognition. Paper presented at the 47th annual meeting of the Midwestern Psychological Association, Chicago, 1975.

Makarenko, A.S. *The road to life.* Vols. I. II. III. Moscow: Foreign Language Publishing House, 1973.

Maletzky, B. Assisted covert sensitization for drug abuse. *The International Journal of the Addictions,* 1974, **9**, 411-429.

Maloney, K.B., & Hopkins, B.L. The modification of sentence structure and its relationship to subjective judgements of creativity in writing. *Journal of Applied Behavior Analysis,* 1973, **6**, 425-433.

Maloney, M., & Ward, M. Ecology: Let's hear from the people. An objective scale for the measurement of ecological attitudes and knowledge. *American Psychologist,* 1973, **28**, 583-586.

Mandelker, A.V., Brigham, T.A., & Bushell, D. The effects of token procedures on a teacher's social contacts with her students. *Journal of Applied Behavior Analysis,* 1970, **3**, 169-174.

Mandell, W., Goldschmidt, P., & Grover, P. *An evaluation of treatment programs for drug abusers.* Baltimore: Johns Hopkins University, 1973.

Mannino, F.V., & Shore, M.F. The effects of consultation: A review of empirical studies. *American Journal of Community Psychology,* 1975, **3**, 1-21.

Markson, E.W., Levitz, G.S., & Gognalons-Caillard, M. The elderly and the community: Reidentifying unmet needs. *Journal of Gerontology,* 1973, **28**, 503-509.

Marlatt, G.A., Demming, B., & Reid, J.B. Loss of control drinking in alcoholics: An experimental analogue. *Journal of Abnormal Psychology,* 1973, **81**, 233-241.

Marler, L. A study of anti-litter messages. *Journal of Environmental Education,* 1970, **3**, 52-53.

Marshall, W.L. The modification of sexual fantasies: A combined treatment approach to the reduction of deviant sexual behavior. *Behaviour Research and Therapy,* 1973, **11**, 557-564.

Martin, W., Jasinski, D., & Mansky, P. Naltrexone, an antagonist for the treatment of heroin dependence. *Archives of General Psychiatry,* 1973, **28**, 784-791.

Martorano, R. Mood and social perception in four alcoholics: Effects of alcohol consumption and assertive training. *Quarterly Journal of Studies on Alcohol,* 1974, **35**, 445-457.

Martorano, R., & Winett, R.A. Use of pseudopatients to evaluate mental health programs. Study in progress, University of Kentucky, 1976.

Masserman, J.H., & Yum, K.S. An analysis of the influence of alcohol on experimental neuroses in cats. *Psychosomatic Medicine,* 1946, **8**, 36-52.

Matlack, D.R. The case of geriatric day hospitals. *Gerontologist,* 1975, **15**, 109-113.

Mattocks, A., & Jew, C. Assessments of an aversive treatment program with extreme acting-out patients in a psychiatric facility for criminal offenders. Unpublished manuscript, Vacaville Medical Facility, 1970.

Matza, D. *Delinquency and drift.* New York: Wiley, 1964.

Matza, D. *Becoming deviant.* Englewood Cliffs, N.J.: Prentice-Hall, 1969.

May, E. Narcotics addiction and control in Great Britain. In P. Wald & P. Hutt (Eds.), *Dealing with drug abuse.* New York: Praeger, 1972.

McBrearty, J.F., Dichter, M., Garfield, Z., & Heath, G.A. Behaviorally oriented program for alcoholism. *Psychological Reports,* 1968, **22**, 287-298.

McCabe, O., Kurland, A., & Sullivan, D. A study of methadone failures in an abstinence program. *The International Journal of the Addictions,* 1974, **9**, 731-740.

McCarthy, E.J. Report of the Senate Special Subcommittee on unemployment problems. In A.M. Okun (Ed.), *The battle against unemployment.* New York: Norton, 1965.

McClannahan, L.E., & Risley, T.R. A store for nursing home residents. *Nursing Homes,* 1973, **22**, 10-11.

McClannahan, L.E., & Risley, T.R. Activities and materials for severely disabled geriatric patients. *Nursing Homes,* 1974a, **23**, 19-23.

McClannahan, L.E., & Risley, T.R. Design of living environments for nursing home residents. *Gerontologist,* 1974b, **14**, 236-240.

McClannahan, L.E., & Risley, T.R. Design of living environments for nursing home residents: Additional strategies for increasing attendance and participation in group activities. *Journal of Applied Behavior Analysis,* 1974c, **7**, 180-184.

McClearn, G.E. The genetic aspects of alcoholism. In P.G. Bourne & R. Fox (Eds.), *Alcoholism: Progress in research and treatment.* New York: Academic Press, 1973.

McConnel, J.V. Criminals can be brainwashed — now. *Psychology Today,* April, 1970, pages 14, 16, 18, 74.

McCord, W., & McCord, J. *Origins of crime.* New York: Columbia University Press, 1959.

McFall, R.M., & Lillesand, D.B. Behavior rehearsal with modeling and coaching in assertion training. *Journal of Abnormal Psychology,* 1970, **76**, 295-303.

McFall, R.M., & Twentyman, C.T. Four experiments on the relative contributions of rehearsal, modeling, and coaching in assertion training. *Journal of Abnormal Psychology,* 1973, **81**, 199-218.

McGlothlin, W. Drug use and abuse. *Annual Review of Psychology,* 1975, **26**, 45-64.

McGovern, K.B., Arkowitz, H., & Gilmore, S.K. The evaluation of social skill training programs for college dating inhibitions. Unpublished manuscript, University of Oregon, 1975.

McGuire, W.J., & Vallance, M. Aversion therapy by electric shock, a simple technique. *British Medical Journal,* 1964, **1**, 151-152.

McKee, J. The Draper experiment: A programmed learning project. In G. Ofiesh & W. Meierhenry (Eds.), *Trends in programmed instruction.* National Education Association, 1964.

McKee, J. Draper experiments in behavior modification. Paper presented at the Behavior Modification Institute, Tuscaloosa, Alabama, May 1969.

McLaughlin, T.F., & Malaby, J. Intrinsic reinforcers in a classroom token economy. *Journal of Applied Behavior Analysis,* 1972a, **5**, 263-270.

McLaughlin, T.F., & Malaby, J. Reducing and measuring inappropriate verbalizations in a token classroom. *Journal of Applied Behavior Analysis,* 1972b, **5**, 329-333.

McNamara, J. The history of United States anti-opium policy. *Federal Probation,* 1973, **37**, 15-21.

McNamee, H.B., Mello, N.K., & Mendelson, J.H. Experimental analysis of drinking patterns of alcoholics, concurrent psychiatric observations. *American Journal of Psychiatry,* 1968, **124**, 1063-1069.

Medland, M.B., & Stachnik, T.J. Good-behavior game: A replication and systematic analysis. *Journal of Applied Behavior Analysis,* 1972, **5**, 45-51.

Meehl, P. Psychology and the criminal law. *University of Richmond Law Review,* 1970, **5**, 1-30.

Mees, H.L. Sadistic fantasies modified by aversion conditioning and substitution: A case study. *Behaviour Research and Therapy,* 1966, **4**, 317-320.

Mehta, N.H., & Mack, C.M. Day care services: An alternative to institutional care. *Journal of the American Geriatric Society,* 1975, **23**, 280-283.

Meichenbaum, D.H., Bowers, K.S., & Ross, R.R. Modification of classroom behavior of institutionalized female adolescent offenders. *Behaviour Research and Therapy,* 1968, **6**, 343-353.

Meichenbaum, D., & Cameron, D. Training schizophrenics to talk to themselves: A means of developing attentional controls. *Behavior Therapy,* 1973, **4**, 515-534.

Melin, G., & Götestam, K. A contingency management program on a drug-free unit for intravenous amphetamine addicts. *Journal of Behavior Therapy and Experimental Psychiatry*, 1973, **4**, 331-337.

Mello, N.K., & Mendelson, J.H. Operant analysis of drinking patterns of chronic alcoholics. *Nature*, 1965, **206**, 43-46.

Melnick, J.A. A comparison of replication techniques in the modification of minimal dating behavior. *Journal of Abnormal Psychology*, 1973, **81**, 51-59.

Mendelson, J.H. Ethanol $-$ 1-C^{14} metabolism in alcoholics and nonalcoholics. *Science*, 1968, **159**, 319-320.

Mendelson, J.H., & Mello, N.K. Experimental analysis of drinking behavior of chronic alcoholics. *Annals of the New York Academy of Sciences*, 1966, **133**, 828-845.

Mennel, R.M. Origins of the juvenile court: Changing perspectives on the legal rights of juvenile delinquents. *Crime and Delinquency*, 1972, **18**, 68-78.

Menninger, K.A. *Man against himself.* New York: Harcourt, Brace, 1938.

Mensh, I.N. Drug addiction. In C.G. Costello (Ed.), *Symptoms of psychopathology.* New York: Wiley, 1970.

Merry, J. The "loss of control" myth. *Lancet*, 1966, **1**, 1257-1268.

Merton, R.K. *Social theory and social structure.* New York: Glencoe Press, 1957.

Meyer, M., Odom, E.E., & Wax, B.S. Birth and life of an incentive system in a residential institution for adolescents. *Child Welfare*, 1973, **52**, 503-509.

Meyers, A.W., Craighead, W.E., & Meyers, H.H. A behavioral-preventive approach to community mental health. *American Journal of Community Psychology*, 1974, **2**, 275-286.

Meyers, J. Consultee-centered consultation with a teacher as a technique in behavior management. *American Journal of Community Psychology*, 1975, **3**, 111-122.

Milakovich, M.E., & Weis, K. Politics and measures of success in the war on crime. *Crime and Delinquency*, 1975, **21**, 1-10.

Milan, M. Behavior modification for the disadvantaged: The token economy as a basis for effective correctional management. Paper presented at the 1972 convention of the American Personnel and Guidance Association, Chicago, March 1972.

Milan, M., & McKee, J. Behavior modification: Principles and applications in corrections. In D. Glaser (Ed.), *Handbook of criminology.* Chicago: Rand McNally, 1974.

Milan, M., Wood, L., Williams, R., Rogers, J., Hampton, L., & McKee, J. *Applied behavior analysis and the imprisoned adult felon project I: The cellblock token economy.* Montgomery, Ala.: Experimental Manpower Laboratory for Corrections, 1974.

Miller, A. *The assault on privacy.* Ann Arbor: University of Michigan Press, 1971.

Miller, B.A., Pokorny, A.D., & Hanson, D.G. A study of dropouts in an inpatient alcoholism treatment program. *Diseases of the Nervous System*, 1968, **29**, 91-99.

Miller, B.A., Pokorny, A.D., Valles, F., & Cleveland, S. Biased sampling in alcoholism treatment research. *Quarterly Journal of Studies on Alcohol*, 1970, **31**, 97-107.

Miller, E.C., Dvorak, B.A., & Turner, D.W. A method of creating aversion to alcohol by reflex conditioning in a group setting. *Quarterly Journal of Studies on Alcohol*, 1960, **21**, 424-431.

Miller, G.A. Psychology as a means of promoting human welfare. *American Psychologist*, 1969, **24**, 1063-1075.

Miller, J., Sensenig, J., Stocker, R., & Campbell, R. Value patterns of drug addicts as a function of race and sex. *The International Journal of the Addictions*, 1973, **8**, 589-598.

Miller, L.K., & Miller, O. Reinforcing self-help group activities of welfare recipients. *Journal of Applied Behavior Analysis*, 1970, **3**, 57-64.

Miller, L.K., & Schneider, R. The use of a token economy in project Head Start. *Journal of Applied Behavior Analysis*, 1970, **3**, 213-220.

Miller, P.M. The use of behavioral contracting in the treatment of alcoholism: A case report. *Behavior Therapy*, 1972, **3**, 593-596.

Miller, P.M. Behavioral treatment of drug addiction: A review. *The International Journal of the Addictions*, 1973a, **8**, 511-520.

Miller, P.M. Behavioral assessment in alcoholism research and treatment: Current techniques. *International Journal of the Addictions*, 1973b, **8**, 831-837.

Miller, P.M. A behavioral intervention program for chronic public drunkenness offenders. *Archives of General Psychiatry*, 1975, **32**, 915-918.

Miller, P.M., Hersen, M., & Eisler, R.M. Relative effectiveness of instructions, agreements, and reinforcement in behavioral contracts with alcoholics. *Journal of Abnormal Psychology*, 1974, **83**, 548-553.

Miller, P.M., Hersen, M., Eisler, R.M., & Hemphill, D.P. Electrical aversion therapy with alcoholics: An analogue study. *Behaviour Research and Therapy*, 1973, **11**, 491-498.

Miller, P.M., Hersen, M., Eisler, R.M., & Hilsman, G. Effects of social stress on operant drinking of alcoholic and social drinkers. *Behaviour Research and Therapy*, 1974, **55**, 279-284.

Miller, W. Lower class culture as a generating milieu of gang delinquency. *Journal of Social Issues*, 1958, **14**, 5-19.

Mischel, W. *Personality and assessment.* New York: Wiley, 1968.

Mischel, W. *Introduction to personality.* (2nd ed.) New York: Holt, Rinehart & Winston, 1976.

Mishara, B.L., & Kastenbaum, R. Wine in the treatment of long-term geriatric patients in mental hospitals. *Journal of the American Geriatric Society*, 1974, **22**, 88-94.

Mitford, J. *Kind and usual punishment: The prison business.* New York: Knopf, 1973.

Monroe, J., Ross, W., & Berzins, J.I. The decline of the addict as "psychopath": Implications for community care. *The International Journal of the Addictions,* 1971, **6**, 601-608.

Moore, D., & Nietzel, M. Generalization and maintenance effects of social learning therapies: Indications of neglected criteria. Unpublished manuscript, University of Kentucky, 1975.

Moos, R., & Insel, P.M. *Issues in social ecology.* Palo Alto, Calif.: National Press Books, 1974.

Morgan, B.S., Blonsky, M.R., & Rosen, H. Employee attitudes toward a hardcore hiring program. *Journal of Applied Psychology,* 1970, **54**, 473-478.

Morris, N., & Hawkins, G. *The honest politician's guide to crime control.* Chicago: The University of Chicago Press, 1970.

Morris, W.W. *Mental health of the older adult.* Proceedings of the University of Iowa's 11th Conference on Gerontology. Iowa City: The Institute of Gerontology, 1967.

Moss, B.B., & Lavery, M.E. Review of a new community health care evaluation and service center. *Gerontologist,* 1974, **14**, 207-209.

Moss, F.E. *Nursing home care in the United States: Failure in public policy.* Introductory report prepared by the Subcommittee on Long-Term Care of the Special Committee on Aging, United States Senate. Washington, D.C.: Government Printing Office, 1974.

Motin, J. Drug-induced attenuation of alcohol consumption. *Quarterly Journal of Studies on Alcohol,* 1973, **34**, 444-472.

Mueller, D.J., & Atlas, L. Resocialization of regressed elderly residents: A behavioral management approach. *Journal of Gerontology,* 1972, **27**, 390-392.

Murrell, S.A. *Community psychology and social systems.* New York: Behavioral Publications, 1973.

Nader, R. *Old age: The last segregation.* New York: Grossman, 1971.

Nagel, W.G. *The new red barn: A critical look at the modern American prison.* New York: Wackor, 1973.

Nathan, P.E. Alcoholism. In H. Leitenberg (Ed.), *Handbook of behavior modification.* New York: Appleton-Century-Crofts, 1976.

Nathan, P.E., & Briddell, D.W. Behavioral assessment and treatment of alcoholism. In B. Kissin & H. Begleiter (Eds.), *The biology of alcoholism.* Vol. 5. New York: Plenum Press, in press.

Nathan, P.E., & Harris, S.L. *Psychopathology and society.* New York: McGraw-Hill, 1975.

Nathan, P.E., & O'Brien, J.S. An experimental analysis of the behavior of alcoholics and nonalcoholics during prolonged experimental drinking. *Behavior Therapy,* 1971, **2**, 455-476.

Nathan, P.E., Titler, N.A., Lowenstein, L.M., Solomon, P., & Rossi, A.M. Behavioral analysis of chronic alcoholism. *Archives of General Psychiatry,* 1970, 22, 419-430.

National Citizens' Committee for Community Relations and the Community Relations Service of the United States Department of Justice. *Putting the hard-core unemployed into jobs.* Washington, D.C.: Government Printing Office, 1967.

National Commission on Marijuana and Drug Abuse. *Drug use in America: Problem in perspective.* Washington, D.C.: Government Printing Office, 1973.

Neikirk, B. Time-of-day electric pricing would vary cost with hour. *Chicago Tribune* (cited in *The Lexington Leader*), June 6, 1975.

Neill, A.S. *Summerhill.* New York: Hart, 1960.

Nelson, R.O. An expanded scope for behavior modification in school settings. *Journal of School Psychology,* 1974, 12, 276-287.

Nettler, G. *Explaining crime.* New York: McGraw-Hill, 1974.

Newbrough, J. Community psychology: A new holism. *American Journal of Community Psychology,* 1973, 1, 201-211.

Newton, J., & Stein, L. Implosive therapy in alcoholism: Comparison with brief psychotherapy. *Quarterly Journal of Studies on Alcohol,* 1974, 35, 1256-1265.

Nietzel, M.T. Psychiatric expertise in and out of court. *Judicature,* 1974, 58, 39-41.

Nietzel, M.T., & Dade, J. Bail reform as an example of a community psychology intervention in the criminal justice system. *American Journal of Community Psychology,* 1973, 1, 238-247.

Nietzel, M.T., Martorano, R., & Melnick, J. The effects of covert modeling with and without reply training on the development and generalization of assertive responses. *Behavior Therapy,* 1977, 8.

Nietzel, M., & Moss, C. The psychologist in the criminal justice system. *Professional Psychology,* 1972, 3, 259-270.

Nietzel, M.T., & Winett, R.A. Demographics, attitudes, and behavioral responses to important environmental events. *American Journal of Community Psychology,* in press.

O'Brien, C.P. The role of conditioning in narcotic addiction. In E. Chirinos (Ed.), *International symposium on behavior modification.* in press.

O'Brien, F., & Azrin, N.H. Interaction-priming: A method of reinstating patient-family relationships. *Behaviour Research and Therapy,* 1973, 11, 133-136.

O'Brien, J., & Raynes, A. Treatment of heroin addiction with behavioral therapy. In W. Keup (Ed.), *Drug abuse: Current concepts and research.* Springfield, Ill.: Thomas, 1972.

O'Brien, J., Raynes, A., & Patch, V. An operant reinforcement system to improve ward behavior in in-patient drug addicts. *Journal of Behavior Therapy and Experimental Psychiatry,* 1971, 2, 239-242.

O'Brien, J., Raynes, A., & Patch, V. Treatment of heroin addiction with aversion therapy, relaxation training, and systematic desensitization. *Behaviour Research and Therapy,* 1972, **10,** 77-80.

O'Connor, R.D. Modification of social withdrawal through symbolic modeling. *Journal of Applied Behavior Analysis,* 1969, **2,** 15-22.

O'Connor, R.D., & Rappaport, J. Application of social learning principles to the training of ghetto blacks. *American Psychologist,* 1970, **25,** 659-661.

Okun, A.M. (Ed.) *The battle against unemployment.* New York: Norton, 1965.

O'Leary, K.D., Becker, W.C., Evans, M.B., & Saudargas, R.A. A token reinforcement program in a public school: A replication and systematic analysis. *Journal of Applied Behavior Analysis,* 1969, **2,** 3-13.

O'Leary, K.D., & Drabman, R.S. Token reinforcement programs in the classroom: A review. *Psychological Bulletin,* 1971, **6,** 379-398.

O'Leary, K.D., Kaufman, K.F., Kass, R.E., & Drabman, R.S. The effects of loud and soft reprimands on the behavior of disruptive students. *Exceptional Children,* 1970, **37,** 145-155.

O'Leary, K.D., & O'Leary, S.G. *Classroom management: The successful use of behavior modification.* Elmsford, N.Y.: Pergamon Press, 1972.

O'Leary, K.D., & Wilson, G. *Behavior therapy: Application and outcome.* Englewood Cliffs, N.J.: Prentice-Hall, 1975.

O'Leary, V.E. The Hawthorne Effect in reverse: Trainee orientation for the hard-core unemployed woman. *Journal of Applied Psychology,* 1972, **56,** 491-494.

Oliver, R. The Virginia program from an administrative perspective. Paper presented at the 82nd annual convention of the American Psychological Association, New Orleans, 1974.

O'Malley, J.E., Anderson, W.H., & Lazare, A. Failure of outpatient treatment of drug abuse. I: Heroin. *American Journal of Psychiatry,* 1972, **128,** 865-868.

Opton, E. Psychiatric violence against prisoners: When therapy is punishment. *Mississippi Law Journal,* 1974, **45,** 605-644.

Orr, D.B. *New directions in employability: Reducing barriers to full employment.* New York: Praeger, 1973.

Oster, C., & Kibat, W.H. Evaluation of a multidisciplinary care program for stroke patients in a day care center. *Journal of the American Geriatric Society,* 1975, **23,** 63-69.

Owen, A., & Winkler, R.C. General practitioners and psychosocial problems: An evaluation using pseudo-patients. *Medical Journal of Australia,* 1974, **2,** 393-398.

Oxberger, L. Revolution in corrections. *Drake Law Review,* 1973, **22,** 250-265.

Packard, R.G. The control of classroom attention: A group contingency for complex behavior. *Journal of Applied Behavior Analysis,* 1970, **3,** 13-28.

Paden, R.C., Himelstein, H.C., & Paul, G.L. Videotape versus verbal feedback in the modification of meal behavior of chronic mental patients. *Journal of Consulting and Clinical Psychology,* 1974, **42,** 623.

Page, S., Caron, P., & Yates, E. Behavior modification methods and institutional psychology. *Professional Psychology,* 1975, **6**, 175-181.

Paine, F.T., Deutsch, D.R., & Smith, R.A. Relationship between family background and work values. *Journal of Applied Psychology,* 1967, **51**, 320-323.

Palmore, E.B., & Manton, K. Ageism compared to racism and sexism. *Journal of Gerontology,* 1973, **28**, 363-369.

Palmore, E.B., & Manton, K. Modernization and status of the aged: International correlations. *Journal of Gerontology,* 1974, **29**, 205-210.

Panyan, M., Boozer, H., & Morris, N. Feedback to attendants as a reinforcer for applying operant techniques. *Journal of Applied Behavior Analysis,* 1970, **3**, 1-4.

Papamarcos, J. System planning amidst roadblocks and confusion. *Power Engineering,* 1975, **79**, 26-35.

Parsonson, B.S., Baer, A.M., & Baer, D.M. The application of generalized correct social contingencies: An evaluation of a training program. *Journal of Applied Behavior Analysis,* 1974, **7**, 427-438.

Patterson, G.R., & Anderson, D. Peers as social reinforcers. *Child Development,* 1964, **35**, 951-960.

Patterson, G.R., Cobb, J.A., & Ray, R.S. A social engineering technology for retraining the families of aggressive boys. In H.E. Adams & I.P. Unikel (Eds.), *Issues and trends in behavior therapy.* Springfield, Ill.: Thomas, 1973.

Patterson, G.R., & Reid, J.B. Intervention for families of aggressive boys: A replication study. *Behaviour Research and Therapy,* 1973, **11**, 383-394.

Pattison, E.M. A critique of alcoholism treatment concepts with special reference to abstinence. *Quarterly Journal of Studies on Alcohol,* 1966, **27**, 49-71.

Paul, G.L. Behavior modification research: Design and tactics. In C.M. Franks (Ed.), *Behavior therapy: Appraisal and status.* New York: McGraw-Hill, 1969a.

Paul, G.L. The chronic mental patient: Current status — future directions. *Psychological Bulletin,* 1969b, **71**, 81-94.

Paul, G.L., & McInnis, T.L. Attitudinal changes associated with two approaches to training mental health technicians in milieu and social learning programs. *Journal of Consulting and Clinical Psychology,* 1974, **42**, 21-33.

Paul, G.L., McInnis, T.L., & Mariotto, M.J. Objective performance outcomes associated with two approaches to training mental health technicians in milieu and social learning programs. *Journal of Abnormal Psychology,* 1973, **82**, 523-532.

Pavlott, J. Effects of reinforcement procedures on negative behaviors in delinquent girls. Unpublished doctoral dissertation, University of Pittsburgh, 1971.

Pedalino, E., & Gamboa, V.U. Behavior modification and absenteeism: Intervention in one industrial setting. *Journal of Applied Psychology,* 1974, **59**, 694-698.

Perkins, M.E., & Bloch, H.I. A study of some failures in methadone treatment.

American Journal of Psychiatry, 1971, **128**, 79-83.

Peterson, D., & Thomas, C. Review of relevant research in correctional rehabilitation. In J. Cull & R. Hardy (Eds), *Fundamentals of criminal behavior and correctional systems.* Springfield, Ill.: Thomas, 1973.

Peterson, T. The Dade County pretrial intervention project: Formalization of the diversion function and its impact on the criminal justice system. *University of Miami Law Review,* 1973, **28**, 86-114.

Petrock, F. Implications of behavior modification for organizational change. In R.A. Winett (chair), *Behavior modification in the community: Progress and problems.* Symposium at the 83rd convention of the American Psychological Association, Chicago, 1975.

Petty, M.M. Relative effectiveness of four combinations of oral and written presentations of job related information to disadvantaged trainees. *Journal of Applied Psychology,* 1974, **59**, 105-106.

Phillips, E.L. Achievement Place: Token reinforcement procedures in a home-style rehabilitation setting for "pre-delinquent" boys. *Journal of Applied Behavior Analysis,* 1968, **1**, 213-223.

Phillips, E.L., Phillips, E.A., Fixsen, D.L., & Wolf, M.M. Achievement Place: Modification of the behaviors of pre-delinquent boys within a token economy. *Journal of Applied Behavior Analysis,* 1971, **4**, 45-59.

Phillips, E.L., Phillips, E.A., Fixsen, D.L., & Wolf, M.M. *The teaching-family handbook.* Lawrence, Kansas: Kansas Printing Service, 1972.

Phillips, E.L., Phillips, E.A., Wolf, M.M., & Fixsen, D.L. Achievement Place: Development of the elected manager system. *Journal of Applied Behavior Analysis,* 1973, **6**, 541-562.

Pierce, C.H., & Risley, T.R. Improving job performance of Neighborhood Youth Corps aides in an urban recreation program. *Journal of Applied Behavior Analysis,* 1974a, **7**, 207-216.

Pierce, C.H., & Risley, T.R. Recreation as a reinforcer: Increasing membership and decreasing disruption in an urban recreation center. *Journal of Applied Behavior Analysis,* 1974b, **7**, 403-412.

Pinkston, E.M., Reese, N.M., LeBlanc, J.M., & Baer, D.M. Independent control of a preschool child's aggression and peer interaction by contingent teacher attention. *Journal of Applied Behavior Analysis,* 1973, **6**, 115-124.

Plant, T.F.A. *Alcohol problems: A report to the nation by the Cooperative Commission on the Study of Alcoholism.* New York: Oxford University Press, 1967.

Poe, W.D. Medical planners and the geriatric imperative. *Journal of the American Geriatric Society,* 1975, **23**, 197-199.

Polakow, R. Covert sensitization treatment of a probationed barbiturate addict. *Journal of Behavior Therapy and Experimental Psychiatry,* 1975, **6**, 53-54.

Polakow, R., & Doctor, R. Treatment of marijuana and barbiturate dependency by contingency contracting. *Journal of Behavior Therapy and Experimental Psychiatry,* 1973, **4**, 375-377.

Polakow, R., & Doctor, R. A behavioral modification program for adult drug offenders. *Journal of Research in Crime and Delinquency,* 1974a, **11**, 63-69.

Polakow, R., & Doctor, R. Establishing behavior therapy in a public agency. Paper presented at the eighth annual convention of the Association for the Advancement of Behavior Therapy, Chicago, 1974(b).

Polakow, R., & Peabody, D. Behavioral treatment of child abuse. *International Journal of Offender Therapy and Comparative Criminology,* 1975, **19**, 100-103.

Polier, J.W. Justice for juveniles. *Child Welfare,* 1973, **52**, 5-13.

Polk, K., Frease, D., & Richmond, F.L. Social class, school experience, and delinquency. *Criminology,* 1974, **12**, 84-96.

Polk, K., & Schafer, W.K. (Ed.) *Schools and delinquency.* Englewood Cliffs, N.J.: Prentice-Hall, 1972.

Pollock, D.D., & Liberman, R.P. Behavior therapy of incontinence in demented inpatients. *Gerontologist,* 1974, **14**, 488-491.

Pomerleau, D., Bobrove, P., & Smith, R. Rewarding psychiatric aides for the behavioral improvement of assigned patients. *Journal of Applied Behavior Analysis,* 1973, **6**, 383-390.

Pommer, D.A., & Streedbeck, P. Motivating staff performance in an operant learning program for children. *Journal of Applied Behavior Analysis,* 1974, **7**, 217-222.

Powell, R.R. Psychological effects of exercise therapy upon institutionalized geriatric mental patients. *Journal of Gerontology,* 1974, **29**, 157-161.

Powell, T.J., & Riley, J.M. The basic elements of community mental health education. *Community Mental Health Journal,* 1970, **6**, 196-202.

Power, C.A., & McCarron, L.T. Treatment of depression in persons residing in homes for the aged. *Gerontologist,* 1975, **15**, 132-135.

Powers, R.B., Osborne, J.G., & Anderson, E.G. Positive reinforcement of litter removal in the natural environment. *Journal of Applied Behavior Analysis,* 1973, **6**, 579-586.

Powers, R., & Powers, E. Responding of retarded children on a backscratch schedule of reinforcement. *Psychological Aspects of Disability,* 1971, **18**, 27-34.

Prentice, N.M. The influence of live and symbolic modeling on promoting moral judgements of adolescent delinquents. *Journal of Abnormal Psychology,* 1972, **80**, 157-161.

President's Commission on Law Enforcement and the Administration of Justice. *Task Force Report: Juvenile Delinquency and Youth Crime.* Washington, D.C.: Government Printing Office, 1967.

President's Council on Aging. *Report to the President.* Washington, D.C.: Government Printing Office, 1963.

Prock, V.N. Effects of institutionalization: A comparison of community, waiting list, and institutionalized aged persons. *American Journal of Public Health,* 1969, **59**, 1837-1844.

Proshansky, H. Unemployment — America's major mental health problem. Paper presented at the annual meeting of the American Psychological Association, Chicago, 1975.

Proshansky, H.M., Ittelson, W.H., & Rivlin, L.G. *Environmental Psychology.* New York: Holt, Rinehart & Winston, 1970.

Pryor, D.H. Somewhere between society and the cemetery: Where we put the aged. *The New Republic,* April 15, 1970, 15-17.

Quay, H. Psychopathic personality as pathological stimulation-seeking. *American Journal of Psychiatry,* 1965, **122,** 180-183.

Quilitch, H.R. Purposeful activity increased on a geriatric ward through programmed recreation. *Journal of the American Geriatrics Society,* 1974, **22,** 226-229.

Quilitch, H.R. A comparison of three staff-management procedures. *Journal of Applied Behavior Analysis,* 1975, **8,** 59-66.

Quilitch, H.R., & Risley, T.R. The effects of play materials on social play. *Journal of Applied Behavior Analysis,* 1973, **6,** 573-578.

Rachman, S.J., & Teasdale, J. Aversion therapy: An appraisal. In C.M. Franks (Ed.), *Behavior therapy: Appraisal and status.* New York: McGraw-Hill, 1969.

Rankin, A. The effects of pre-trial detention. *New York University Law Review,* 1964, **39,** 642-646.

Rao, D.B. Day hospitals and welfare homes in the care of the aged. *Journal of the American Geriatric Society,* 1971, **19,** 781-787.

Rappaport, J., & Chinsky, J.M. Models for delivery of service from a historical and conceptual perspective. *Professional Psychology,* 1974, **5,** 42-50.

Rappaport, J., Davidson, W., Wilson, M. & Mitchell, A. Alternatives to blaming the victim or the environment: Our places to stand have not moved the earth. *American Psychologist,* 1975, **30,** 525-528.

Raskin, D. International issues in drug abuse. *The International Journal of the Addictions,* 1974, **9,** 365-372.

Rathus, S.A. An experimental investigation of assertive training in a group setting. *Journal of Behavior Therapy and Experimental Psychiatry,* 1972, **3,** 81-86.

Rathus, S.A. Instigation of assertive behavior through videotape-mediated assertive models and directed practice. *Behaviour Research and Therapy,* 1973, **11,** 57-65.

Ray, E., & Kilburn, K. Behavior modification techniques applied to community behavior problems. *Criminology,* 1970, **8,** 173-184.

Raymond, M. The treatment of addiction by aversion conditioning with apomorphine. *Behaviour Research and Therapy,* 1964, **1,** 287-291.

Raymond, M.J. Case of fetishism treated by aversion therapy. *British Medical Journal,* 1965, **2,** 854-857.

Regester, D.C. Changes in autonomic responsivity and drinking behavior of alcoholics as a function of aversion therapy. *Dissertation Abstracts International,* 1971, **32,** 1225.

Reichel, W. New models in geriatrics and long-term care. *Journal of the American Geriatric Society*, 1973, **21**, 259-260.

Reichenfeld, H.F., Csapo, K.G., Carriere, L., & Gardner, R.C. Evaluating the effect of activity programs on a geriatric ward. *Gerontologist*, 1973, **13**, 305-310.

Reid, D.H., Luyben, P.L., Rawers, R.J., & Bailey, J.S. The effects of prompting and proximity of containers on newspaper recycling behavior. *Environment and Behavior*, 1976, **8**, 471-482.

Reid, E. Women at a standstill: The need for radical change. *International Labor Review*, 1975, **III**, 459-468.

Reimringer, M.J., Morgan, S., & Bramwell, P. Succinylcholine as a modifier of acting-out behaviour. *Clinical Medicine*, July 1970, 28-29.

Reingold, J., Wolk, R., & Schwartz, S. A gerontological sheltered workshop: The aged person's attitude about money. *Journal of the American Geriatric Society*, 1971, **19**, 315-331.

Reiss, M.L., Piotrowski, W.D., and Bailey, J.S. Behavioral community psychology: Encouraging low-income patients to seek dental care for their children. *Journal of Applied Behavioral Analysis*, 1976, **9**, 387-398.

Remnet, V.L. A group program for adaptation to a convalescent hospital. *Gerontologist*, 1974, **14**, 336-341.

Renn, D.K. The right to treatment and the juvenile. *Crime and Delinquency*, 1973, **19**, 477-484.

Renner, K.E. Some issues surrounding the academic sheltering of community psychology. *American Journal of Community Psychology*, 1974, **2**, 95-106.

Report of the National Advisory Commission on Civil Disorders. Washington, D.C.: Government Printing Office, 1968.

Reppucci, N., & Saunders, J. Social psychology of behavior modification: Problems of implementation in natural settings. *American Psychologist*, 1974, **29**, 649-660.

Resnick, L.B., Wang, M.C., & Kaplan, J. Task analysis in curriculum designs: A hierarchical sequenced introductory mathematics curriculum. *Journal of Applied Behavior Analysis*, 1973, **6**, 679-709.

Rice, P.R. Educo-therapy: A new approach to delinquent behavior. *Journal of Learning Disabilities*, 1970, **3**, 16-23.

Richards, S.A., & Jaffee, C.L. Blacks supervising whites: A study of interracial difficulties in working together in a simulated organization. *Journal of Applied Psychology*, 1972, **56**, 234-240.

Richette, L.A. *The throwaway children*. Philadelphia: Lippincott, 1969.

Riessman, F. A neighborhood based mental health approach. In E.L. Cowen, E.A. Gardner, & M. Zax (Eds.), *Emergent approaches to mental health problems*. New York: Appleton-Century-Crofts, 1967.

Rimm, D.C., & Masters, J.C. *Behavior therapy: Techniques and empirical findings*. New York: Academic Press, 1974.

Rinn, R.C., & Vernon, J.C. Process of evaluation of outpatient treatment in a community mental health center. *Journal of Behavior Therapy and Experimental Psychiatry*, 1975, **6**, 5-11.

Rinn, R.C., Vernon, J.C., & Wise, M.J. Training parents of behaviorally disordered children in groups: A three years' program evaluation. *Behavior Therapy*, 1975, **6**, 378-387.

Rioch, M.J., Elkes, C., Flint, A.A., Usdansky, B.S., Newman, R.G., & Silber, E. NIMH pilot study in training of mental health counselors. *American Journal of Community Psychology*, 1963, **33**, 678-689.

Risley, T.R., Clark, H., & Cataldo, M.F. Behavioral technology for the normal, middle-class family. In L.A. Hamerlynck, L.C. Handy, & E.J. Mash (Eds.), *Parenting: The change, maintenance, and directions for healthy family behaviors*, in press.

Robens, L. *Human engineering*. London: Jonathan Cape, 1970.

Robertshaw, C.S., Kelly, T.J., & Hicbert, H.D. Contingent time off to increase verbal behavior: A case report. *Journal of Clinical Psychology*, 1973, **41**, 459-461.

Robinson, R.A. The prevention and rehabilitation of mental illness in the elderly. *Interdisciplinary Topics in Gerontology*, 1969, **3**, 89-102.

Robison, J., & Smith, G. The effectiveness of correctional programs. *Crime and Delinquency*, 1971, **17**, 67-80.

Roe, A. Community resources centers. *American Psychologist*, 1970, **25**, 1033-1040.

Rose, S.D., Sundel, M., Delange, J., Corwin, L., & Palumbo, A. The Hartwig Project: A behavioral approach to the treatment of juvenile offenders. In R. Ulrich, R. Stachnik, & J. Mabry (Eds.), *Control of human offenders*. Vol. 2. New York: Scott, Foresman, 1970.

Rosen, E., Fox, R.E., & Gregory, I. *Abnormal psychology*. Philadelphia: Saunders, 1972.

Rosen, H., & Turner, J. Effectiveness of two orientation approaches in hard-core unemployed and absenteeism. *Journal of Applied Psychology*, 1971, **55**, 296-301.

Rosenblum, G. The new role of the clinical psychologist in a community mental health center. *Community Mental Health Journal*, 1968, **4**, 403-410.

Rosenhan, D.L. On being sane in insane places. *Science*, 1973, **179**, 250-258.

Rosenthal, D. Heredity in criminality. Paper presented at the annual meeting of the American Association for the Advancement of Science, 1973.

Rosenthal, R., & Rosnow, R. *Artifact in behavioral research*. New York: Academic Press, 1969.

Rosenzweig, N. Some differences between elderly people who use community resources and those who do not. *Journal of the American Geriatric Society*, 1975, **23**, 224-233.

Rosin, A.J. Why were they in hospital so long? *Gerontologia Clinica*, 1970, **12**, 40-48.

Rostow, C.D., & Smith, C.E. Effects of contingency management of chronic patients on ward control and behavioral adjustment. *Journal of Behaviour Therapy and Experimental Psychiatry*, 1975, **6**, 1-4.

Rouse v. Cameron, 373 F. 2nd 451, 452 (D.C. Cir. 1966).

Rubin, B.K., & Stolz, S.B. Generalization of self-referent speech established in a retarded adolescent by operant procedures. *Behavior Therapy*, 1974, **5**, 93-106.

Ryan, W. *Blaming the victim.* New York: Vintage, 1971.

Rychlak, J. *Introduction to personality and psychotherapy.* Boston: Houghton Mifflin, 1973.

Sage, W. Crime and the clockwork lemon. *Human Behavior*, September 1974, 16-23.

Sajwaj, T., Twardosz, S., & Burke, M. Side effects of extinction procedures in a remedial preschool. *Journal of Applied Behavior Analysis*, 1972, **5**, 163-175.

Salzberg, B.H., Wheeler, A.J., Devar, L.T., & Hopkins, B.L. The effect of intermittent feedback and intermittent contingent access to play on printing of kindergarten children. *Journal of Applied Behavior Analysis*, 1971, **4**, 163-171.

Sanchez v. Ciccone, No. 20182-4, 3061-4 (W. D. Mo. 1973).

Sanders, M.G. Alcoholic cardiomyopathy: A critical review. *Quarterly Journal of Studies on Alcohol*, 1970, **31**, 324-386.

Sanders, R.M., & Hanson, P.J. A note on a simple procedure for redistributing a teacher's student contacts. *Journal of Applied Behavior Analysis*, 1971, **4**, 157-161.

Sanderson, R.E., Campbell, D., & Laverty, S.G. An investigation of a new aversive conditioning treatment for alcoholism. *Quarterly Journal of Studies on Alcohol*, 1963, **24**, 261-275.

Santogrossi, D.A., O'Leary, K.D., Romanczyk, R.G., & Kaufman, K.F. Self evaluation by adolescents in a psychiatric hospital school token economy. *Journal of Applied Behavior Analysis*, 1973, **6**, 277-287.

Santore, A.F., & Diamond, H. The role of a community mental health center in developing services to the aging. *Gerontologist*, 1974, **14**, 201-206.

Sarason, I. The evolution of community psychology. *American Journal of Community Psychology*, 1973, **1**, 91-97.

Sarason, S.B. *The creation of settings and the future societies.* San Francisco: Jossey-Bass, 1972.

Sarason, S.B. *The psychological sense of community: Prospects for a community psychology.* San Francisco: Jossey-Bass, 1974.

Sashkin, M., Morris, W.C., & Horst, L. A comparison of social and organizational change models: Information flow and data use processes. *Psychological Review*, 1973, **80**, 510-526.

Saunders, A. Behavior therapy in prisons: Walden II or clockwork orange. Eighth annual convention of Association for Advancement of Behavior Therapy, Chicago, 1974.

Scarpitti, F.R., & Stephenson, R.M. Juvenile court dispositions: Factors in the decision-making process. *Crime and Delinquency*, 1971, **17**, 142-151.

Schaefer, H.H., Sobell, M.B., & Mills, K.C. Baseline drinking behavior in alcoholics and social drinkers: Kinds of drinks and sip magnitude. *Behaviour Research and Therapy*, 1971, **9**, 23-27.

Schafer, S. *The victim and his criminal: A study in functional responsibility.* New York: Random House, 1968.

Schilder, P. The psychogenesis of alcoholism. *Quarterly Journal of Studies on Alcohol*, 1941, **2**, 277-283.

Schnelle, J.F., Kirchner, R.E., McNees, M.P., & Lawler, J.M. Social evaluation research: The evaluation of two police patrolling strategies. *Journal of Applied Behavior Analysis*, 1975, **8**, 353-366.

Schnelle, J.F., & Lee, J.F. A quasi-experimental retrospective evaluation of a prison policy change. *Journal of Applied Behavior Analysis*, 1974, **7**, 483-494.

Schnelle, J.F., McNees, M.P., Gendrich, J., & Hannah, J.T. An outpatient therapy information system based on applied behavioral analysis design and measurement standards. Unpublished manuscript, Luton Mental Health Center, Nashville, Tennessee, 1975.

Schnelle, J.F., Weathers, M.T., Hannah, J.T., & McNees, M.P. Community social evaluation: A multiple baseline analysis of the effect of a legalized liquor law in four middle Tennessee counties. *Journal of Community Psychology*, 1975, **3**, 224-230.

Schoen, K. PORT: A new concept of community-based correction. *Federal Probation*, September 1972, **36**, 35-40.

Schoenfeldt, L.F. Utilization of manpower: Development and evaluation of an assessment-classification model for matching individuals with jobs. *Journal of Applied Psychology*, 1974, **59**, 583-595.

Schofield, W. *Psychotherapy: The purchase of friendship.* Englewood Cliffs, N.J.: Prentice-Hall, 1964.

Schonfield, D. Future commitments and successful aging. I. The random sample. *Journal of Gerontology*, 1973a, **28**, 189-196.

Schonfield, D. Future commitments and successful aging. II. Special groups. *Journal of Gerontology*, 1973b, **28**, 197-201.

Schulberg, H.C. State planning for community mental health programs: Implications for psychologists. *Community Mental Health Journal*, 1965, **1**, 37-42.

Schultz, J.L. The cycle of juvenile court history. *Crime and Delinquency*, 1973, **19**(4), 457-476.

Schur, E.M. *Crimes without victims.* Englewood Cliffs, N.J.: Prentice-Hall, 1965.

Schur, E.M. Reactions to deviance: A critical assessment. *American Journal of Sociology*, 1969, **75**, 309-322.

Schur, E.M. *Radical non-intervention: Rethinking the delinquency problem.* Englewood Cliffs, N.J.: Prentice Hall, 1973.

Schwartz, G. Biofeedback as therapy: Some theoretical and practical issues. *American Psychologist,* 1973, **28**, 666-673.

Schwartz, M., & Henderson, G. The culture of unemployment: Some notes on Negro children. In A.B. Shostak & W. Comberg (Eds.), *Blue-collar world: Studies of the American worker.* Englewood-Cliffs, N.J.: Prentice-Hall, 1964.

Schwitzgebel, R. *Streetcorner research.* Cambridge, Mass.: Harvard University Press, 1964.

Schwitzgebel, R.L. Short-term operant conditioning of adolescent offenders on socially relevant variables. *Journal of Abnormal Psychology,* 1967, **72**, 134-142.

Schwitzgebel, R. Electronic alternatives to imprisonment. *Lex et Scientia,* 1968, **5**, 99.

Schwitzgebel, R.L. Preliminary socialization for psychotherapy of behavior-disordered adolescents. *Journal of Consulting and Clinical Psychology,* 1969, **33**, 71-77.

Schwitzgebel, R.K. Limitations on the coercive treatment of offenders. *Criminal Law Bulletin,* 1972, **8**, 267-320.

Schwitzgebel, R.K. A conceptual model for the protection of prisoners' rights. Paper presented at the 82nd annual convention of the American Psychological Association, New Orleans, 1974a.

Schwitzgebel, R. The right to effective mental treatment. *California Law Review,* 1974b, **62**, 936-951.

Schwitzgebel, R., & Kolb, D.A. Inducing behavior change in adolescent delinquents. *Behavior Research and Therapy,* 1964, **1**, 297-304.

Scott, E., & Scott, K. An overview of crime: A smorgasbord of causes and solutions. In E. Scott & K. Scott (Eds.), *Criminal rehabilitation within and without the walls.* Springfield, Ill.: Thomas, 1973.

Scott, J.W., & Bushell, D., Jr. The length of teacher contacts and students' off-task behavior. *Journal of Applied Behavior Analysis,* 1974, **7**, 39-44.

Sears, D.W. Elderly housing: A need determination technique. *Gerontologist,* 1974, **14**, 182-187.

Seashore, S.E., & Bowers, D.G. Durability of organizational change. *American Psychologist,* 1970, **25**, 227-233.

Seaver, W.B., & Patterson, A.H. Decreasing fuel oil consumption through feedback and social commendation. Unpublished manuscript, The Pennsylvania State University, 1975.

Seidman, E., & Rappaport, J. The educational pyramid: A paradigm for training, research, and manpower utilization in community psychology. *American Journal of Community Psychology,* 1974, **2**, 119-130.

Serber, M., & Keith, C. The Atascadero project: Model of a sexual retraining program for incarcerated homosexual pedophiles. *Journal of Homosexuality,* 1974, **1**, 87-97.

Severy, L.J. Exposure to deviance committed by valued peer group and family members. *Journal of Research in Crime and Delinquency*, 1973, **10**, 35-46.

Sewell, D.O. *Training the poor: A benefit-cost analysis of manpower programs in the U.S. antipoverty programs.* Kingston, Ontario: Industrial Relations Centre of Queen's University, 1971.

Shadel, C.A. Aversion treatment of alcohol addiction. *Quarterly Journal of Studies on Alcohol,* 1944, **5**, 216-228.

Shaefer, H.H., & Martin, P.L. Behavior therapy for "apathy" of hospitalized schizophrenics. *Psychological Reports,* 1966, **19**, 1147-1158.

Shah, S.A. A behavioral conceptualization of the development of criminal behavior therapeutic principles, and applications. A Report to the President's Commission on Law Enforcement and the Administration of Justice, 1966.

Shah, S.A. A behavioral approach to outpatient treatment of offenders. In H. Rickard (Ed.), *Unique programs in behavior readjustment.* Elmsford, N.Y.: Pergamon Press, 1970.

Shah, S.A. Perspectives and directions in juvenile corrections. *Psychiatric Quarterly,* 1973, **47**, 12-36.

Shanas, E. *The health of older people: A social survey.* Cambridge, Mass.: Harvard University Press, 1962.

Shanas, E. Factors affecting care of the patient: Clients, government policy, role of the family and social attitudes. *Journal of the American Geriatric Society,* 1973, **21**, 394-397.

Shapiro, M. Legislating the control of behavior control: Autonomy and the coercive use of organic therapies. *Southern California Law Review,* 1974, **47**, 237-356.

Shaw, C.R., & McKay, H.D. *Juvenile delinquency and urban areas.* Chicago: University of Chicago Press, 1942.

Shean, G.D., & Zeidberg, Z. Token reinforcement therapy: A comparison of matched groups. *Journal of Behavior Therapy and Experimental Psychiatry,* 1971, **2**, 94-105.

Sherman, T.M., & Cormier, W.H. An investigation of the influence of student behavior on teacher behavior. *Journal of Applied Behavior Analysis,* 1974, **7**, 11-21.

Sherwood, S., Morris, J.N., & Barnhart, E. Developing a system for assigning individuals into an appropriate residential setting. *Journal of Gerontology,* 1975, **30**, 331-342.

Shimoni, N. Development and evaluation of a model of school psychological services – A systems approach. Unpublished doctoral dissertation, University of North Carolina at Chapel Hill, 1973.

Shireman, G., Mann, K., Larsen, C., & Young, T. Findings from experiments in treatment in the correctional institution. *Social Science Review,* 1972, **46**, 38-59.

Shore, H. What's new about alternatives. *Gerontologist,* 1974, **14**, 6-11.

Shore, M. Psychological theories of the causes of antisocial behavior. *Crime and Delinquency,* 1971, **17**, 956-968.

Short, J.F. *Gang delinquency and delinquent subcultures.* New York: Harper & Row, 1968.

Shuman, S. The placebo cure for criminality. *Wayne Law Review,* 1973, **19**, 847-872.

Sidman, M. *Tactics of scientific research.* New York: Basic Books, 1960.

Sielaft, T.J. Modification of work behavior. *Personnel Journal,* 1974, **9**, 513-517.

Silberman, C. *Crisis in the classroom.* New York: Random House, 1970.

Silbert, J.D., & Sussman, A. The rights of juveniles confined in training schools. *Crime and Delinquency,* 1975, **20**, 373-388.

Silver, C.P. A jointly sponsored geriatric social club and day hospital. *Gerontologia Clinica,* 1970, **12**, 235-240.

Silverstein, S.J., Nathan, P.E., & Taylor, H.A. Blood alcohol estimation and controlled drinking by chronic alcoholics. *Behavior Therapy,* 1974, **5**, 1-15.

Silverstone, B., & Winter, L. The effects of introducing a heterosexual living space. *Gerontologist,* 1975, **17**, 83-85.

Simmons, L. As cited in P.E. Slater. Cross cultural views of the aged. In R. Kastenbaum (Ed.), *New thoughts on old age.* New York: Springer, 1964. Pp. 229-236.

Simmons, L., & Gold, M. The myth of international control: American foreign policy and the heroin traffic. *The International Journal of the Addictions,* 1973, **8**, 779-800.

Skinner, B.F. *Science and human behavior.* New York: Macmillan, 1953.

Skinner, B.F. *Beyond freedom and dignity.* New York: Knopf, 1971.

Slack, C.W. Experimenter-subject psychotherapy: A new method of introducing intensive office treatment for unreachable cases. *Mental Hygiene,* 1960, **44**, 238-256.

Sloan, H.N., & Ralph, J.L. A behavior modification program in Nevada. *International Journal of Offender Therapy and Comparative Criminology,* 1973, **17**, 290-296.

Slocum, J.W., & Strawser, R.H. Racial differences in job attitudes. *Journal of Applied Psychology,* 1972, **56**, 28-32.

Smart, R.G. Effects of alcohol on conflict and avoidance behavior. *Quarterly Journal of Studies on Alcohol,* 1965, **26**, 187-205.

Smart, R., & Fejer, D. Drug use among adolescents and their parents: Closing the generation gap in mood modification. *Journal of Abnormal Psychology,* 1972, **79**, 153-160.

Smith, C. Free-bus experiment a success in Seattle. Associated Press in *The Louisville Courier-Journal,* February 16, 1975.

Smith, D., Gay, G., & Ramer, B. Adolescent heroin abuse in San Francisco.

Proceedings of the third national conference on methadone treatment, November, 1971.

Smith, J.J. A medical approach to problem drinking. *Quarterly Journal of Studies on Alcohol*, 1949, **10**, 251-257.

Smith, K.J., & Lipman, A. Constraint and life satisfaction. *Journal of Gerontology*, 1972, **27**, 77-82.

Smith, M.B., & Hobbs, N. The community and the community mental health center. *American Psychologist*, 1966, **21**, 499-509.

Smith, P.M., & Austrin, H.R. Socialization as related to delinquency classification. *Psychological Reports*, 1974, **34**, 677-678.

Sobell, M.B., Schaeffer, H.H., & Mills, K.C. Differences in baseline drinking between alcoholics and normal drinkers. *Behaviour Research and Therapy*, 1972, **10**, 257-269.

Sobell, M.B., & Sobell, L.C. Individualized behavior therapy for alcoholics: Rationale procedures, preliminary results and appendix. *California Mental Health Research Monograph*, No. 13, Sacramento, California, 1972.

Sobell, M.B., & Sobell, L.C. Alcoholics treated by individualized behavior therapy: One year treatment outcome. *Behaviour Research and Therapy*, 1973a, **11**, 599-618.

Sobell, M.B., & Sobell, L.C. Evidence of controlled drinking by former alcoholics: A second year evaluation of individualized behavior therapy. Paper presented at the 81st convention of the American Psychological Association. Montreal, 1973b.

Sobell, M.B., & Sobell, L.C. Individualized behavior therapy for alcoholics. *Behavior Therapy*, 1973c, **4**, 49-72.

Sobell, L.C., Sobell, M.B., & Christelman, W.C. The myth of "one drink." *Behaviour Research and Therapy*, 1972, **10**, 119-125.

Soden, E. The need for realistic treatment of alcohol and drug addiction. *Federal Probation*, 1973, **37**, 40-42.

Solomon, R.L. Punishment. *American Psychologist*, 1964, **19**, 239-253.

Solomon, R.W., & Wahler, R.G. Peer reinforcement control of classroom problem behavior. *Journal of Applied Behavior Analysis*, 1973, **6**, 49-56.

Sommer, R. *Tight spaces: Hard architecture and how to humanize it*. Englewood Cliffs, N.J.: Prentice-Hall, 1974.

Sommer, R., & Ross, H. Social interaction on a geriatric ward. *International Journal of Social Psychology*, 1958, **3**, 128-133.

Spece, R. Conditioning and other technologies used to "treat?" "rehabilitate?" "demolish?" prisoners and mental patients. *Southern California Law Review*, 1972, **45**, 616-684.

Spence, D.L., Cohen, S., & Kowalski, C. Mental health, age, and community living. *Gerontologist*, 1975, **17**, 77-82.

Spergel, I.A. Community-based delinquency-prevention programs: An overview. *Social Service Review*, 1973, **47**, 16-31.

Spevack, M., Pihl, R., & Rowan, T. Behavior therapies in the treatment of drug abuse: Some case studies. *Psychological Record,* 1973, **23**, 179-184.

Spreitzer, E., & Snyder, E.E. Correlates of life satisfaction among the aged. *Journal of Gerontology,* 1974, **29**, 454-458.

Staats, A.W., & Butterfield, W.H. Treatment of non-reading in a culturally deprived juvenile delinquent: An application of reinforcement principles. *Child Development,* 1965, **3**, 925-942.

Staats, A.W., Finley, J.R. Minke, K.A., & Wolf, M.M. Reinforcement variables in the control of unit reading responses. *Journal of the Experimental Analysis of Behavior,* 1964, **7**, 139-149.

Staats, A.W., Staats, C.K., Schultz, R.E., & Wolf, M. The conditioning of textual responses using "extrinsic" reinforcers. *Journal of the Experimental Analysis of Behavior,* 1962, **5**, 33-40.

Stahl, J.R., Thomson, L.E., Leitenberg, H., & Hasazi, J.E. Establishment of praise as a conditioned reinforcer in socially unresponsive psychiatric patients. *Journal of Abnormal Psychology,* 1974, **83**, 488-496.

Stamford, B.A. Physiological effects of training upon institutionalized geriatric men. *Journal of Gerontology,* 1972, **27**, 451-455.

Stamford, B.A. Effects of chronic institutionalization on the physical working capacity and trainability of geriatric men. *Journal of Gerontology,* 1973, **28**, 441-446.

Steffen, J. Electromyographically induced relaxation in the treatment of chronic alcoholism. *Journal of Consulting and Clinical Psychology,* 1975, **43**, 275.

Steffen, J., Nathan, P.E., & Taylor, H. Tension-reducing effects of alcohol: Further evidence and some methodological considerations. *Journal of Abnormal Psychology,* 1974, **83**, 542-547.

Steffy, R.A., Hart, J., Craw, M., Torney, D., & Marlett, N. Operant behavior modification techniques applied to a ward of severely regressed and aggressive patients. *Journal of the Canadian Psychiatric Association,* 1969, **14**, 59-67.

Stein, K., & Rozynko, V. Psychological and social variables and personality patterns of drug abusers. *The International Journal of the Addictions,* 1974, **9**, 431-446.

Stein, T.J. Some ethical considerations of short-term workshops in the principles and methods of behavior modification. *Journal of Applied Behavior Analysis,* 1975, **8**, 113-115.

Steiner, C.M. The alcoholic game. *Quarterly Journal of Studies on Alcohol,* 1969, **30**, 920-938.

Steinfeld, G. The use of covert sensitization with institutionalized narcotic addicts. *The International Journal of the Addictions,* 1970, **5**, 225-232.

Steinfeld, G., Rautio, E., Rice, A., & Egan, M. The use of covert sensitization with narcotic addicts (further comments). Danbury, Conn.: Federal Correction Institute, Narcotics Unit, 1973.

Steketee, J.P. Community and behavioral approaches to delinquency: The court's perspective. Paper presented at American Psychological Association Convention, Montreal, Canada, 1973.

Stephenson, R.M., & Scarpitti, F.R. Essexfields: A non-residential experiment in group centered rehabilitation of delinquents. *American Journal of Correction,* 1969, 12-13.

Stevens, R.S. Reasons for admitting patients to geriatric hospitals. *Gerontologia Clinica,* 1970, **12**, 219-228.

Stolz, S.B., Wienckowski, L.A., & Brown, B.S. Behavior modification: A perspective on critical issues. *American Psychologist,* 1975, **30**, 1027-1048.

Stone, B., Winkler, R.C., & Hewson, D.M. An evaluation of a psychosexual counseling course for general practitioners using pseudo-patients. Unpublished manuscript, University of New South Wales, Sydney, Australia, 1975.

Stuart, R.B. Operant-interpersonal treatment for marital discord. *Journal of Consulting and Clinical Psychology,* 1969, **33**, 675-682.

Stuart, R.B. Behavioral contracting within the families of delinquents. *Journal of Behavior Therapy and Experimental Psychiatry,* 1971, **2**, 1-11.

Stuart, R.B. Notes on the ethics of behavior research and intervention. In L.A. Hamerlynck, L.C. Handy, & E.J. Mash (Eds.), *Behavioral change: Methodology, concepts and practice.* Champaign, Ill.: Research Press, 1973.

Stuart, R.B. Teaching facts about drugs: Pushing or preventing. *Journal of Educational Psychology,* 1974, **66**, 189-201.

Sulzer, E. Behavior modification in adult psychiatric patients. In L.P. Ullmann & L. Krasner (Eds.), *Case studies in behavior modification,* New York: Holt, Rinehart & Winston, 1965.

Suratt, P.P., Ulrich, R.E., & Hawkins, R.P. An elementary student as a behavioral engineer. *Journal of Applied Behavior Analysis,* 1969, **2**, 85-92.

Susman, J. Juvenile justice: Even-handed or many-handed? *Crime and Delinquency,* 1973, **19**, 493-507.

Sutherland, E.H., & Cressey, D.R. *Principles of criminology.* Philadelphia: Lippincott, 1960.

Sutker, P., Allain, A., & Moan, C. Addict attitudes toward methadone maintenance: A preliminary report. *The International Journal of the Addictions,* 1974, **9**, 337-344.

Sykes, G. The future of criminality. *American Behavioral Scientist,* 1972, **15**, 403-419.

Syme, L. Personality characteristics and the alcoholic: A critique of current studies. *Quarterly Journal of Studies on Alcohol,* 1957, **18**, 288-302.

Tait, D.C., & Hodges, E.F. Follow-up study of predicted delinquents. *Crime and Delinquency,* 1971, **17**, 202-212.

Tchobanian, R. Trade unions and the humanization of work. *International Labor Review,* 1975, **III**, 199-218.

Tharp, R.G., & Wetzel, R.J. *Behavior modification in the natural environment.* New York: Academic Press, 1969.

Thiman, J. Conditioned reflex treatment of alcoholism: I. *New England Journal of Medicine,* 1949a, **17**, 368-370.

Thiman, J. Conditioned reflex treatment of alcoholism: II. *New England Journal of Medicine,* 1949b, **17**, 408-410.

Thompson, G.B. Work versus leisure roles: An investigation of morale among employed and retired men. *Journal of Gerontology,* 1973, **28**, 339-344.

Thompson, I., & Rathod, N. Aversion therapy for heroin dependence. *Lancet,* 1968, **2**, 382-384.

Thomson, N., Fraser, D., & McDougall, A. The reinstatement of speech in near-mute schizophrenics by instructions, imitative prompts and reinforcement. *Journal of Behavior Therapy and Experimental Psychiatry,* 1974, **5**, 83-89.

Thoresen, C., & Mahoney, M. *Behavioral self-control.* New York: Holt, Rinehart & Winston, 1974.

Thorne, G.L., Tharp, R.G., & Wetzel, R.J. Behavior modification techniques: New tools for probation officers. *Federal Probation,* 1967, **31**, 21-27.

Tiffany, D.W., Cowan, J.R., & Tiffany, P.M. *The unemployed: A social-psychological portrait.* Englewood-Cliffs, N.J.: Prentice-Hall, 1970.

Timbers, G.D., Phillips, E.L., Fixsen, D.L., & Wolf, M.M. Modification of the verbal interaction behavior of a pre-delinquent youth. Presented at the American Psychological Association Convention, Washington, D.C., September 1971.

Time, September 16, 1974.

Tobias, L.L., & MacDonald, M.L. Withdrawal of maintenance drugs with long-term hospitalized mental patients: A critical review. *Psychological Bulletin,* 1974, **81**, 107-125.

Tomaino, L. Social work and the prevention of youth offenses. *Child Welfare,* 1968, **47**, 85-94.

Tomlinson, J.R. Implementing behavior modification programs with limited consultation time. *Journal of School Psychology,* 1972, **10**, 379-386.

Tomlinson, K.Y. Our shameful nursing homes. *Reader's Digest,* October 1972.

Torok, L. A convict looks at crime and criminals. *Catholic Viewpoints,* 1971, **27**, 17.

Triandis, H.C., Feldman, J.M., Weldon, D.E., & Harvey, W.M. Designing pre-employment training for the hard to employ: A cross-cultural psychological approach. *Journal of Applied Psychology,* 1974, **59**, 687-693.

Triandis, H.C., & Malpass, R.S. Studies of black and white interaction in job settings. *Journal of Applied Social Psychology,* 1971, **1**, 101-117.

Trotter, S. ACLU scores token economy. *APA Monitor,* August 1974, **5**, 1, 7.

Trotter, S. Token economy program perverted by prison officials. *APA Monitor,* February 1975, **6**, 10.

Tucker, S.M., Combs, M.E., & Woolrich, A.M. Independent housing for the elderly: The human element in design. *Gerontologist,* 1974, **15**, 73-76.

Turner, A.J. Behavioral community mental health centers: Development, management, and preliminary results. In R.A. Winett (chair), *Behavior modification in the community: Progress and problems.* Symposium presented at the 83rd convention of the American Psychological Association, 1975.

Turner, A.J., & Goodson, W.H. Catch a fellow worker doing something good today. Unpublished manuscript, Huntsville-Madison County Mental Health Center, Huntsville, Alabama, 1975.

Turner, A.J., & Pyfrom, C. Evaluation and its use in a comprehensive community mental health center. Unpublished manuscript, Huntsville-Madison County Mental Health Center, 1974.

Turner, H. (Ed.) *Psychological functioning of older people in institutions and in the community.* New York: National Council on Aging, 1967.

Tuso, M.A., & Geller, E.S. Applied behavior analysis for ecological rebalance: A tutorial review. *Journal of Applied Behavior Analysis,* 1976, **9**, 526.

Tuso, M.A., Witmer, J.F., & Geller, E.S. *Littering behavior as a function of response priming and environmental litter.* Paper presented at the meeting of the Midwestern Psychological Association, Chicago, May 1975.

Twain, D., McGee, R., & Bennett, L.A. Functional areas of psychological activity. In S.L. Brodsky (Ed.), *Psychologist in the criminal justice system.* Urbana, Ill.: University of Illinois Press, 1973.

Twardosz, S., Cataldo, M.F., & Risley, T.R. An open environment design for infant and toddler day care. *Journal of Applied Behavior Analysis,* 1974, **1**, 529-546.

Twentyman, C.T., & McFall, R.M. Behavioral training of social skills in shy males. *Journal of Consulting and Clinical Psychology,* 1975, **43**, 384-395.

Tyler, V.O. Application of operant token reinforcement to academic performance of an institutionalized delinquent. *Psychological Reports,* 1967, **21**, 249-260.

Tyler, V.O., & Brown, G.D. The use of swift, brief isolation as a group control device for institutionalized delinquents. *Behaviour Research and Therapy,* 1967, **5**, 1-9.

Tyler, V.O., & Brown, G.D. Token reinforcement of academic performance with institutionalized delinquent boys. *Journal of Educational Psychology,* 1968, **59**, 164-168.

Ullman, A.D. Sociocultural backgrounds of alcoholism. *Annual American Academy of Political Social Sciences,* 1958, **35**, 48-54.

Ullmann, L.P. *Institution and outcome: A comparative study of psychiatric hospitals.* New York: Pergamon Press, 1967.

Ullmann, L.P., & Krasner, L. *Case studies in behavior modification.* New York: Holt, Rinehart & Winston, 1965.

Ullmann, L.P., & Krasner, L. *A psychological approach to abnormal behavior.* Englewood Cliffs, N.J.: Prentice-Hall, 1969.

Ullmann, L.P., & Krasner, L. *A psychological approach to abnormal behavior.* (2nd ed.). Englewood Cliffs, N.J.: Prentice-Hall, 1975.

Underwood, B.J. *Psychological research.* New York: Appleton-Century-Crofts, 1957.

United States Congress. *The older American worker: Age discrimination in employment.* Report of the Secretary of Labor under Section 715 of the Civil Rights Act of 1964. June 1965.

U.S. Department of Health, Education, and Welfare. *Working with older people: A guide to practice.* Volume II (USPHS Pub. No. 1459). Washington, D.C. GPO, 1970.

Vaillant, G.E. The natural history of narcotic drug addiction. *Seminars in Psychiatry,* 1970, **2,** 486-498.

VanHouten, R., Hill, S., & Parsons, M. An analysis of a performance feedback system: The effects of timing and feedback, public posting, and praise upon academic performance. *Journal of Applied Behavior Analysis,* 1975, **8,** 449-457.

VanHouten, R.V., Morrison, E., Jarvis, R., & McDonald, M. The effects of explicit training and feedback on compositional response rate in elementary school children. *Journal of Applied Behavior Analysis,* 1974, **7,** 547-555.

VanHouten, T., & Sullivan, K. Effects of an audio cueing system on the rate of teacher praise. *Journal of Applied Behavior Analysis,* 1975, **8,** 197-202.

Voetglin, W.L., Lemere, F., & Bros, W.R. Conditioned reflex therapy of alcoholic addiction: III. An evaluation of present results in light of previous experience with this method. *Quarterly Journal of Studies on Alcohol,* 1940, **1,** 501-515.

Voetglin, W.L., Lemere, F., Bros, W.R., & O'Hallaren, P. Conditioned reflex therapy of chronic alcoholics: IV. A preliminary report on the value of reinforcement. *Quarterly Journal of Studies on Alcohol,* 1941, **2,** 505-511.

Vogler, R.E., Compton, J., & Weissbach, T. Integrated behavior change techniques for alcoholics. *Journal of Consulting and Clinical Psychology,* 1975, **43,** 233-243.

Vogler, R.E., Lunde, S.E., Johnson, G.R., & Martin, P.L. Electrical aversion conditioning with chronic alcoholics. *Journal of Consulting and Clinical Psychology,* 1970, **34,** 302-307.

Vogler, R.E., Lunde, S.E., & Martin, P.L. Electrical aversion conditioning with chronic alcoholics: Follow-up and suggestions for research. *Journal of Consulting and Clinical Psychology,* 1971, **36,** 450-454.

Von Holden, M. A behavioral modification approach to disciplinary segregation. Paper presented at the 99th Congress of Corrections, Minneapolis, August 1969.

Vorenberg, J., & Lukoff, I. Addiction, crime, and the criminal justice system. *Federal Probation,* 1973, **37,** 3-7.

Wahler, R.G. Some structural aspects of deviant child behavior. *Journal of Applied Behavior Analysis,* 1975, **8,** 27-42.

Wald, P., & Hutt, P. The drug abuse survey project: Summary of findings, conclusions, and recommendations. In P. Wald & P. Hutt (Eds.), *Dealing with drug abuse.* New York: Praeger, 1972.

Waldo, G. Myths, misconceptions, and the misuse of statistics in correctional research. *Crime and Delinquency,* 1971, **17**, 57-66.

Waldo, G.P., & Dinitz, S. Personality attributes of the criminal: An analysis of research studies: 1950-1965. *Journal of Research on Crime and Delinquency,* 1967, **4**, 185-202.

Waldorf, D. Social control in therapeutic communities for the treatment of drug addicts. *The International Journal of the Addictions,* 1971, **6**, 29-44.

Walker, H.M., & Buckley, N.K. Programming generalization and maintenance treatment effects across time and across settings. *Journal of Applied Behavior Analysis,* 1972, **5**, 209-224.

Walker, H.M., Hops, H., & Johnson, S.M. Generalization and maintenance of classroom treatment effects. *Behavior Therapy,* 1975, **6**, 188-200.

Wallace, C.J., & Davis, J.R. Effects of information and reinforcement on the conversational behavior of chronic psychiatric patient dyads. *Journal of Consulting and Clinical Psychology,* 1974, **42**, 656-662.

Wallgren, H., & Barry, H. *Actions of alcohol.* Amsterdam: Elsevier, 1970.

Webb, E., Campbell, D., Schwartz, R., & Sechrest, L. *Unobtrusive measures: Nonreactive research in the social sciences.* Chicago: Rand McNally, 1966.

Weber, L. *The English infant school and informed education.* Englewood Cliffs, N.J.: Prentice-Hall, 1971.

Weiler, D. A public school voucher demonstration: The first year at Alum Rock; Summary and Conclusions, a report prepared for The National Institute of Education, Santa Monica: Rand Corporation, June 1974.

Weinman, G., Gelbart, P., Wallace, M., & Post, M. Inducing assertive behavior in chronic schizophrenics: A comparison of socioenvironmental, desensitization, and relaxation therapies. *Journal of Consulting and Clinical Psychology,* 1972, **39**, 246-252.

Wenk, E.A. Schools and delinquency prevention. *Crime and Delinquency Literature,* 1974, **6**, 236-258.

Wetzel, R. Use of behavioral techniques in a case of compulsive stealing. *Journal of Consulting Psychology,* 1966, **30**, 367-374.

Wexler, D. Therapeutic justice. *Minnesota Law Review,* 1972, **57**, 289-338.

Wexler, D. Token and taboo: Behavior modification, token economies and the law. *California Law Review,* 1973, **61**, 81-109.

Wexler, D. Of rights and reinforcers. *San Diego Law Review,* 1974a, **11**, 957-971.

Wexler, D.B. Mental health law and the movement toward voluntary treatment. *California Law Review,* 1974b, **62**, 671-692.

White House Conference on Aging. *Aging in the States.* Washington, D.C.: Government Printing Office, 1971.

Whitlock, C., & Bushell, D. Some effects of "backup" reinforcers on reading behavior. *Journal of Experimental Child Psychology,* 1967, **5**, 50-57.

Wikler, A. On the nature of addiction and habituation. *British Journal of Addiction,* 1961, **57**, 73-74.

Wikler, A. Conditioning factors in opiate addiction and relapse. In D. Wilner & G. Kassebaun (Eds.), *Narcotics.* New York: McGraw-Hill, 1965.

Wikler, A. Dynamics of drug dependence: Implications of a conditioning theory for research and treatment. *Archives of General Psychiatry,* 1973, **28**, 611-616.

Wikler, A., & Pescor, F.T. Classical conditioning of a morphine abstinence phenomenon, reinforcement of opiate drinking behavior and "relapse" in morphine-addicted rats. *Psychopharmacologia,* 1967, **10**, 225-284.

Wilkinson, R. *The prevention of drinking problems.* New York: Oxford University Press, 1970.

Willems, E.P. Behavioral technology and behavioral ecology. *Journal of Applied Behavior Analysis,* 1974, **7**, 151-166.

Williams, H.R. Low and high methadone maintenance in the out-patient treatment of the hard core heroin addict. *The International Journal of the Addictions,* 1970, **5**, 439-447.

Williams, J.R., & Gold, M. From delinquent behavior to official delinquency. *Social Problems,* 1972, **20**, 209-229.

Williams, L., Martin, G.L., McDonald, S., Hardy, L., & Lambert, Sr., L. Effects of a backscratch contingency of reinforcement for table serving on social interaction with severely retarded girls. *Behavior Therapy,* 1975, **6**, 220-229.

Williams, R.J. Alcoholics and metabolism. *Scientific American,* 1948, **179**, 50-53.

Williams, R.J. Biochemical individuality and cellular nutrition: Prime factors in alcoholism. *Quarterly Journal of Studies on Alcohol,* 1959, **20**, 452-463.

Wilson, A. Disulfiram implantation in alcoholism treatment. *Journal of Studies on Alcohol,* 1975, **36**, 555-565.

Wilson, G.T., & Davison, G.C. Aversion techniques in behavior therapy: Some theoretical and methodological considerations. *Journal of Consulting and Clinical Psychology,* 1969, **33**, 327-329.

Wilson, G.T., Leaf, R., & Nathan, P.E. The aversive control of excessive drinking by chronic alcoholics in a laboratory setting. *Journal of Applied Behavior Analysis,* 1975, **8**, 13-26.

Wilson, G.T., & Rosen, R.C. Training controlled drinking in an alcoholic through a multifaceted behavioral treatment program: A case study. In J.D. Krumboltz & C.E. Thoresen (Eds.), *Counseling methods.* New York: Holt, Rinehart & Winston, 1975.

Wilson, J.W. Starting a geriatric day care center within a state hospital. *Journal of the American Geriatric Society,* 1973, **21**, 175-179.

Wiltz, N.A., & Patterson, G.R. An evaluation of parent training procedures designed to alter inappropriate aggressive behavior of boys. *Behavior Therapy,* 1974, **5**, 215-221.

Wincze, J.P., Leitenberg, H., & Agras, W.S. The effects of token reinforcement and feedback on the delusional verbal behavior of chronic paranoid schizophrenics. *Journal of Applied Behavior Analysis,* 1972, **5**, 247-265.

Winett, R.A. Behavior modification and open education. *Journal of School Psychology,* 1973, **12**, 207-214.

Winett, R.A. Behavior modification and social change. *Professional Psychology,* 1974, **5**, 244-250.

Winett, R.A. Disseminating a behavioral approach to energy conservation. *Professional Psychology,* 1976a, **7**, 222-228.

Winett, R.A. Environmental design: An expanded behavioral research framework for school consultation and educational innovation. *Professional Psychology,* 1976b, **7**, 631-636.

Winett, R.A., Battersby, C., & Edwards, S.M. The effects of architectural change, individualized instruction and group contingencies on the behavior and academic production of sixth graders. *Journal of School Psychology,* 1975, **13**, 28-40.

Winett, R.A., Calkins, D., Douglas, C., & Prus, J. Community psychologist as a resource linker in the schools. *Journal of Community Psychology,* 1975, **3**, 85-87.

Winett, R.A., Deitchman, E., Woods, M., & Solernou, J. An inservice course for teachers as a method of consultation. *Teacher Educator,* 1976, in press.

Winett, R.A., & Edwards, S.M. An evaluation plan for educational innovations. *Journal of Community Psychology,* 1974, **2**, 345-351.

Winett, R.A., Moffatt, S.A., & Fuchs, W.L. Social issues and research strategies in day care. *Professional Psychology,* 1975, **6**, 145-154.

Winett, R.A., & Nietzel, M.T. Behavioral ecology: Contingency management of consumer energy use. *American Journal of Community Psychology,* 1975, **3**, 123-133.

Winett, R.A., Richards, C.S., Krasner, L., & Krasner, M. Child monitored token reading program. *Psychology in the Schools,* 1971, **5**, 259-262.

Winett, R.A., & Roach, A.M. The effects of reinforcing academic behavior on social behavior. *The Psychological Record,* 1973, **23**, 391-396.

Winett, R.A., & Winkler, R.C. Current behavior modification in the classroom: Be still, be quiet, be docile. *Journal of Applied Behavior Analysis,* 1972, **5**, 499-504.

Winkler, R.C. Management of chronic psychiatric patients by a token reinforcement system. *Journal of Applied Behavior Analysis,* 1970, **3**, 47-55.

Winkler, R.C. Research into mental health practice using pseudo-patients. *Medical Journal of Australia,* 1974, **2**, 599-603.

Winkler, R.C. Battalio, R.C., Kagel, J.H., Fisher, E.B., Miles, C.G., Basman, R.L., & Krasner, L. Income, consumption and saving as a function of economic structure in applied and research token economies. Unpublished manuscript, Texas A and M University, 1975.

Wisocki, P. The successful treatment of a heroin addict by covert conditioning techniques. *Journal of Behavior Therapy and Experimental Psychiatry,* 1973, **4**, 55-61.

Witmer, J.F., & Geller, E.S. Facilitating paper recycling: Prompting versus reinforcement effects. *Journal of Applied Behavior Analysis,* 1976, **9**, 315-322.

Wolfbein, S.L. *Employment, unemployment, and public policy.* New York: Random House, 1965.

Wolpe, J. *Psychotherapy by reciprocal inhibition.* Stanford: Stanford University Press, 1958.

Wolpe, J. Conditioned inhibition of craving in drug addiction: A pilot experiment. *Behaviour Research and Therapy,* 1965, **2**, 285-287.

Woody, R.H. Process and behavioral consultation. *American Journal of Community Psychology,* 1975, **3**, 277-286.

Work in America: Report of a Special Task Force to the Secretary of Health, Education, and Welfare. Cambridge, Mass: Upjohn Institute for Employment and MIT Press, 1973.

Wortman, P. Evaluation research: A psychological perspective. *American Psychologist,* 1975, **30**, 562-575.

Wyatt v Aderholt, 503 F. 2d 1305 (5th Cir. 1974).

Wyatt v. Stickney, 344 F. Supp. 373, 380 (M. D. Alabama, 1971).

Yablonsky, L. *The tunnel back: Synanon.* New York: Macmillan, 1965.

Yates, A.J. *Behavior therapy.* New York: Wiley, 1970.

Young, E.R., Rimm, D.C., & Kennedy, T.D. An experimental investigation of modeling and verbal reinforcement in the modification of assertive behavior. *Behaviour Research and Therapy,* 1973, **11**, 317-319.

Zax, M., & Cowen, E.L. Research on early detection and prevention of emotional dysfunction in young school children. In C.D. Spielberger (Ed.), *Current topics in clinical and community psychology.* Vol. 1. New York: Academic Press, 1969.

Zax, M., & Cowen, E.L. *Abnormal psychology: Changing conceptions.* New York: Holt, Rinehart & Winston, 1972.

Zax, M., & Specter, G.A. *An introduction to community psychology.* New York: Wiley, 1974.

Zeisel, H. F.B.I. statistics: A detective story. *American Bar Association Journal,* 1973, **59**, 510-512.

Zifferblatt, S.M., & Hendricks, C. Applied behavioral analysis of social problems – Population change, a case in point. *American Psychologist,* 1974, **29**, 649-660.

Zigler, E., Abelson, W.D., & Seitz, V. Motivational factors in the performance of economically disadvantaged children on the Peabody Picture Vocabulary test. *Child Development,* 1973, **44**, 299-303.

Zinberg, N., & Robertson, J. *Drugs and the public.* New York: Simon & Schuster, 1972.

Zusman, J. Some explanations of the changing appearance of psychotic patients: Antecedents of the social breakdown syndrome complex. In E.M. Gruenberg (Ed.), *Evaluating the effectiveness of community mental health programs.* New York: Milbank Memorial Fund, 1966.

NAME INDEX

Abel, G., 129
Abelson, H., 145
Abelson, W.D., 41
Abraham, K., 187
Adam, E.E., 309
Adams, G.M., 295
Adams, K.A., 62
Adams, S., 100
Adler, A., 187
Agras, S., 282
Albahary, R., 173, 174
Albee, G.W., 4, 62, 346, 347, 348
Alden, L., 348
Alexander, J.F., 62, 79, 85, 89
Alexander, R.A., 300
Alford, H., 283
Alford, J., 191
Al-Issa, I., 221
Allain, A., 151
Allen, G.J., 279
Allen, R.P., 200, 212
Allen, S., 151
Alpern, M., 249
Alpert, M., 222, 282
Altman, J., 152
Alvord, J.R., 78, 85
Amen, G., 149
Amir, M., 99
Anant, S.S., 159, 161, 196, 197
Anderson, D., 115
Anderson, E.G., 317, 325, 335
Anderson, J., 274, 275
Anderson, L., 222
Anderson, L.S., 1
Anderson, L.T., 282
Anderson, W.H., 151
Ankus, M., 297

Antunes, G., 61
Arehart, J.L., 152
Argyle, M., 300, 304, 309
Arie, T., 293
Arkowitz, H., 274, 275, 276, 279
Arnon, D., 149, 181
Aron, W., 150
Arthur, G.L., 297
Arvey, R.D., 300, 303
Ashem, B., 161, 197
Atlas, L., 288, 296
Atthowe, J.M., 4, 26, 30, 143, 226,
    229, 239, 240, 241, 242, 259,
    264, 280
Atwater, J.A., 77
Austrin, H.R., 62
Axelrod, S., 52
Ayala, H.E., 76
Ayllon, T., 31, 32, 33, 41, 42, 252
Azrin, N.H., 104, 189, 214, 216, 217,
    221, 224, 226, 252, 275, 305

Baden, M.M., 183
Baer, A.M., 50
Baer, D.M., 35, 49, 50
Bahn, A.K., 229
Bailey, J., 99
Bailey, J.S., 5, 16, 53, 75, 76, 84,
    249, 252, 253, 320, 325, 326
Baker, R.D., 36
Baker, S., 103
Ballard, K.D., 22
Bander, K.W., 279
Bandura, A., 2, 3, 99, 115, 136, 138,
    139, 155, 186, 187, 189
Barbee, J.R., 305
Bard, M., 346

Barlow, D., 129
Barnes, J.A., 293, 294
Barnhart, E., 293
Barrera, F., 69, 82
Barrish, H.H., 24
Barrow, G.M., 287
Barry, H., 183, 190
Barry, J.R., 300
Bartels, B.D., 348
Bartlett, E.R., 280
Baskin, A., 15
Basmann, R.L., 262
Bass, B.M., 300
Bass, H., 152
Bassett, J., 102, 130
Bathurst, W., 149
Battalio, R.C., 262, 329, 330
Battersby, C., 24, 32, 33
Bauman, G., 346
Beasley, R.W., 61
Beatty, R.W., 308
Beaubrun, M., 192
Becker, H., 64, 99
Becker, J.M., 302
Becker, W., 19
Bednar, R.L., 70, 83, 180
Behling, M., 43
Bell, B.D., 289
Bell, W.G., 288
Bellack, L., 15, 229, 263
Bender, L., 99
Bengston, V.L., 286
Benjamin, L., 308
Benne, K.D., 230
Bennett, C.C., 1
Bennett, L.A., 348
Bennis, W.G., 230
Berck, D., 80
Bereiter, C., 14
Berg, W.E., 288
Bergler, E., 187
Berman, Y., 99
Berni, R., 297
Bernstein, D.A., 100
Berwick, P., 133
Berzins, J.I., 129, 180, 181, 182
Betts, D., 293, 298
Biase, D., 150
Bigelow, G., 171, 172, 173, 174, 179, 211, 212, 214
Birkett, D.P., 293, 294
Birnbaum, B., 132
Birnbom, F., 293, 298

Blachly, P.H., 160
Blackford, L., 145
Blake, B.G., 194, 196
Blanchard, E., 102, 129, 130
Blane, H.T., 190
Bloch, H.L., 171
Blonsky, L.E., 291
Blonsky, M.R., 308
Bloom, B.L., 1
Bloom, R., 300
Bloomfield, H.H., 267
Blum, E., 190
Blum, R.H., 183
Boblitt, W.E., 282
Bobrove, P., 245, 247
Boehm, V.R., 300, 305
Bolin, D.C., 234
Bolman, W.M., 346
Bolstad, S.R., 21, 30
Boltuch, B., 293, 294
Bootzin, R.R., 26, 229
Boozer, H., 245
Boren, J., 103
Bornstein, P., 144, 264, 280
Bottrell, J., 128
Boudin, H., 164, 165, 166, 175, 180, 182
Bourestom, N.C. 288, 293
Bourne, P., 191
Bowcock, J., 191
Bower, R., 150
Bowers, D.G., 230
Bowers, K.S., 70
Bowles, P.E., 50
Boyd, R., 287
Boyd, S.B., 40
Brakel, S., 127
Bramwell, P., 112
Brantley, J., 164, 166, 180, 182
Braukmann, G.J., 76, 84, 90, 96, 353
Braun, S.H., 11, 94, 144
Braunstein, L., 183
Braverman, J., 284
Brayfield, A.H., 229
Brecher, E., 145, 150
Breuing, M.K., 35
Briddell, D.W., 185, 196, 203, 220, 225
Brigham, T.A., 35, 40
Brill, L., 151, 152
Briscoe, N., 5, 252, 253
Broden, M., 49
Brodsky, S., 102, 141
Brody, E.M., 297
Bronfenbrenner, U., 44, 261

Brook, R., 150
Bros, W.R., 191, 192
Brotman, H.B., 286
Brown, A.S., 296
Brown, B., 152
Brown, B.S., 4
Brown, C.C., 36
Brown, G.D., 68, 69, 73, 82, 83
Brown, K.M., 249
Brown, R.E., 50, 52
Bruce, C., 49
Brunn, K., 187
Buckholdt, D., 32
Buckley, N.K., 26, 27, 29
Buehler, R.E., 71
Bugge, I., 144, 264, 280
Burchard, J.D., 68, 69, 73, 82, 83
Burgess, R.L., 313, 314, 315, 321
Burke, M., 30, 32
Burrill, R.H., 297
Burvill, P.W., 288, 293
Bushell, D., 35, 36, 41
Butler, A.K., 297
Butler, R.N., 289, 293
Butterfield, W.H., 36, 67, 82

Caddy, G., 201, 202, 221
Cahoon, D., 154
Caird, F.I., 286
Caldwell, L.R., 280
Calkins, D., 16
Callahan, E.J., 117
Callner, D., 175, 179, 283
Cameron, D., 272, 273, 282
Campbell, D., 193, 209
Campbell, D.T., 55, 87, 131, 235, 336
Campbell, J.P., 230
Campbell, R., 181
Cantrell, M.L., 53
Cantrell, R.P., 52
Caplan, G., 346, 348
Caplan, H., 139
Cappell, H., 188
Caron, P., 126
Carriere, L., 295
Carter, V., 49
Cartwright, D., 180
Casriel, D., 149
Cataldo, M.F., 47, 256, 339, 341
Catlin, R., 164, 166, 174, 175, 180,
    182
Caudill, B., 189

Cautela, J., 161, 196, 197, 294, 297
Cayner, J.J., 282
Chafetz, M.E., 183, 185, 188
Chaffee, J.L., 323, 324, 325, 326
Chapanis, A., 298
Chapman, C., 318, 319
Chatfield, S., 125
Cheek, F., 173, 174
Chein, L., 154
Chin, R., 230
Chinlund, S., 153
Chinsky, J.M., 4, 127, 229, 292
Christelman, W.C., 200
Christensen, A., 274, 275
Cicchetti, D.V., 287
Claeson, L.E., 196
Clancy, J., 193
Clarfield, S.P., 346
Clark, H.B., 17, 40, 50, 256, 258
Clark, J.V., 274
Clark, R., 100
Clark, R.N., 313, 314, 315, 320, 321
Clegg, R., 123
Clemente, F., 285
Clements, C., 101, 102
Clements, C.B., 294
Clements, H., 100, 123
Clore, G.L., 282
Cloward, R.D., 17, 61, 99
Cobb, J.A., 29, 232
Coghlan, A., 167, 168, 170
Cohen, H.L., 63, 66, 72, 83
Cohen, J., 146, 153, 175
Cohen, J., 308
Cohen, M., 200, 211, 212, 214
Cohen, R., 145
Cohen, S., 283
Coleman, J., 115
Coleman, J.V., 281
Coleman, R., 71, 83
Collier, W., 149, 180
Collins, R.W., 297
Colman, A., 103
Colthart, S.M., 297
Combs, M.E., 298
Compton, S., 210, 226
Cone, J.D., 27, 310, 319, 328, 329,
    330, 339, 344
Conger, J.J., 187
Conrad, J., 137
Cooper, M.L., 49
Cooper, S., 1
Copeland, R.E., 50, 52

Cordua, G., 31
Corey, J.R., 36
Cormier, W.H., 17
Corwin, L., 78
Cossairt, A., 18, 49, 50
Costello, R.M., 190, 191, 197, 199
Cowan, J.R., 304
Cowen, E.L., 1, 3, 4, 34, 60, 62,
    123, 186, 228, 229, 230, 260,
    346, 347, 355
Cox, T., 180
Craig, M., 62
Craighead, E., 15, 345
Cranston, S.S., 49
Craw, M., 280
Cressey, D., 99, 137
Cressler, D.L., 242, 243, 244
Cristler, C., 49
Cromwell, P., 123
Crosby, C., 154
Csapo, K.G., 295
Curran, J., 279
Curtiss, K.A., 18, 19
Cutler, R., 167
Cutler, S.J., 286, 288
Cutter, H.S., 200, 297

Dade, J., 124
Daffron, W.C., 303
Daily, D., 150
Dale, F., 151
Dale, R., 151
Damich, E., 132, 133, 134, 137
Davidson, L.M., 308
Davidson, W.S., 57, 77, 78, 80, 84,
    85, 94, 126, 198, 199, 348, 352
Davies, D.L., 200
Davis, C., 336
Davis, F., 49
Davis, J.R., 272
Davis, W.J., 62
Davison, G.C., 2, 134, 198, 228, 229
Davol, G., 144, 280
DeAngelis, G., 180
DeCarlo, T.J., 286
Dederich, C., 150
DeGrazia, F., 125
Deitchman, R., 51
Delange, J., 78
DeLong, J., 146, 148, 149, 151,
    152, 153
Delquadri, J., 23
Demming, B., 200

Demone, H.W., 185, 188
DeRisi, W.J., 74, 83, 126
Dermody, H.E., 63
Deslauriers, B.C., 334, 335, 336
Deutsch, D.R., 300
Devar, L.T., 35
deVries, H.A., 295
Diamond, H., 290, 291
Dichter, M., 219
Dineen, J.P., 17
Dinitz, S., 61
Dirks, S., 113
D'Lugoff, B., 173, 174, 179
Doctor, R., 118, 119, 120, 122, 166,
    168, 171
Dodge, M.C., 312
Dohrenwend, E., 167, 168, 170
Doke, L.A., 47
Dolch, E.W., 36
Dole, V., 151
Donnan, H.H., 297
Donner, L., 161, 197
Dorr, D., 62, 346
Dorsey, J.R., 346
Douglas, C., 16
Douglass, E.B., 292
Drabman, R.S., 15, 20, 21, 26, 29,
    36, 41
Dreher, G., 286
Droppa, D., 161, 179
Dulany, D., 138
Dunette, M.D., 230
Dunn, A., 296
DuPont, R.L., 151
Dvorak, B.A., 192
Dwarshuis, L., 181, 348

Edgerton, R.B., 187
Edlund, C.V., 41
Edwards, S., 14, 24, 32, 33
Egan, M., 161
Eimers, R.C., 52
Eisler, R.M., 187, 189, 195, 213,
    263, 269, 270, 271, 272, 277, 283
Elkes, C., 348
Elkins, R., 198
Elliot, D.S., 60
Emerson, M., 49
Empey, L.T., 60
Emrick, C.D., 190
Englemann, S., 14
Epstein, L.H., 117

Epstein, N., 62, 191
Erickson, L.M., 281
Erickson, M.L., 60
Eriksson, J., 167, 168, 169, 179
Erwin, W.S., 292
Estes, C.L., 290
Estes, W.K., 142
Esser, P.H., 190
Evans, M.B., 19
Everett, P.B., 333, 334, 335, 336, 338
Eysenck, H., 99, 115

Faillace, L.A., 200, 212
Fairweather, G.W., 13, 14, 96, 122,
    242, 243, 244, 310, 316
Falkowski, W., 195
Farrar, C.H., 193
Farris, J.C., 321
Faust, F.L., 64
Feigenbaum, E.M., 286
Fejer, D., 155
Feldman, J.M., 299, 300, 303
Feldman, R.A., 59
Feldstein, M.S., 301, 309
Fenichel, O., 154
Fensterheim, H., 283
Ferguson, R.H., 299, 300, 301, 309
Ferritor, D.C., 32
Field, M., 287
Filipezak, J., 63, 72, 83
Fineman, K.R., 68, 82
Finfrock, S.R., 35
Finkestein, M., 293
Finley, J.R., 36
Finnie, W.C., 312, 313
Fisher, E.B., 262
Fishman, S., 157, 158, 175
Fiske, D., 87, 180
Fixsen, D.L., 44, 45, 46, 76, 77,
    84, 353
Flanagan, B.A., 129
Flax, N., 59
Fletcher, C.R., 287
Flint, A.A., 348
Flores, T., 305
Fodor, I.E., 69, 82
Foote, C., 124
Fordyce, W.E., 297
Foshee, T.J., 249
Fowler, R.W., 297
Fox, R., 49

Fox, R.E., 186
Fox, V., 97
Foy, D.W., 269, 272
Franks, C., xxviii, 2, 183, 186, 190,
    198, 199, 225
Fraser, D., 281
Frease, D., 61
Freed, E.X., 188
Frekany, G.J., 295
Freud, S., 99, 187
Friedlander, F., 307, 308
Friedman, P.H., 279
Fromm, E., 187
Fuchs, W., 46, 257
Furness, J.M., 71
Furst, P.W., 62

Gaitz, C.M., 287
Galassi, J.P., 265
Galassi, M.D., 265
Gamboa, V.U., 309
Gambrill, E.D., 265, 279
Gardner, E.A., 60
Gardner, J.M., 249, 250
Gardner, R.C., 295
Gardner, W., 100
Garetz, D., 287
Garetz, F.K., 287
Garfield, Z., 219
Garfinkel, H., 64
Garlington, W.K., 283
Garton, K.L., 35
Gay, G., 149
Gazda, G.M., 190
Gearing, F., 151
Geddy, P., 283
Geiger, O.G., 297
Gelbart, P., 275
Geller, E.S., 107, 108, 111, 126, 313,
    320, 321, 322, 323, 324, 325, 326
Gentile, J.R., 86
Gerard, D., 154
Gerard, D.L., 190
Gilligan, J., 263
Gilmore, S.K., 279
Gilner, F.H., 266, 267
Ginsberg, A.B., 287
Glaser, D., 100
Glass, E., 131
Glickman, H., 273, 282
Glicksman, M., 167, 168, 169, 176, 177

Glueck, E., 61, 62
Glueck, S., 61, 62
Glynn, T., 22
Glynn, P., 22
Gobert, J., 132, 139
Goedhart, A., 276
Goetz, E.M., 35
Goffman, E., 126, 341
Gognalons-Caillard, M., 293
Gold, J., 288
Gold, M., 60, 61
Gold, M., 147
Gold, S., 167
Goldenberg, I., 61
Goldiamond, I., 130
Goldschmidt, P., 152
Goldsmith, J.B., 268
Goldsmith, L., 49
Goldstein, A., 152
Goldstein, A.P., 2, 267, 276, 277, 278
Goldstein, S., 293
Goldstein, S.C., 287
Goldston, S., 308
Goodale, J.G., 300, 301, 303, 309
Goodman, M., 59
Goodman, P.S., 304, 307
Goodson, W.H., 233
Goodwin, D., 183
Goodwin, L., 354
Gordon, M.E., 303
Gordon, W.W., 191
Gorham, D.C., 280
Gormally, J., 279
Gorodesky, M., 181
Götestam, K., 167, 168, 170
Gottman, J., 86, 131
Gottesman, L.E., 288, 293
Graubard, P.S., 17, 34, 35
Grauer, H., 293, 298
Graves, H.R., 59
Gray, B.B., 36
Greathouse, L., 70
Green, D.P., 46
Green, D.R., 283
Green, L.W., 280
Greenberg, S., 307, 308
Greenwood, C.R., 15, 16, 23, 29
Gregory, I., 186
Grey, A.L., 63
Griffin, C.L., 346
Griffiths, R.R., 211, 212
Gripp, R.F., 263, 280
Gross, N., 224

Grossman, H., 62
Grover, P., 152
Gruver, G.G., 62
Gubrium, J.F., 293
Guerney, B.G., 348
Guild, J., 23, 191
Gurian, B.S., 290, 291
Gutride, M.E., 267, 269

Haber, W., 302
Haberman, P.W., 183
Hall, R.V., 18, 49, 52
Hallam, R., 195
Halleck, S.L., 94
Hamblin, R.L., 32
Hamburg, S., 214
Hamill, C.M., 293
Hampton, L., 102
Hanlon, T., 152
Hannah, J.T., 55, 231
Hanson, D.G., 224
Hanson, P.J., 40
Hardy, L., 281
Harris, A., 172
Harris, R., 97
Harris, R., 288, 290
Harris, S.L., 145, 154, 185
Harris, V.W., 16, 24, 40, 348
Harrison, H., 102
Harry, J., 61
Harshberger, D., 127, 240, 259, 260, 261
Hart, B.M., 38
Hart, J., 280
Hartman, C., 222
Harvey, W.M., 300, 303
Hasazi, J.E., 281
Haskett, G.J., 37, 38, 39
Hassol, L., 1
Hauserman, N., 43, 44
Hawkins, G., 97, 99, 100, 183
Hawkins, R., 15
Hayden, M.L., 31
Hayes, S.G., 310, 319, 328, 329,
    330, 339, 344
Haynes, S.N., 282
Hayward, S.C., 333
Hazell, K., 287
Heap, R.F., 282
Heath, G.A., 219
Hedberg, A.G., 209
Hedquist, F.J., 279

Heldman, A., 139
Heller, K., 2
Hemphill, D.P., 195, 220
Hendee, J.C., 313, 314, 320, 321
Henderson, G., 300
Hendricks, G., 3, 341, 342, 343
Herbert, E.W., 31
Herman, C.P., 188
Herman, S.H., 24
Herring, J., 80
Hersch, C., 5, 229, 230
Hersen, M., 187, 189, 195, 213, 263,
    270, 272, 277, 282
Hershenson, D.B., 187
Hewson, D.M., 237
Hicbert, H.D., 280
Hickey, T., 298
Higgins, R.L., 188, 225
Hijazi, Y., 150, 180
Hill, C.E., 279
Hill, M.J., 190
Hill, S., 25
Hilsman, G., 187
Hilts, P., 136
Himelstein, H.C., 273
Himes, J., 300, 305
Hindelang, M., 100, 129
Hitler, A., 139
Hitz, D., 186
Hobbs, N., 1, 229
Hodges, E.F., 62
Hoffman, D., 5, 252
Holahan, C., 280
Holland, J.G., 93, 107
Hollingshead, A.B., 299
Holz, W.C., 104
Holzberg, J.D., 348
Holzinger, R., 193
Hommen, D., 346
Hopkins, B.L., 18, 35, 49, 280
Hops, H., 23, 28, 29
Hord, J.E., 282
Horst, L., 230
Horton, G.O., 52
Horton, L.E., 73, 83
Hoyer, F.W., 296
Hoyer, W.J., 296
Hsu, J., 194
Hubben, J., 276
Huber, H., 203
Huddleston, C.M., 53
Hudson, J.H., 286

Hulin, C.L., 300, 309
Hunt, G.M., 189, 214, 216, 217, 221,
    224, 226
Hunt, R.G., 230
Hunter, G.F., 267
Hurvitz, N., 229
Hutt, P., 146, 147

Inghram, R., 164
Ingram, R.E., 323
Insel, P.M., 46, 262, 340
Irvine, R.E., 292
Irwin, J., 59
Ittelson, W.H., 262, 310, 343
Iwata, B.A., 249
Izzo, L.D., 62, 346

Jackson, B.T., 116
Jackson, C., 31
Jacobs, J., 127
Jaffe, J.H., 151, 152
Jaffee, C.L., 300, 308
James, H., 59
Jarvik, L., 99
Jarvis, R., 35
Jasinski, D., 152
Jeffrey, C., 127
Jellinek, E.H., 185, 200
Jesness, C.F., 72, 74, 83
Jew, C., 114
Johnson, D., 107, 111
Johnson, E.H., 299
Johnson, G.R., 195
Johnson, L.A., 297
Johnson, M., 16
Johnson, M.B., 277
Johnson, S.M., 21, 28, 30
Johnson, V.S., 319
Jones, F.H., 52
Jones, R., 28, 283
Jordan, V.E., 60
Judge, T.G., 286

Kafer, R.A., 296
Kagel, J.H., 220, 262, 329
Kahn, R.L., 287, 288, 292
Kale, R.J., 280
Kalish, R.A., 285

Kandel, H., 41, 42
Kaplan, J., 39
Kaplan, S.J., 305
Karen, A., 149
Karlin, R., 203
Karoly, P., 140
Kass, R.E., 41
Kastenbaum, R., 296, 297
Katon, R., 151
Katz, I., 308
Kaufman, K.F., 19, 41
Kaye, J.H., 280
Kazdin, A.E., 3, 11, 18, 25, 26, 28,
    136, 138, 143, 229, 264, 270, 278,
    279, 281, 283, 311
Keil, E.C., 305
Keith, C., 113
Kellam, A.M., 116
Kelly, A.M., 280, 289
Kelly, D.H., 61
Kelly, J.G., 1, 4, 48, 228
Kelly, K., 41
Kennedy, T.D., 275
Kepner, E., 219
Kessler, M., 346, 347
Keve, P., 122
Kibat, W.H., 293
Kielser, D., 181
Kifer, R.E., 46, 76, 283
Kilano, J.R., 282
Kilburn, K., 127
Killinger, G., 123
Killingsworth, C.C., 300, 301
Kirby, F.D., 40
Kirigin, K.A., 76, 77, 84
Kirkpatrick, J.J., 303
Kirschner, N., 55, 266
Kirtner, W., 180
Kissin, B., 181
Kittrie, N.N., 183
Kivens, L., 234
Kleban, M.H., 297
Klein, D.C., 1, 229
Klein, M.W., 62
Klein, R.D., 86
Kleinman, M., 181
Klodin, V., 99
Knapczyk, D.R., 40
Knapp, R.H., 348
Knight, R.P., 187
Koegel, R., 55
Kohlenberg, R., 116, 316, 331

Kolb, D.A., 79, 85
Kolton, M., 181
Kostka, M.P., 265
Kowalski, C., 283
Kraft, T., 162, 163, 178, 221
Kramer, J., 264
Krasnegor, L., 165
Krasner, L., v, xx, xvii, 2, 3, 11,
    15, 55, 64, 100, 126, 136, 145,
    154, 183, 190, 216, 261, 262, 280, 281,
    295, 309, 345, 355
Krasner, M., 15
Kreling, B., 346
Krueger, A., 71, 83
Ksander, M., 293
Kurland, A., 151, 152
Kushner, M., 116
Kuypers, J.A. 286

LaHart, D.E., 320
Lahey, B.B., 36, 38
Lair, C.V., 297
Lambert, L., 281
Lana, R.E., 86
Landau, H., 273
Langley, M.H., 59
LaRosa, J., 150
LaRosa, J., 150
Larsen, C., 100
Laster, R., 97, 125
Laverty, S.G., 193, 199
Lavery, M.E., 289
Lawler, J.M., 55
Lawrence, C., 172, 179
Laws, D., 129
Lawton, M.P., 297
Layman, D., 31, 41, 42
Lazare, A., 151
Lazarus, A.A., 219
Leaf, R., 196
LeBlanc, J.M., 49
Lee, J.F., 55, 131
Lee, R., 154
Leeke, W., 100, 123
Lefcourt, H., 137
Lehr, U., 286
Lehrman, N.S., 263
Leitenberg, H., 117, 281, 282, 357
LeLaurin, K., 46
Lemere, F., 186, 191, 192
Lemert, E.M., 64, 99

Lenfestey, W., 37, 38, 39
Lennard, H., 151
Leonard, L.E., 289
Leopold, R.L., 229
Lerner, E., 287
Leslie, D.K., 295
Lesser, E., 157, 158, 175
Lester, D., 185
Levinson, P., 106, 107
Levitan, S.A., 302
Levitt, E.L., 63
Levitz, G.S., 293
Lewinsohn, P.M., 263, 286
Lewis, M.A., 46, 283
Lewis, S., 181
Lewis, S., 292
Ley, R., 301
Libb, J.W., 294
Liberman, R., 159, 160, 178
Liberman, R.P., 298
Libet, J.M., 263
Libo, L., 357, 358
Libow, L.S., 286
Liebson, I., 171, 172, 200, 211, 212
Lichtman, C.M., 230
Likert, R., 230
Lillesand, D.B., 265, 274
Lindesmith, A., 147
Lindquist, C., 264
Lindsey, R., 337
Lipman, A., 286
Lipsius, S., 150
Litow, L., 23, 24
Litz, M.C., 265
Livingston, G., 40
Lloyd, K.E., 282
Lobitz, G.K., 30
Logan, D., 222
Lombroso, C., 99
Lomont, J.F., 266, 267, 269
London, P., 2, 89
Long, J., 55
Long, J.D., 24
Longin, H.E., 274
Longwell, B., 180
Lorenze, E.J., 293
Lorion, R.P., 228, 233
Lovaas, O., 55, 100
Lovibond, S.H., 201, 202, 221
Lovitt, T.C., 18, 19
Lowenstein, L.M., 188
Lowenthal, M.F., 286
Lubetkin, B., 157, 158, 175, 222

Luger, M., 60
Lukoff, I., 152
Lunde, S.E., 195
Luyben, P.D., 325, 326

MacAndrew, C., 187
MacCalden, M., 336
Maccoby, M., 187
MacCulloch, M.J., 193
MacCulloch, M.L., 193
MacDonald, M.L., 263, 264, 265, 267,
    268, 270, 279, 284, 285, 286, 288,
    289, 291, 293, 294, 296, 297, 308
Mack, C.M., 292, 293
Macleod, R.D., 286, 288
Macrae, J.W., 40, 50
MacPhillamy, D.J., 286
Maddox, G.L., 292, 297
Madill, M.F., 193
Madonia, A.J., 346
Magnum, G.L., 303, 309
Maher, B., 139
Mahoney, M.J., 3, 18, 129, 139, 140
Makarenko, A.S., 45
Malaby, J., 24
Maley, R., 127, 240, 259, 260, 261
Malm, U., 196
Maloney, D.M., 76
Maloney, K.B., 35
Maloney, M., 337, 345
Maletzky, B., 159, 161, 179
Malpass, R., 308
Mandelker, A.V., 40
Mandell, W., 152
Mann, D., 61
Mann, K., 100
Mannino, F.V., 48, 347
Mansky, P., 152
Manton, D., 286
Margaro, P.A., 263, 280
Mariotto, M., 250
Markson, E.W., 293
Marlatt, G.A., 188, 189, 200, 275
Marler, L., 312
Marlett, N., 280
Marshall, W.L., 117
Marston, A.R., 265, 273, 275
Martens, J., 276
Martin, G.L., 281
Martin, L.K., 193
Martin, P.L., 195, 280
Martin, W., 152

Martorano, R., 178, 220, 239
Masters, J.C., 2, 3, 142, 228
Masserman, J.H., 187
Matlack, D.R., 292, 293
Matsunaga, G., 346
Matsuyama, S., 99
Mattocks, D., 114
Matza, D., 64
Matzger, A., 149
May, E., 153
Maynard, H., 242
McBrearty, J.F., 219
McCabe, O., 151, 152
McCarron, L.T., 297
McCarthy, E.J., 299, 300
McClannahan, L.E., 295, 296
McClearn, G.E., 189
McConnell, J.V., 92
McCord, J., 63
McCord, W., 63
McCourt, J.F., 297
McDonald, M., 35
McDonald, S., 281
McDougall, A., 281
McFall, R.M., 264, 265, 266, 268, 269,
    273, 274, 275, 279
McGee, R., 348
McGlothlin, W., 145, 146, 149, 151
McGovern, K.B., 279
McGrath, R., 264
McGuire, W.J., 193
McInnis, T., 250
McKay, H.D., 61
McKee, J., 101, 102, 104, 105, 106
McLaughlin, T.F., 24
McNamara, J., 146, 148
McNamee, H.B., 188, 200
McNees, M.P., 36, 55, 231
Medland, M.B., 24
Meehl, P., 100
Mees, H.L., 116
Mehta, N.H., 292, 293
Meichenbaum, D.H., 69, 83, 272,
    273, 282
Melin, G., 167, 168, 170
Mello, N.K., 188, 225
Melnick, J., 178, 279
Mendelson, J.H., 185, 188, 225
Mennel, R.M., 58
Menninger, K.A., 187
Mensh, I.N., 154
Mercatoris, M., 15

Merry, J., 200
Merton, R.K., 61, 99
Meyer, M., 90
Meyers, A.W., 333, 345
Meyers, H.H., 345
Meyers, J., 348
Milakovich, M.E., 58
Milan, M., 102, 104, 105, 106, 130
Miles, C.G., 262
Miller, A., 128
Miller, B.A., 224
Miller, D., 251
Miller, E.C., 192
Miller, G.A., 229
Miller, J., 181
Miller, L.K., 34, 251
Miller, M.B., 17
Miller, P.M., 179, 187, 189, 195,
    213, 217, 220, 225, 270, 272,
    277, 283
Miller, W., 99
Mills, K.C., 200, 203
Minke, K.A., 36
Mischel, W., 3
Mishara, B.L., 296
Mitchell, A., 126
Mitchell, M.A., 49
Mitford, J., 136
Moffatt, S., 46, 257
Moan, C., 151
Moore, C.H., 282
Moore, D., 226
Monroe, J., 181
Moos, R., 46, 262, 340
Morgan, B.S., 308
Morgan, S., 112
Morris, J.N., 293
Morris, N., 97, 99, 100, 183, 245
Morris, U., 133
Morris, W.C., 230
Morris, W.W., 284
Morrison, E., 35
Mortimer, R., 193
Mosher, D.L., 279
Moss, B.B., 289
Moss, C.S., 141
Moss, F.E., 284, 293, 285
Moss, M., 297
Motin, J., 191
Mueller, D.J., 296
Murrell, S., 261
Mussio, S.J., 300

Nader, R., 285
Nagel, W.G., 59
Nathan, P.E., 145, 154, 184, 185, 186, 188, 196, 197, 200, 201, 203, 209, 220, 225
Neale, J.M., 2, 228
Neikirk, B., 332
Neill, A.S., 45
Nelson, R.O., 50, 51
Nelson, S., 139
Nerviano, V., 224
Nettler, G., 97, 99
Newbrough, J., 357, 358
Newman, R.G., 348
Newton, J., 221
Nietzel, M.T., 124, 139, 141, 178, 226, 311, 316, 327, 328, 329, 331, 332, 333
Nixon, R.M., 58

Oakes, C., 287
O'Brien, C.P., 155, 156, 160
O'Brien, F., 275
O'Brien, J., 166, 168, 171, 172
O'Brien, J.S., 188
O'Connor, R.D., 25, 304, 346
Odom, E.E., 90
Ohlin, L., 61, 99
O'Hollaren, P., 192
Okun, A.M., 299, 301
O'Leary, K.D., 3, 19, 20, 26, 41, 49, 126, 183, 189, 200, 225
O'Leary, S.G., 3, 26, 49
O'Leary, V.E., 306, 307, 308
Oliver, R., 108, 126
Oliver, R.C., 293
Olsen, W.T., 288
O'Malley, J.E., 151
Opton, E., 102, 112, 132, 135, 137, 141
Orebaugh, A.L., 322
Orr, D.B., 309
Osborne, J.G., 317
Oster, C., 293
Otis, M., 279
Ottomanelli, G., 167
Owen, A., 235
Owen, M., 49
Oxberger, L., 124

Packard, R.G., 23
Paden, R.C., 273

Page, S., 126
Paine, F.T., 300
Palmore, E.B., 286
Palumbo, A., 78
Panyan, M., 49, 245
Papamarcos, J., 332
Paransky, H., 304, 307
Parks, J., 190
Parsons, B.V., 79, 85, 89
Parsons, M., 25
Parsonson, B.S., 50
Patch, V., 166, 171, 172
Patterson, A.H., 330
Patterson, G.R., 71, 115, 232, 283, 348
Pattison, E.M., 200
Paul G.L., 115, 130, 177, 250, 263, 264, 267, 270, 273, 279, 280, 284
Pavlott, J., 71, 83
Peabody, D., 118
Pedalino, E., 309
Perkins, M.E., 171
Pescor, F.T., 156
Peterson, C.L., 117
Peterson, D., 99
Peterson, T., 125
Petrock, F., 251
Petty, M.M., 303
Phillips, E.A., 44, 76, 353
Phillips, E.L., 44, 46, 53, 74, 76, 77, 84, 282
Phillips, T., 316, 331
Pierce, C.H., 255
Pihl, R., 158, 160
Pinkston, E.M., 31, 49
Pinkston, S., 269, 271, 277
Piotrowski, W.D., 253
Plant, T.F., 299
Plaska, T., 297
Plutchik, R., 273
Poe, W.D., 288
Pokorny, A.D., 224
Pokracki, F., 346
Polakow, R., 118, 119, 120, 121, 129, 130, 142, 166, 168, 171, 172, 177
Polier, J.W., 59
Polk, K., 60, 61
Pollock, D.D., 297
Pomerleau, O.F., 245, 247
Pommer, D.A., 247
Porcia, E., 49
Post, D.S., 321
Post, M., 275

Powell, B.J., 193
Powell, R.R., 295
Powell, T.J., 229
Power, C.A., 297
Powers, E., 281
Powers, R., 281
Powers, R.B., 317, 325, 335
Pratt, D.M., 346
Prentice, N.M., 62
Prock, V.N., 293
Proctor, W., 316, 331
Proshansky, H.M., 262, 299, 310, 340
Prus, J., 16
Pryor, D.H., 284
Pumroy, D.K., 23, 24
Pyfrom, C., 234

Quarrington, B., 297
Quay, H., 99
Quilitch, H.R., 39, 55, 247, 294, 295

Rabon, D., 49
Rachman, S.J., 195, 199
Rainey, L., 279
Ralph, J.L., 72, 83
Ramer, B., 149
Rankin, A., 124
Rao, D.B., 292
Rappaport, J., 4, 80, 126, 127, 143,
    229, 292, 304, 346, 348, 352, 354,
    355, 357
Rappeport, M., 145
Raskin, D., 147
Rathod, N., 159, 160, 175
Rathus, S.A., 265, 266, 279
Rautio, E., 161
Rawers, R.J., 325
Ray, E., 127
Ray, R.S., 232
Raymond, M.J., 117, 158, 160, 175, 191
Raynes, A., 166, 171, 172
Redlich, F.C., 299
Reese, N.M., 49
Regan, E., 164
Regester, D.C., 194
Reichel, W., 287
Reichenfeld, H.F., 295
Reid, D.H., 325
Reid, E., 308
Reid, J.B., 200, 283

Reidel, R.G., 296
Reimringer, M.J., 112
Reingold, J., 293
Reinhorz, H.Z., 346
Reiss, M.L., 253, 254
Remnet, V.L., 293
Renn, D.K., 59
Renner, K.E., 358
Reppucci, N., 4, 13, 15, 91
Resnick, L.B., 39, 40
Rhyne, L., 264
Rice, A., 161
Rice, P.R., 69, 82
Richards, C.S., 15
Richards, S.A., 300, 308
Richette, L.A., 59
Richmond, F.L., 61
Riessman, F., 348
Riley, J.M., 299
Rimm, D.C., 2, 3, 142, 228, 275
Rinn, R.C., 231, 232, 233
Rioch, M.J., 348
Risley, T.R., 17, 39, 46, 47, 230, 255,
    256, 258, 260, 295, 296, 318, 319, 341
Rivlin, L.G., 262, 310
Roach, A., 32
Robens, L., 309
Roberts, M., 32, 33
Robertshaw, C.S., 280
Robertson, J., 148
Robinson, M.R., 78, 85
Robinson, R.A., 287, 291, 292, 293
Robison, J., 100
Robson, R.T., 303, 309
Rodin, A.H., 86
Roe, A., 229
Rogers, J., 102
Romanczyk, R.G., 19
Rooney, W.M., 274
Roosa, J.B., 283
Rose, S.D., 78, 84
Rosen, E., 186
Rosen, H., 306, 307, 308
Rosen, R.C., 220
Rosenberg, C., 293
Rosenberg, H., 17
Rosenblum, G., 1, 229
Rosenfeld, E., 154
Rosenhan, D.L., 235, 237
Rosenthal, D., 99
Rosenthal, R., 87
Rosenstiel, A.K., 161

Rosenzweig, N., 292
Rosin, A.J., 293
Rosnow, R., 87
Ross, H., 296
Ross, R.R., 70
Ross, S.M., 283
Ross, W., 181, 182
Rossi, A.M., 188
Rostow, C.D., 280
Rotter, J., 170
Rowan, T., 158, 160
Rozynko, V., 181
Rubin, B.K., 281
Rubin, R.D., xxviii
Ruiz, M., 164
Rychlak, J., 139

Saenger, G., 190
Sage, W., 112, 129, 142
Sajwaj, T., 30, 31
Salipant, P., 304, 307
Salzberg, B.H., 35
Sanders, O.H., 122, 242
Sanders, M.G., 183
Sanders, R.M., 40
Sanderson, R.E., 193
Santogrossi, D.A., 19
Santore, A.F., 290, 291
Sarason, I., 355, 357, 358
Sarason, S.B., 229, 255, 350
Sashkin, M., 230
Saudargas, R.A., 19
Saunders, A., 106, 131, 134, 135, 141
Saunders, J., 4, 13, 15, 91
Saunders, M., 24
Scarpitti, F.R., 59
Schaaf, W., 276
Schaefer, H.H., 200, 203
Schafer, S., 97, 125
Schafer, W.K., 60, 61
Schilder, P., 187
Schneider, R., 34
Schnelle, J.F., 55, 131, 231
Schrayer, D., 145
Schochet, B.V., 347
Schoen, K., 122, 141
Schoenfeldt, L.F., 309
Schofield, W., 177
Schonfield, D., 286
Schulberg, H.C., 229
Schultz, J.L., 58, 59
Schur, E.M., 58, 64, 81, 124

Schutte, R.C., 35
Schutz, R.E., 36
Schwaab, E.L., 200
Schwartz, G., 3
Schwartz, M., 300
Schwartz, R., 235
Schwartz, S., 293
Schwitzgebel, R., 66, 79, 85, 127, 128, 132
Schwitzgebel, R.K., 100, 134, 136
Scott, E., 287
Scott, J.W., 41
Scott, K., 287
Sears, D.W., 292
Seashore, S.E., 230
Seaver, W.B., 330
Sechrest, L.B., 2, 235
Seidman, E., 80, 348, 355, 356, 357
Seitz, V., 41
Sensenig, J., 181
Serber, M., 113
Settin, J.M., 294
Severy, L.J., 61, 280
Sewell, D.D., 301, 302, 303, 304
Shaefer, H.H., 280
Shadel, C.A., 192
Shah, S.A., 57, 66, 99, 115, 127, 140
Shainline, A., 62
Shamow, J., 36
Shanas, E., 288, 293
Shapiro, M., 132, 137, 139, 140
Shaw, C.R., 61
Shean, G.D., 280
Shee, S.M., 21
Sherman, T.M., 16, 17, 24, 40, 348
Sherwood, S., 293
Shields, F., 40
Shimoni, N., 53
Shireman, C., 100
Shore, H., 292, 293
Shore, M., 99
Shore, M.F., 48
Short, J.F., 61
Shuman, S., 100
Sidman, M., 81, 86, 329, 334
Sielaft, T.J., 309
Silber, E., 348
Silberman, C., 34
Silbert, J.D., 92
Silver, C.P., 293
Silverstein, S.J., 201
Silverstone, B., 296
Simmons, J., 55
Simmons, L., 147

Simmons, L., 285
Simpson, S.C., 296
Sisson, J., 190
Skinner, B.F., 2, 137, 139
Skinner, K.K., 266
Slack, C.W., 66
Sloan, H.N., 15, 72, 83
Slocum, J.W., 309
Smart, R., 155
Smart, R.G., 187
Smith, C., 335
Smith, C.E., 280
Smith, D., 149
Smith, G., 100
Smith, G., 164
Smith, J.J., 185
Smith, K.J., 286
Smith, L., 32
Smith, M.B., 1, 229
Smith, P.M., 62
Smith, R.A., 300
Smith, R.H., 245
Snyder, E.E., 285
Sobell, L.C., 188, 200, 203, 204, 205,
    206, 207, 208, 209, 211, 221, 225, 226
Sobell, M.B., 188, 200, 203, 204, 205, 206,
    207, 208, 209, 211, 221, 225, 226
Soden, E., 152
Solernou, J., 51
Solomon, P., 188
Solomon, R.W., 15, 142
Sommer, R., 262, 296, 340, 341
Spece, R., 112, 113, 114, 132, 134
Specter, G.A., 1, 11, 55, 240, 250,
    262, 346
Spector, N.J., 266
Speers, W., 212
Spence, D.L., 283
Spergel, I.A., 60
Spevack, M., 158, 160, 162, 163
Spinetta, J.J., 298
Spitalnik, R., 15, 20
Spreitzer, E., 285
Staats, A.W., 36, 67, 82
Staats, C.K., 36
Stachnik, T.J., 24
Stahl, J.R., 281
Stamford, B.A., 294, 295
Stancyk, S.E., 36
Standen, J., 172, 174
Stanford, A.G., 220
Stanley, J., 131

Stans, A., 35
Steffen, J., 188, 221
Steffy, R.A., 280
Stein, K., 181
Stein, L., 221
Stein, T.J., 14, 51
Steiner, C.M., 190
Steinfeld, G., 159, 161, 176, 178
Steinke, G.V., 279
Steketee, J.P., 65
Stephenson, R.M., 59
Stevens, R.S., 293
Stocker, R., 181
Stolz, S.B., 4, 281
Stone, B., 237
Strang, C.D., 296
Strawser, R.H., 309
Streedbeck, P., 247
Stuart, R.B., 78, 84, 89, 94, 134,
    153, 215
Sullivan, D., 151
Sullivan, K., 25, 52
Sulzer, E., 218, 226, 348
Summers, G.F., 285
Sundel, M., 78
Suratt, P.P., 15
Susman, J., 59
Sussman, A., 92
Sutherland, E.H., 99
Sutker, P., 151
Sutton, W., ix
Sykes, G., 127
Syme, L., 186

Tait, D.C., 62
Taubman, M.T., 77
Taylor, H., 188, 201
Tchobanian, R., 309
Teasdale, J., 199
Terrell, D.L., 346
Tharp, R.G., 3, 18, 49, 53, 63, 66,
    78, 84, 126, 348
Thiman, J., 192
Thomas, C., 99
Thomas, J.D., 18, 22
Thompson, G.B., 286
Thompson, I., 159, 169, 175
Thomson, C.L., 49
Thomson, L.E., 281
Thomson, N., 281
Thoresen, C., 3, 18, 129, 139, 140
Thorne, G.L., 63, 66

Tiffany, D.W., 304
Tiffany, P.M., 304
Timbers, G.D., 76
Titler, N.A., 188
Tobias, L.L., 263
Tomaino, L., 63
Tomarchio, T., 172, 174
Tomlinson, J.R., 51
Tomlinson, K.Y., 285, 288
Tornatzky, L, 14, 122, 242
Torney, D., 280
Torok, L., 99
Triandis, H.C., 300, 303, 308
Trickett, E., 181
Tromontana, J., 24
Trost, M.A., 62, 346
Trotter, S.M., 111, 126, 137
Tu, J., 353
Tucker, B., 49
Tucker, S.M., 298
Turner, A.J., 230, 233, 234
Turner, D.W., 192
Turner, H., 295
Turner, J., 306, 307
Turner, J., 348
Tuso, M.A., 313, 320
Twain, D., 348
Twardosz, S., 30, 47, 339, 341
Twentyman, C.T., 264, 265, 266, 269, 279
Tyler, J.D., 348
Tyler, V.O., 68, 69, 73, 82, 83

Ullman, A.D., 184
Ullman, L.P., viii, xi, xiii, xvi, xix, xxii,
    xxiv, xxvi, 2, 3, 11, 55, 64, 100,
    126, 136, 145, 154, 183, 190, 216,
    261, 262, 263, 281, 295, 309, 345
Ulrich, R.E., 15
Umberger, D.L., 303
Underwood, B.J., 81
Usdansky, B.S., 348

Vaillant, G.E., 176, 180
Valentine, V., 164
Vallance, M., 193
VanBelle, H.A., 276
VanderHoff, E., 193
VanderWater, S.L., 193
Van Dusen, W., 193
VanHouten, R., 25, 35, 52
Vernon, J.C., 231, 232

Voetglin, W.L., 191, 192
Vogler, R., 195, 210, 221, 226
Von Holden, M., 102
Vorenberg, J., 152
Voss, H., 60

Wagner, B., 270, 272
Wahler, R.G., 15, 26, 31
Wald, P., 146, 147
Waldo, G.P., 62, 97
Waldorf, D., 150
Walen, S.R., 143
Walker, H.M., 26, 27, 28, 29, 30
Wallace, C.J., 272
Wallace, M., 275
Wallgren, H., 183, 190
Walters, R., 115
Wang, M.C., 39
Ward, M., 337, 345
Warner, A., 151
Wax, B.S., 90
Weathers, M.T., 55
Webb, E., 235
Weber, L., 52
Weiler, D., 55, 141
Weinberg, S., 70
Weinhold, B.K., 279
Weinman, G., 275
Weis, K., 58
Weissbach, T., 210
Weldon, D., 300, 303
Wenk, E.A., 62
Wetzel, R.J., 3, 18, 49, 53, 63, 66,
    68, 78, 82, 84, 126, 348
Wexler, D., 132, 133, 134, 136
Wneelan, P.A., 280
Wheeler, A.J., 35
Whitehead, P., 150
Whitlock, C., 36
Wienckowski, L.A., 4
Wiersma, H., 276
Wikler, A., 155, 156
Wile, R., 190
Wilkinson, R., 183
Willard, D., 49
Willems, E.P., 26, 30, 259, 261, 334
Williams, H.R., 152
Williams, J.R., 60
Williams, L., 281
Williams, R., 102
Williams, R.J., 185, 200

Williams, R.L., 24, 30
Wiltz, N.A., 348
Wilson, A., 191
Wilson, A.B., 346
Wilson, G.T., 126, 183, 189, 196, 198,
    200, 220, 226, 228
Wilson, J.W., 293
Wilson, M., 126
Wilson, V., 131
Wiltz, N.A., 348
Wincze, J.P., 282
Winett, R.A., 3, 4, 10, 11, 14, 15, 16,
    18, 24, 32, 33, 34, 46, 51, 55,
    137, 239, 244, 257, 311, 316, 327,
    328, 329, 330, 331, 332, 333, 345
Winkel, G., 262
Winkler, R.C., 11, 32, 34, 137, 235,
    236, 238, 262, 282, 329
Winter, L., 296
Wise, M.J., 232
Wisocki, P., 171, 172, 175, 178
Witmer, J.F., 313, 322, 323, 324
Wodarski, J.S., 59
Wolf, M.M., 24, 36, 44, 45, 53, 76,
    77, 353
Wolfbein, S.L., 301
Wolford, T.R., 77, 84
Wolk, R., 293

Wolpe, J., 157, 158, 175, 178
Wood, L., 102
Woods, M., 51
Woody, R.H., 347
Woolridge, A.M., 298
Woolridge, R.L., 53
Wortman, P., 131
Wylie, R.G., 321

Yablonsky, L., 150
Yates, A.J., 65, 126
Young, E.R., 275
Young, T., 100
Yum, K.S., 182

Zax, M., 1, 3, 4, 11, 34, 55, 60, 186,
    228, 229, 230, 240, 250, 262, 346, 347
Zeidberg, J., 288
Zeiger, J., 288
Zeisel, H., 97
Zelhart, P.F., 70
Zifferblatt, S.M., 3, 341, 342, 343
Zigler, E., 41
Zimmerman, R., 167
Zinberg, N., 147
Zusman, J., 264, 280

SUBJECT INDEX

Abstinence
vs. controlled drinking, 190, 199,
200-201, 204, 206-208, 224, 225
vs. controlled drug use, 148, 150, 165
Academic skills
creativity, 35-36
homework and question asking, 40-41
language development, 38-39
mastery curriculum, 39
reading, 36-37
self-paced learning, 39
writing, 34-35
Acceptability for Psychotherapy Scale,
182
Achievement Place, 353
follow-up evaluation of, 77
and juvenile delinquency, 74-77, 90
and peer control, 44-46
Adjective Checklist Mood Scale, 223
Adult corrections
behavioral interventions for
aversion therapies, 112-114,
141-143
conceptual adequacy of, 128-130
ecological conventionality of,
123-128
ethics of, 136-144
institutional programs, 101-115
legal challenges to, 131-136
methodological evaluations of,
130-131
nonresidential behavior therapy,
115-118
probation, 118-121
programmed instruction, 101-102
overview of, 6-7

Adult crime
cost of, 97, 99
rates of, 97-99
and recidivism rates, 100
theories of, 99
Aging
behavioral interventions for, 294-298
day care centers for, 292-293
home services for, 287,290
assistance services, 288
health services, 288-289
psychological services, 289
institutional treatments for, 293-298
milieu therapy, 293-294
reality orientation, 293-294
sheltered workshops, 293-294
multiservice centers for, 290-292
overview of, 9
and Principle of Least Intervention,
287-288, 292
social problems of, 285-287, 298
Aid to Families with Dependent Children,
252
Alcoholics Anonymous, 150, 174, 190,
200, 204-205
Alcoholism
anxiety reduction techniques for
221-222
assertion training for, 222-223
aversion methods for, 191-199
broad spectrum approaches for, 199-
214
classification of, 184-185
and crime, 183
impact of, 183-184
moderation training for

BAL discrimination, 201-203
environmental approaches, 211-214
multimodal approaches, 203-211
operant approaches for, 214-218
overview of, 7-8
rates of, 183
theories of, 185-190
American Civil Liberties Union (National Prison Project), 107, 131, 134, 137
American Enterprise Institute, 301, 302
American Psychological Association, 321
ethical standards of, xvi
Amphetamines, 145, 158, 160, 164, 166, 167, 168, 170, 173
Anomie theory, 61
Atascadero State Hospital, 112-114, 129

Barbiturates, 145, 153, 155, 162, 164, 165, 166, 168, 171, 172, 173
Behavior Research Project, 78-79
Behavioral community psychology, ix, xix, xx, xxi-xxiv, 5, 10, 11, 48, 97, 244, 298, 310, 345, 358-359
ethics of, xxiv, xxv, 11
and social change, 3-4
Behavioral contracting
and adult probation, 118-121
and drug use, 162-168
and juvenile delinquency, 78
Broad spectrum behavior therapy, 8
and adult offenders, 115-118
and alcoholism, 199-214
Bureau of Narcotics and Dangerous Drugs, 147

California Institute for Women, 112
California Youth Authority, 72
Cambridge-Sommerville Youth Study, 63
Cellblock Token Economy, 104-106
Center for Studies of Crime and Delinquency, 57
Child abuse, 119
Children as change agents
effects on peers, 14-17
effects on teachers, 17-18
Clockwork Orange, 140
Cocaine, 145-146, 159

Community corrections, 123-128
bail reform, 124-125
decriminalization, 123-125, 127
deinstitutionalization, 123, 127
work release programs, 123
Community mental health
behavioral community mental health, 230-235
and behavioral innovation, 239-240, 260
and community organization, 251-256
and experimental social innovation, 243-245
and organizational change, 245-251
overview of, 8
and pseudo-patient methodology, 235-239
and the public health model, 256-259, 261-262
Community psychology
and the applied behavioral paradigm, vii, xiii-xviii, 2-6, 326, 345-358
definitions of, 1-2, 261
training models for, 355-358
Connecticut State Prison, 112
Consultation
and behavioral workshops, 50-52
and continuing education programs, 48
types of, 347-349
with school personnel, 48-50, 52, 53
Contingency Management Program, 6, 126, 131, 137
compared to START, 107-111
Goochland County State Farm, 108
Richmond State Penitentiary, 108
St. Brides Correctional Unit, 108
Control Unit Treatment Program, 131
Courier Journal, The, 316, 326
Covert modeling, 178, 278-279

Day Top Village, 150
Demerol, 157, 158
Dissemination
and community mental health, 229, 234, 239-245, 257, 259
and community psychology, 353-354
and environmental protection, 326
and juvenile delinquency interventions, 94, 96
and school interventions, 14

Diversion
  of adult offenders, 125, 127
  of juvenile delinquents, 64, 65, 80
Draper Correctional Center (Experimental
    Manpower Laboratory for
    Corrections), 6, 101, 102, 104-
    106, 130
Drinamyl, 162, 163
Drug abuse
  behavioral approaches to, 156-175
    aversion techniques, 157-162
    contingency management, 162-
      170
    evaluations of, 175-182
    extinction, 170
    multimodal treatments, 170-175
    systematic desensitization, 162-
      163
    token economies, 168-170
  civil commitment for, 149, 176
  and crime, 146, 152
  crisis intervention for, 153-154
  detoxification, 148-149, 171, 176,
    177
  educational programs for, 153
  and health problems, 146
  legal controls of, 146-148
  moral controls of, 148
  overview of, 7
  rates of, 145-146
  theories of, 154-156
  therapeutic communities, 149-151
  and the withdrawal syndrome, 151-
    152, 155, 176

Educational Pyramid, 355-356
Ego Strength Scale, 181
Electronic rehabilitation system, 127-128
Environmental problems
  architecture, 339-341
  energy use and peaking, 326-333
  littering, 312-320
    antecedent approaches to, 313-
      320
    marked item technique, 319-320
    reinforcement approaches to,
      313-320
  and mental health, 310
  overview of, 11
  population change, 341-343
  recycling, 320-326

transportation, 333-338

Federal Bureau of Investigation, 57, 97
Federal Bureau of Prisons, 97, 107, 131,
    134

Gaites-MacGinitie Achievement Test, 70
Generalization
  and aging problems, 298
  and alcoholism interventions, 209,
    224, 226-227
  of community mental health
    programs, 239-245
  and drug abuse interventions, 177-
    178
  and juvenile delinquency interven-
    tions, 88
  and interventions for psychiatric
    residents, 283
  response, 25, 31-34
  stimulus, 25-30
Group contingencies
  applied to school problems, 22-24
  good behavior game, 24, 35

Hallucinogens, 145, 159, 161, 162, 163,
    167
Hardening the target, 127
Head Start, 34, 38
Health, Education and Welfare,
    Department of, 92, 99
Heroin addiction, 145, 146, 148, 151,
    152, 153, 157, 158, 159, 160,
    161, 165, 166, 167, 171, 172,
    173, 176
  and the conditioned abstinence
    syndrome, 155-156, 160
  heroin maintenance, 153
  methadone, 151, 174, 176, 177
    action of, 151
    attrition rates, 152
    dosage levels, 151
    evaluation of, 151-152
    and polydrug abuse, 152, 171-
      172
    opiate antagonists, 152-153, 177
Huber Act, 123
Huntsville Madison County Mental
    Health Center, 230-235, 245, 260

Hyperactivity
    behavioral approaches to, 41-42
    use of Ritalin for, 41-42

Identification with Addicts Scale, 182
Informed consent, 96, 113-114, 133-
    134, 140, 167, 237, 238
Internal Revenue Service (IRS), 147
Interpersonal Checklist, 267
Iowa Security Medical Facility, 112

Job Opportunities in the Business Sector,
    302
Johnny Cake Child Study Center, 257
Joint Commission on Correctional
    Manpower and Training, 63
Joint Commission on Mental Health of
    Children, 63
Journal of Applied Psychology, 304
Juniper Gardens, 255, 318
Justice, Department of, 147
Juvenile crime and delinquency
    behavioral approaches to
        community based nonresidential
            programs, 77-80
        community based residential
            programs, 74-77
        compared to client-centered and
            psychodynamic therapies, 79-80
        compared to transactional analysis,
            72-73
        early history of, 65-67
        ethical evaluations of, 92-96
        institutional programs for, 67-74
        methodological evaluations of,
            81-89
        theoretical evaluations of, 89-91
    behavioral theories of, 89-91
    community based interventions for,
        60-62
    rates of, 57-58
    and status offenses, 58
    theories of, 61-62
Juvenile Delinquency Control Act, 99
Juvenile justice system
    criticisms of, 59-60
    history of, 58-59
    Illinois Juvenile Courts, 58
    Juvenile Court Act, 58
    overview of, 6

Labor, Department of, 99, 299
Law Enforcement Assistance Adminis-
    tration (LEAA), 92, 99, 136, 147
Living Environments Group, 47-48, 341

MAAC Behavioral Adjustment Scale, 223
Maintenance
    and aging problems, 298
    and alcoholism interventions, 209,
        224, 226-227
    of community mental health
        programs, 239-245
    and drug abuse interventions, 177-178
    and interventions for psychiatric
        residents, 283
Manpower Development and Training
    Act, 301, 302, 303, 307
Manpower Improvement through
    Community Effort, 303
Marijuana, 145, 159, 161, 168
Medical model
    characteristics of, ix-xiii
    criticisms of, ix-xiii
    and psychoanalysis, xiii
Methamphetamines, 145
Metropolitan Readiness Test, 41
Miasma, x, xi, xvii
MMPI, 182, 267
Model Cities Program, 99
Morphine, 152, 157, 158

Narcotic Addict Rehabilitation Act, 149
National Advisory Commission on Civil
    Disorders, 299
National Commission on Marijuana and
    Drug Abuse, 145
National Institute of Mental Health
    (NIMH), 145, 230
National Training School for Boys CASE
    Program, 66, 72
Neighborhood Youth Corps, 255
Nonprofessionals
    and adult offenders, 123
    and aging programs, 298
    and drug abuse programs, 181-182
    and juvenile delinquency, 62-63, 65
Numorphan, 171
Nursing homes, 284-285

Omnibus Crime Control and Safe Streets
  Act, 99
Open classrooms, 37-38, 46
Operations Re-Entry, 240-241
Opportunities Industralization Center,
  304

Paraprofessionals, xx, 3, 10, 11, 51
  in alcoholism interventions, 211, 214
  in community mental health programs,
    228, 250-251, 260
  in drug abuse interventions, 165, 168,
    182
PASS, 29
Patient uniformity myth, 181
Phenobarbitol, 163
Phoenix House, 150
Physeptone, 158, 160
Planned Activity Check Evaluation, 248
PORT, 122
Post Behavior Therapy Club, 162, 178
Prevention, 355
  of adult crime, 127-128
  of alcoholism, 211
  and community mental health, 229,
    260, 261
  of juvenile delinquency, 62
  of school problems, 55
  types of, 346-347
Primary Mental Health Project, 346
Primary prevention, xx, 346
Pseudo-addicts, 160
Psychological sense of community, vii,
  350-353
Psychiatric residents
  characteristics of, 263-264
  moral treatment for, 263
  overview of, 8-9
  social skill (assertion) training,
    264-281
    behavioral treatment packages
      for, 265-270
    comparisons of alternative
      interventions for, 273-280
    and control of inappropriate
      behavior, 282-283
    and intervention priming, 275
    and physical appearance, 282
    single intervention elements for,
      270-273
    token economies for, 280-281
Psychostimulants, 145, 167

Quasi-experimental designs
  in adult corrections, 131
  in school interventions, 55

Racial integration, 43-44
Right-to-be-different (refuse treatment)
  and adult offenders, 133-134, 137
  and juvenile delinquency, 92
Right-to-treatment
  and adult offenders, 132-133
  and juvenile delinquency, 92
Rotter I-E Scale, 170

School problems
  overview of, 5-6
  summary of behavioral interventions
    for, 53-54
Scrambled Sentences Test, 223
Sedatives, 145, 174
Self control
  applied to school problems, 18-22
  to promote generalization, 20-22
Sexual Reorientation Program, 113
Social change, 230, 345, 349, 353, 354,
    355, 359
  and activism, 349-350
  person vs. system oriented inter-
    ventions, 1, 355, 358
Stanford-Binet IQ Test, 41
START, 6, 106-107, 131, 134-135
  compared to the Contingency
    Management Program, 107-111
Supreme Court, 59, 132
Synanon, 149, 150
Systems-ecological perspective
  and adult offenders, 127
  in classrooms, 26, 30-31, 55
  in community mental health, 228,
    259-260, 262
  and day care centers, 46-48
  and environmental problems, 334
Symbolic modeling, 25

Time series analyses, 86, 131
Token economies
  in classrooms, 24-25
  and drug abuse, 168-170
  prosthetic vs. therapeutic, 26
  and social skills training, 280-281
Tranquilizer abuse, 159, 161, 174

Tutoring, 14
  advantages of, 17
  cross-age, 16-17
  peer, 16
  and triadic consultation, 18
Two-factor learning theory, 142

Unemployment
  behavioral interventions for, 304-307
  effects of, 299-301
  and employment maintenance
    programs, 306-308
  and Federal Manpower programs,
    301-304
  macroeconomic interventions for,
    309
  overview of, 9
  rates of, 299
  types of, 301

Vacaville Rehabilitation Center, 112-
    114, 129
Victim compensation and restitution pro-
    grams, 97, 125
Victimless crimes, 124
Voucher programs
  in prisons, 55
  in schools, 141

Walter Reed Project, 103
Wisconsin State Penitentiary, 112

YAVIS syndrome, 3, 181

TITLES IN THE PERGAMON GENERAL PSYCHOLOGY SERIES (Continued)

Vol. 38. W.R. BALLER—*Bed Wetting: Origins and Treatment*
Vol. 40. T.C. KAHN, J.T. CAMERON, & M.B. GIFFEN—*Psychological Methods in Evaluation and Counseling*
Vol. 41. M.H. SEGALL—*Human Behavior and Public Policy: A Political Psychology*
Vol. 42. G.W. FAIRWEATHER *et al.*—*Creating Change in Mental Health Organizations*
Vol. 43. R.C. KATZ & S. ZLUTNICK—*Behavior Therapy and Health Care: Principles and Applications*
Vol. 44. D.A. EVANS & W.L. CLAIBORN—*Mental Health Issues and the Urban Poor*
Vol. 45. K.P. HILLNER—*The Psychology of Learning*
Vol. 46. T.X. BARBER, N.P. SPANOS & J.F. CHAVES—*Hypnosis, Imagination and Human Potentialities*
Vol. 47. B. POPE—*Interviewing*
Vol. 48. L. PELTON—*The Psychology of Nonviolence*
Vol. 49. K.M. COLBY—*Artificial Paranoia—A Computer Simulation of Paranoid Processes*
Vol. 50. D.M. GELFAND & D.P. HARTMANN—*Child Behavior Analysis and Therapy*
Vol. 51. J. WOLPE—*Theme and Variations: A Behavior Therapy Casebook*
Vol. 52. F.H. KANFER & A.P. GOLDSTEIN—*Helping People Change: A Textbook of Methods*
Vol. 53. K. DANZIGER—*Interpersonal Communication*
Vol. 54. P.A. KATZ—*Towards the Elimination of Racism*
Vol. 55. A.P. GOLDSTEIN & N. STEIN—*Prescriptive Psychotherapies*
Vol. 56. M. HERSEN & D.H. BARLOW—*Single-Case Experimental Designs: Strategies for Studying Behavior Changes*
Vol. 57. J. MONAHAN—*Community Mental Health and the Criminal Justice System*
Vol. 58. R.G. WAHLER, A.E. HOUSE & E.E. STAMBAUGH III—*Ecological Assessment of Child Behavior: A Clinical Package for Home, School, and Institutional Settings*
Vol. 59. P.A. MAGARO—*The Construction of Madness — Emerging Conceptions and Interventions into the Psychotic Process*
Vol. 60. P.M. MILLER—*The Behavioral Treatment of Alcoholism*
Vol. 61. J.P. FOREYT—*Behavioral Treatment of Obesity*
Vol. 62. A. WANDERSMAN, P. POPPEN & D.F. RICKS—*Humanism and Behaviorism: Dialogue and Growth*
Vol. 63. M. NIETZEL, R. WINETT, M. MACDONALD & W. DAVIDSON—*Behavioral Approaches to Community Psychology*
Vol. 64. J. FISCHER & H. GOCHROS—*Handbook of Behavior Therapy with Sexual Problems*
Vol. I: General Procedures
Vol. II: Approaches to Specific Problems
Vol. 65. M. HERSEN & A. BELLACK—*Behavioral Assessment: A Practical Handbook*
Vol. 66. M.M. LEFKOWITZ, L.D. ERON, L.O. WALDER & L.R. HUESMANN—*Growing Up To Be Violent: A Longitudinal Study of the Development of Aggression*
Vol. 67. T.X. BARBER—*Pitfalls in Human Research: Ten Pivotal Points*
Vol. 68. I. SILVERMAN—*The Human Subject in the Psychological Laboratory*
Vol. 69. G.W. FAIRWEATHER & L.G. TORNATZKY—*Experimental Methods for Social Policy*
Vol. 70. A.S. GURMAN & A.M. RAZIN—*Effective Psychotherapy*
Vol. 71   J.L. MOSES & W.C. BYHAM—*Applying the Assessment Center Method.*